Quick Reference

NEUROSCIENCE

THIRD EDITION

for Rehabilitation Professionals

The Essential Neurologic Principles
Underlying Rehabilitation Practice

Quick Reference

NEUROSCIENCE

THIRD EDITION

for Rehabilitation Professionals

The Essential Neurologic Principles
Underlying Rehabilitation Practice

Sharon A. Gutman, PhD, OTR, FAOTA
Associate Professor of Rehabilitation and Regenerative Medicine
Programs in Occupational Therapy
Columbia University Medical Center
New York, New York

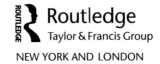
Routledge
Taylor & Francis Group

NEW YORK AND LONDON

First published 2017 by SLACK Incorporated

Published 2024 by Routledge
605 Third Avenue, New York, NY 10158

and by Routledge
4 Park Square, Milton Park, Abingdon, Oxon OX14 4RN

Routledge is an imprint of the Taylor & Francis Group, an informa business

Library of Congress Cataloging-in-Publication Data

Names: Gutman, Sharon A., author.
Title: Quick reference neuroscience for rehabilitation professionals : the
  essential neurologic principles underlying rehabilitation practice /
  Sharon Gutman.
Other titles: Neuroscience for rehabilitation professionals
Description: Third edition. | Thorofare, NJ : Slack Incorporated, [2017] |
  Includes bibliographical references and index.

9781630911522 (paperback : alk. paper)

Subjects: | MESH: Nervous System--anatomy & histology | Nervous
  System--physiopathology | Rehabilitation | Outlines
Classification: LCC RC343 (print) | NLM WL 18.2 | DDC
  616.8--dc23
LC record available at https://lccn.loc.gov/2016017165

ISBN: 9781630911522   (pbk)
ISBN: 9781003526216   (ebk)

DOI: 10.4324/9781003526216

Contents

ABOUT THE AUTHOR

Sharon A. Gutman, PhD, OTR, FAOTA is an Associate Professor of Rehabilitation and Regenerative Medicine in the Occupational Therapy Programs at Columbia University in New York, New York. Dr. Gutman has a background in neuroscience and has worked with a wide array of populations as an occupational therapist, including traumatic brain injury, psychiatric disability, autism spectrum disorder, developmental delay, and homelessness. In the past 2 decades, she has taught courses and written journal articles and books regarding the fundamentals of clinical neuroscience and the neurologic basis of pathological conditions. Dr. Gutman served as the editor of the *American Journal of Occupational Therapy* between 2008 and 2014.

FOREWORD

Neuroscience is an extremely important foundational science for the rehabilitation professions. An introduction to neuroscience must include an understanding of neuroanatomy, neurophysiology, and neuropathology. In addition, application of neuroanatomy and neurophysiology to understand clinical diagnostic tests is absolutely essential to rehabilitation professionals. While there are many textbooks available, there is a dire need for a comprehensive, concise, and easy to comprehend text for students in rehabilitation. *Quick Reference Neuroscience* by Sharon A. Gutman is an outstanding text that fulfills the need of rehabilitation professionals.

As an occupational therapist and neuroscientist, I have taught topics in neuroscience to rehabilitation students and conducted clinical neuroscience research for over 15 years. During this time I have come across numerous textbooks, most of which are not written with rehabilitation students in mind. The third edition of *Quick Reference Neuroscience* by Sharon A. Gutman improves on the previous edition of the textbook, which was an invaluable resource for rehabilitation students. This edition is very well organized into 3 main sections: neuroanatomy; function of the neurological system underlying physical, psychological, cognitive, and visual perceptual disorders; and clinical neuropathology related to aging, memory, and addiction. An additional section discusses common neurodiagnostic tests administered in clinical neurology.

There are several unique aspects of this text that make this edition outstanding. First, the material is presented in a simple bulleted format, which organizes the material and makes it easy to access. Second, the illustrations, painstakingly drawn by Dr. Gutman, bring the text to life. The figures will allow readers to visualize abstract neuroanatomical structures that are often difficult to conceptualize. Third, text boxes help translate neuroscience principles to common neurological disorders. Finally, and perhaps most importantly, the textbook reviews material that is most pertinent to rehabilitation professionals in their daily clinical practice.

Potential audiences for this text include students enrolled in neuroscience or neurorehabilitation courses in occupational and physical therapy programs. Given that the book is easy to understand and comprehensive, both students and faculty will benefit from the text. Similarly, clinicians working in the area of neurological rehabilitation will utilize this text as it establishes the clinical relevance of neuroscience.

Dr. Gutman should be congratulated for the enhancements made to this major contribution to the neuroscience literature.

Ashwini K. Rao, EdD, OTR, FAOTA
Associate Professor of Rehabilitation and Regenerative Medicine
Program in Physical Therapy
Gertrude H. Sergievsky Huntington's Disease Center of Excellence
Columbia University Medical Center
New York, New York

INTRODUCTION

The third edition of *Quick Reference Neuroscience* continues to meet a need in the rehabilitation professions that has gone unfilled—the availability of a source that simplifies and thoroughly breaks down neuroscience information into the essential principles that can be used to understand neurological conditions and principles underlying rehabilitation evaluation and practice. Although many excellent textbooks exist that provide exhaustive neuroscience information, much of that information may be extraneous to a practicing therapist who needs to quickly review a specific neuroscience concept to better explain that information to a patient, or it may be extraneous to a student needing to learn the critical neuroscience principles supporting a specific rehabilitation intervention. We are all on information overload and need resources that quickly but fully provide condensed information in a user-friendly, easy-to-use format. The discipline of neuroscience has exploded in the past 2 decades as imaging technologically has facilitated knowledge of the brain in ways previously unimaginable. Much of this newly gained knowledge of brain function relates to molecular and cellular levels—levels of brain analysis of which highly competent rehabilitation therapists do not require in-depth understanding. In fact, much of the molecular and cellular understanding of brain function is not directly used by therapists to treat patients in clinical rehabilitation settings. While it is important to have some understanding of the cellular brain processes underlying behavior, our need as rehabilitation professionals to use this information in practice is not the same as that of a neurologist, neurosurgeon, or neuropathologist. Rehabilitation practitioners are under overwhelming productivity demands for patient care and for evidence dissemination (ie, reading journal articles and using relevant research evidence in practice). Students in rehabilitation health care programs are similarly under tremendous pressure to master a large body of relevant coursework and fieldwork education in a limited amount of time. It seems imprudent to further add to student and practitioner requirements the need to memorize cellular neuroscience information that will not be used in practice.

Quick Reference Neuroscience is a condensed textbook for the practitioner and student who are learning or reviewing the most relevant body of neuroscience supporting rehabilitation therapy. The book is divided into 3 overarching sections: the first addresses neuroanatomy; the second addresses the function of neurological systems underlying physical, psychological, cognitive, and visual perceptual disorders; and the third addresses clinical neuropathology related to aging, addiction, memory, and the neurological substrates of sex and gender.

A separate section describes the common neurodiagnostic tests that therapists do not administer but must have knowledge of when results are discussed at treatment team meetings.

Text is presented in a bulleted format with key information explained in understandable language used by the therapist rather than the neuroscientist. Large-scale color illustrations allow readers to easily visualize neuroanatomical structures and systems that are difficult to see in photos or imaging scans. Text boxes are used in each section to help readers apply key neuroscience concepts to the understanding of common neurological disorders and treatment. Such disorders are the very ones that rehabilitation professionals will observe in clinical settings. All section questions encourage readers to apply neuroscience information to clinical reasoning and problem solving. The most important characteristic about this textbook is its relevance to the specific body of neuroscience that rehabilitation professionals use on a daily basis. This book does not contain neuroscience information that students must memorize for a test and then forget. All presented information is directly relevant to clinical practice, and students and therapists will find that they review this information over the years, whether their careers address the treatment of physical dysfunction, psychiatric disorders, or learning and cognitive disabilities.

Learning is facilitated when information is presented at the learner's pace, ability, and motivational level. *Quick Reference Neuroscience* is an attempt to transform dense information that is not easily related to clinical rehabilitation into an easy-to-understand resource that is directly related to a learner's career goals. This textbook has now gone into its third edition primarily because it facilitates learning, and students and practitioners find the book approachable and readable. Educators, too, have told me that the book has helped them understand how best to identify and teach the most pertinent neuroscience information to student rehabilitation professionals. I invite students, clinicians, and educators to read and use this book as a resource in your curricula, clinical settings, and careers.

Sharon A. Gutman, PhD, OTR, FAOTA
Associate Professor of Rehabilitation and Regenerative Medicine
Programs in Occupational Therapy
Columbia University Medical Center
New York, New York

Directional Terminology

DIRECTIONAL TERMINOLOGY

Anterior or Ventral
- Refers to the front of the organism. Ventral means the "belly" of a 4-legged animal.[1-6]

Posterior or Dorsal
- Refers to the back of the organism.[1-6]

Superior
- Refers to the direction above. One structure is above another.[1-6]

Inferior
- Refers to the direction below. One structure is below another.[1-6]

Rostral
- Refers to the head of the organism. Also refers to structures that are above others.[1-6]

Caudal
- Refers to the tail of the organism. Also refers to structures that are below others.[1-6]

Medial
- Refers to structures that are close to the midline of the body.[1-6]

Lateral
- Refers to structures that are further from the midline of the body.[1-6]

PLANES OF THE BRAIN

Midsagittal
- The midsagittal plane divides the left and right cerebral hemispheres. This plane divides the brain in half and runs along the medial longitudinal fissure.[1-6]

Sagittal (also called *Parasagittal*)
- The sagittal planes run parallel to the midsagittal plane.[1-6]

Coronal (also called *Frontal* or *Transverse*)
- The coronal planes run perpendicular to the sagittal planes. Coronal planes divide the anterior aspect of the brain from the posterior aspect.[1-6]

Horizontal
- The horizontal planes divide the superior aspect of the brain from the inferior aspect.[1-6]

Gutman SA. *Quick Reference Neuroscience for Rehabilitation Professionals: The Essential Neurologic Principles Underlying Rehabilitation Practice, Third Edition* (pp 2-3).
© 2017 Taylor & Francis Group.

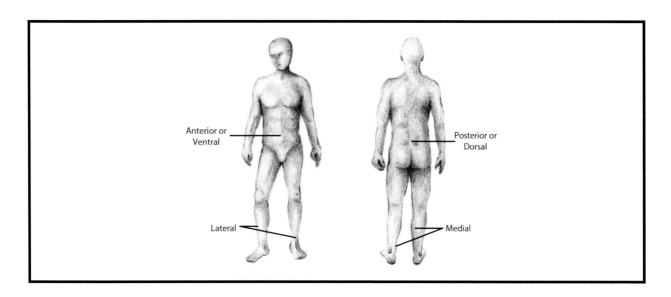

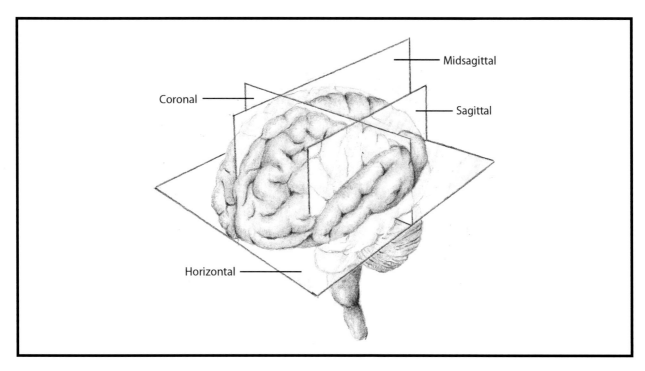

REFERENCES

1. Haines DE. *Neuroanatomy in Clinical Context: An Atlas of Structures, Sections, and Systems.* 9th ed. Philadelphia, PA: Wolters Kluwer, Lippincott, Williams, and Wilkins; 2014.

2. Notle J. *The Human Brain: An Introduction to Its Functional Anatomy.* 6th ed. St. Louis, MO: Mosby; 2008.

3. Woolsey TA, Hanaway J, Gado MH. *The Brain Atlas: A Visual Guide to the Human Central Nervous System.* 3rd ed. New York, NY: Wiley; 2007.

4. Hendelman W. *Atlas of Functional Neuroanatomy.* 3rd ed. Boca Raton, FL: CRC Press; 2015.

5. England M, Wakeley J. *Color Atlas of the Brain and Spinal Cord.* 2nd ed. St. Louis, MO: Mosby; 2005.

6. Felten DL, Shetty A. *Netter's Atlas of Neuroscience.* 2nd ed. Philadelphia, PA: Saunders; 2010.

Division of the Nervous System

- The nervous system is divided into the following[1-6]:
  - Central nervous system (CNS)
  - Peripheral nervous system (PNS)
- The CNS is composed of the following[1-6]:
  - Brain
  - Spinal cord
- The PNS is composed of the following[1-6]:
  - Cranial nerves (CN)
  - Autonomic nervous system (ANS)
  - Somatic nervous system (SNS)
- The brain has 6 major component parts[1-6]:
  1. Cerebral lobes
  2. Cerebellum
  3. Basal ganglia
  4. Diencephalon
  5. Brainstem
  6. Limbic system
- The ANS is composed of the following[1-6]:
  - Parasympathetic nervous system
  - Sympathetic nervous system
- The SNS is responsible for the innervation of skeletal muscles.[1-6]

Gutman SA. *Quick Reference Neuroscience for Rehabilitation Professionals:*
The Essential Neurologic Principles Underlying Rehabilitation Practice,
Third Edition (pp 4-7).
© 2017 Taylor & Francis Group.

Autonomic Nervous System

Innervation of Visceral Muscles and Glands
- Cardiac muscle
- Lungs
- Gastrointestinal tract
- Secretory glands

Parasympathetic Nervous System
- Homeostasis
- Slowing body down
- Decreased blood pressure
- Decreased heart rate
- Peristalsis

Sympathetic Nervous System
- Arousal
- Fight/flight
- Increased blood pressure
- Increased heart rate
- Cessation of peristalsis

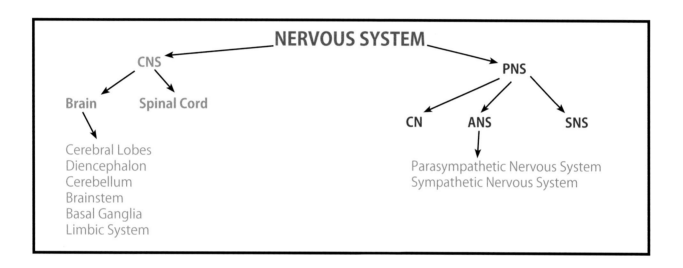

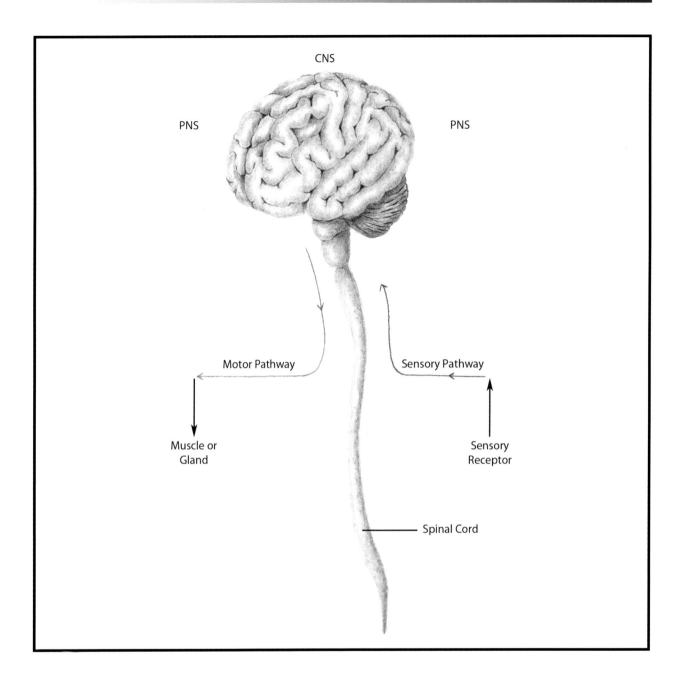

REFERENCES

1. Haines DE. *Neuroanatomy in Clinical Context: An Atlas of Structures, Sections, and Systems.* 9th ed. Philadelphia, PA: Wolters Kluwer, Lippincott, Williams, and Wilkins; 2014.
2. Notle J. *The Human Brain: An Introduction to Its Functional Anatomy.* 6th ed. St. Louis, MO: Mosby; 2008.
3. Woolsey TA, Hanaway J, Gado MH. *The Brain Atlas: A Visual Guide to the Human Central Nervous System.* 3rd ed. New York, NY: Wiley; 2007.
4. Hendelman W. *Atlas of Functional Neuroanatomy.* 3rd ed. Boca Raton, FL: CRC Press; 2015.
5. England M, Wakeley J. *Color Atlas of the Brain and Spinal Cord.* 2nd ed. St. Louis, MO: Mosby; 2005.
6. Felten DL, Shetty A. *Netter's Atlas of Neuroscience.* 2nd ed. Philadelphia, PA: Saunders; 2010.

Gross Cerebral Structures

GROSS CEREBRAL STRUCTURES

Gyri (s., Gyrus)

- Gyri are the wrinkles, or folds, on the surface of the cerebral hemispheres.[1-6]

Sulci (s., Sulcus)

- Sulci are the valleys, or crevices, between the gyri.[1-6]

Convolutions

- Convolutions are the collective name for the gyri and sulci. They are the raised and depressed surfaces of the brain.
- Because brain growth is confined by the skull, the brain folds in on itself as it grows.
- Theorists surmise that the more gyri and sulci one has, the larger one's brain surface is and the more brain capacity one has for brain functions.
- Human brain convolutions are unique—like a fingerprint. However, there are certain sulci and gyri that are common in all human brains.[1-6]

Fissure

- A fissure is a deep groove in the surface of the brain.
- A fissure is deeper than a sulcus; a finger can be inserted into a fissure during dissection. A sulcus is shallow.[1-6]

Medial Longitudinal Fissure

- The medial longitudinal fissure separates the right and left cerebral hemispheres.
- This fissure runs along the midsagittal plane.[1-6]

Central Sulcus (also called the *Sulcus of Rolando*)

- The central sulcus separates the frontal and parietal lobes.
- It also separates the primary motor cortex (M1) from the primary somatosensory cortex (SS1).[7,8]

Precentral Gyrus

- The precentral gyrus is the *primary motor cortex* (M1). This area handles voluntary motor movement.
- It is located just anterior to the central sulcus.[9]

Postcentral Gyrus

- The postcentral gyrus is the *primary somatosensory cortex* (SS1). It is located just posterior to the central sulcus.
- This is the part of the brain that mediates the detection of physical sensation.[10]

Lateral Fissure (also called *Fissure of Sylvius*)

- This fissure separates the temporal lobe from the frontal lobe.[11]

Gutman SA. *Quick Reference Neuroscience for Rehabilitation Professionals: The Essential Neurologic Principles Underlying Rehabilitation Practice, Third Edition* (pp 8-36).
© 2017 Taylor & Francis Group.

CEREBRAL LOBES

- Each hemisphere has 4 separate lobes.

Frontal Lobes

- The borders of the frontal lobes are the lateral fissure and the central sulcus.
- The frontal lobes mediate cognition (intelligence, problem solving, and short-term memory), expressive language, motor planning, mathematical calculations, and working memory.
- The prefrontal lobe mediates executive functions (organization, planning, sequencing, and motivation), self-insight, and regulation of emotions.
- The frontal lobes develop mostly after birth. Development is not thought to be complete until late adolescence or early adulthood.[12]

Parietal Lobes

- The parietal lobes sit just posterior to the frontal lobes.
- The central sulcus divides the parietal lobes from the frontal lobes.
- The posterior border is the parieto-occipital sulcus and can be seen on a midsagittal cross-section.
- The inferior border is the temporal lobe and the lateral fissure.
- Their functions are sensory detection, perception, and interpretation.[13]

Temporal Lobes

- The temporal lobes are the most inferior or caudal lobes.
- They have a poorly defined posterior border, the anterior occipital lobe.
- Their functions are audition (hearing), comprehension of language, and long-term memory.[14]

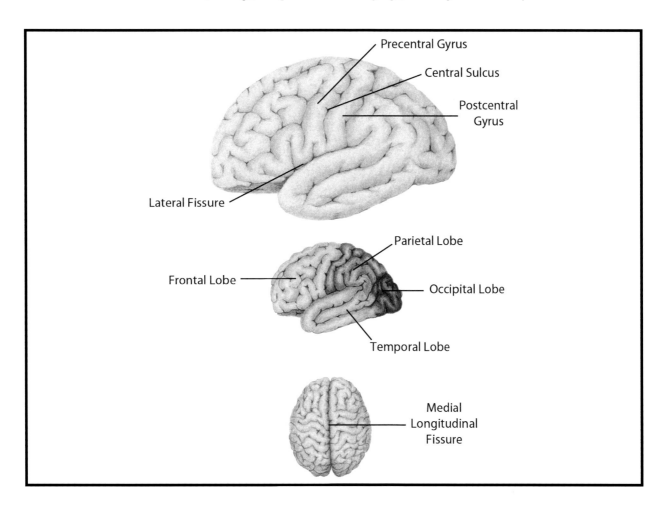

Occipital Lobes

- The occipital lobes are the most posterior lobes.
- They are responsible for the interpretation of visual stimuli from the optic pathways.[15]

Insula

- The insula is a portion of the cerebral cortex that lies deep in the lateral fissure.
- It is covered from view by the frontal, parietal, and temporal lobes.
- Some sources consider the insula a fifth lobe; others consider the insula an extension of the temporal lobe and limbic structures.
- The insula has a role related to basic survival mechanisms such as taste (gustation), sensation of the viscera, and autonomic and homeostasis functions.
- Because of its connections to the limbic system, the insula also functions in emotional processing, including empathy, self-awareness, and emotional regulation.
- The insula appears to become active during the experience of addictive cravings and visceral pain.
- Although not fully understood, the insula appears to have a role in language processing through its pathways to the temporal lobe structures.[16]

RIGHT VS LEFT HEMISPHERES

Right Hemisphere

- The right hemisphere is largely responsible for the interpretation of perceptual and spatial information (eg, reading maps, creating music or art).
- It is responsible for the interpretation of information that requires abstraction as opposed to concrete cognitive processes.
- It is also responsible for the interpretation of tonal inflections in language (as opposed to the concrete meaning of words).
- This hemisphere is responsible for taking the literal interpretation of a story and forming abstract symbolism and metaphors.
- It is responsible for the interpretation of the emotional messages underlying the concrete meaning of words.
- The right hemisphere controls movement on the left side of the body.
- It receives sensory information from the left side of the body.[17]

Left Hemisphere

- In people who are right-hand dominant, the left hemisphere is usually dominant.
- The left hemisphere plays a large role in human language (the expression and interpretation of written and spoken words).
- People with aphasia (language dysfunction) have often sustained left hemisphere damage.
- This hemisphere controls movement on the right side of the body.
- It receives sensory information from the right side of the body.[18]

GRAY MATTER VS WHITE MATTER

- The cerebral hemispheres consist of gray and white matter.

Gray Matter

- Areas where gray matter covers part of the central nervous system (CNS) are called the *cortex* (pl., *cortices*).
- Humans have a cerebral cortex and a cerebellar cortex.
- Gray matter sits on the surface of the cerebrum and the cerebellum.
- Gray matter extends deep within the CNS and forms nuclei body such as the red nucleus and basal ganglia.
- It has a grayish or beige appearance because it consists of nerve cell bodies (nuclei).
- The gray matter is non-myelinated brain matter. Myelin is a lipid that insulates a nerve and increases conduction velocity.[1-6]

Ganglia

- Ganglia are collections of neural cell bodies (or nuclei) usually located outside of the CNS, or in the peripheral nervous system (PNS).
- Example: Dorsal root ganglia
- The dorsal root ganglia contain the cell bodies of the sensory spinal nerves.[1-6]

White Matter

- White matter is located beneath the gray matter, in the internal regions of the cerebrum and cerebellum.
- White matter consists of myelinated fiber tracts or neuronal axons.[1-6]

Commissure

- A commissure is any collection of axons (white matter) that connect one side of the nervous system to the other.[1-6]
- Example: Corpus callosum and the pyramidal decussation

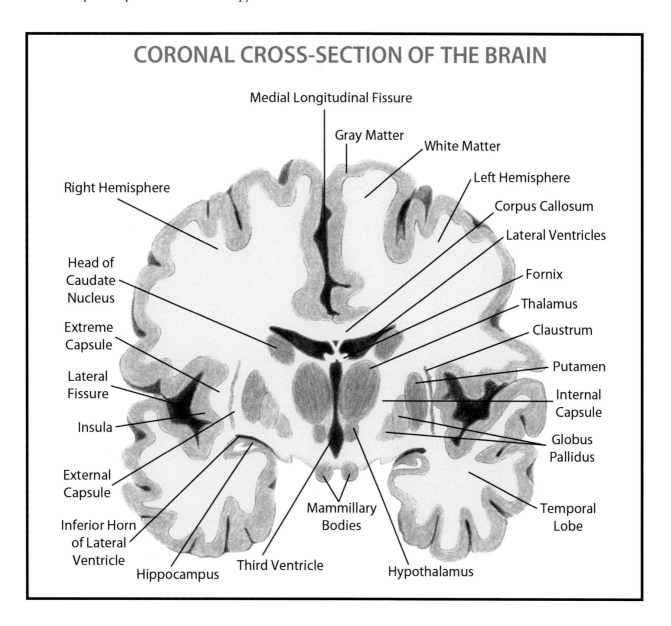

CORONAL CROSS-SECTION OF THE BRAIN

DIENCEPHALON

- In phylogenetic terms, the diencephalon is considered to be an old part of the brain, while the cortex is considered to be a newer brain region.
- The diencephalon consists of 4 structures[19]:
  1. Thalamus
  2. Hypothalamus
  3. Epithalamus
  4. Subthalamus

Thalamus

- Thalamus means "egg-shaped." There are 2 thalamic lobes, 1 in each hemisphere.
- The 2 halves of the thalamus form the lateral walls of the third ventricle. A flattened gray band called the *inter-thalamic adhesion* connects the thalamic lobes.
- The thalamus contains 26 pairs of nuclei. These primarily receive sensory data from the sensory systems. These nuclei then relay the sensory data to specific parts of the cerebral hemispheres.
- All sensory information, except olfaction, travels through the thalamus before it reaches the cortex and is consciously interpreted. The thalamus can be considered a gateway to the cortex.
- However, the thalamus does not passively relay sensory information. It is a dynamic structure that works collaboratively with the cortex in feedforward, feedback, and loop circuits.
- The thalamus receives motor information from the cerebral hemispheres and relays it to the motor receptors, again, in a dynamic process in which the thalamus and cortex work collaboratively.
- The thalamus has a role in sleep-wake cycles and consciousness/alertness.
- It works with the reticular formation to alert the brain to important incoming sensory information and to calm the organism during anxiety. The thalamus acts as a screen for information traveling to the cortex, inhibiting less important information that can be handled at a subcortical level and alerting the cortex to important information that must be dealt with at a conscious level.
- Important thalamic nuclei include the following:
  - *Lateral geniculate nucleus*: responsible for visual processing
  - *Medial geniculate nucleus*: responsible for auditory processing
  - *Ventrolateral nucleus*: responsible for the organization of motor responses
  - *Ventral posterolateral nucleus*: responsible for tactile-sensory processing
- These nuclei have pathways leading to and from the thalamus and traveling to and from specific sensory and motor systems.
- This allows such functions (eg, vision and audition) to be handled at both a conscious and unconscious level. For example, a cortically blind person may not identify the presence of a visual object but may negotiate his or her body movements to accurately avoid contact with the object. Similarly, a person with cortical hearing loss may startle in response to the slam of a door, even though the sound of the slammed door was never consciously interpreted.[20]

Hypothalamus

- The hypothalamus is located just anterior and inferior to the thalamus.
- There are 2 hypothalamic lobes, 1 in each hemisphere.
- Functions include the following[21]:
  - Regulates the autonomic nervous system (ANS)
  - Releases hormones from the pituitary gland, adrenal glands, and pineal gland
  - Regulates temperature
  - Regulates hunger and thirst
  - Regulates sleep-wake cycles (circadian rhythms) and fatigue
  - Works collaboratively with the limbic system in the expression of emotions

Epithalamus

- The epithalamus is located just posterior to the thalamus and just anterior to the pineal gland.
- This is a very small structure composed of the habenula (a nucleus at the posterior of the epithalamus), pineal gland, stria medullaris (a fiber bundle containing afferent fibers), and habenular commissure (a commissure located in front of the pineal gland that connects the habenular nuclei in each hemisphere).
- This region of the brain connects limbic system structures with other brain regions.
- Epithalamic function includes the secretion of melatonin through the pineal gland, which regulates circadian rhythms.[22]

Subthalamus

- The subthalamus is a deep structure and is considered a thalamic nuclei group located caudal to the thalamus.
- The subthalamus contains cells that use dopamine.
- It is a key structure connecting feedback and feedforward circuits of the thalamus and basal ganglia.
- The subthalamus is larger than the epithalamus, and it can be identified in certain coronal cross-sections.
- The function of this structure is not well understood, but some researchers believe it to be a component of the basal ganglia that may function in action selection.
- There is some evidence that the subthalamic nucleus has a role in impulse control.[23]
- The borders of the epithalamus and subthalamus are not distinct.

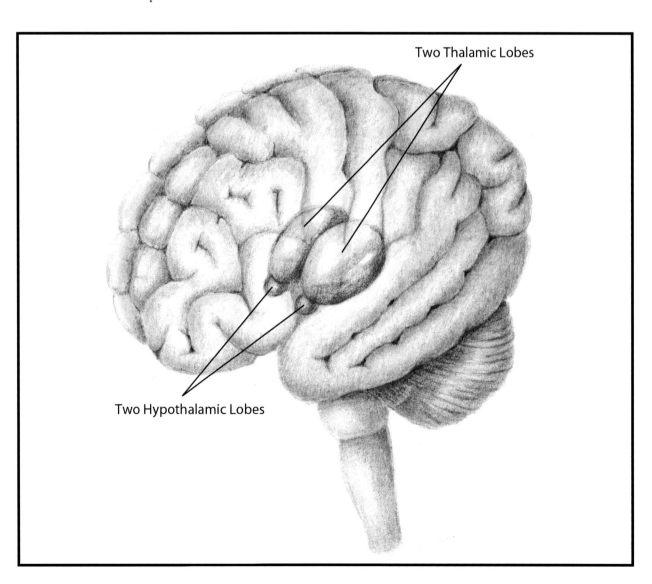

Two Thalamic Lobes

Two Hypothalamic Lobes

OTHER STRUCTURES OF THE DIENCEPHALON

Pituitary Gland

- There is only one pituitary gland in the body.
- The pituitary gland is an endocrine gland that secretes hormones that regulate growth, reproductive activities, and metabolic processes.
- These hormones include the following:
  - Growth hormone (GH)
  - Prolactin (PRL), for lactation
  - Luteinizing hormone (LH), for reproduction
  - Follicle stimulating hormone (FSH), for reproduction
  - Thyroid stimulating hormone (TSH), for metabolism
  - Adrenocorticotrophic hormone (ACTH), for the regulation of stress
- The pituitary works collaboratively with the hypothalamus. The synthesis and secretion of these hormones are controlled by neuropeptides released from the hypothalamus.[24]

Infundibulum

- The infundibulum is the stalk that extends from the hypothalamus and holds the pituitary gland.[25]

Pineal Gland

- The pineal gland is a midline structure located just posterior to the thalamus.
- There is only one pineal gland in the body.
- The pineal gland is innervated by the ANS and is considered to be an endocrine gland. It secretes melatonin, which functions in circadian rhythms (sleep-wake cycles).
- The pineal gland influences the pituitary gland's release of FSH and LH, which are sex hormones.[26]

Posterior Commissure

- The posterior commissure connects the right and left halves of the diencephalon.
- It is located just above the superior colliculi.
- This structure allows communication between the hemispheres if the corpus callosum is lesioned or removed because of pathology.[27]

Anterior Commissure

- The anterior commissure connects the olfactory bulb to the amygdala and may have a role in olfaction.
- It is located in the anterior thalamus and passes through the head of the caudate nucleus.
- This structure allows communication between the hemispheres if the corpus callosum is lesioned.
- There is some evidence that this commissure may function in pain perception.[27,28]

Interthalamic Adhesion

- The interthalamic adhesion is a flattened band of fibers that may allow communication between the 2 thalamic lobes.
- It is located centrally in the thalamus and is present in only 70% to 80% of humans.[29,30]

Septum Pellucidum

- The septum pellucidum is a sheath-like cover that extends over the medial wall of each lateral ventricle.
- The function of this structure is not well understood.[31]

STRUCTURES LOCATED NEAR THE DIENCEPHALON (BUT NOT PART OF THE DIENCEPHALON)

Corpus Callosum

- The corpus callosum is the largest commissure in the brain.
- It allows the right and left cerebral hemispheres to communicate with each other.
- This structure arches around the anterior horn of the lateral ventricles.[32]

Optic Chiasm

- A chiasm is a crossing-over point.
- The optic chiasm is a cross-shaped connection located between the optic nerves.
- It is a midline structure specifically located at the base of the brain just superior to the pituitary gland.[33]

Internal Capsule

- The internal capsule is a large fiber bundle that connects the cerebral cortex with the diencephalon.
- All descending motor messages from the motor cortex travel through the internal capsule to the thalamus, brainstem, spinal cord, and the skeletal muscles.
- Sensory information from the sensory receptors ascends in the spinal cord, through the brainstem, to the thalamus, through the internal capsule, to the SS1.[34]

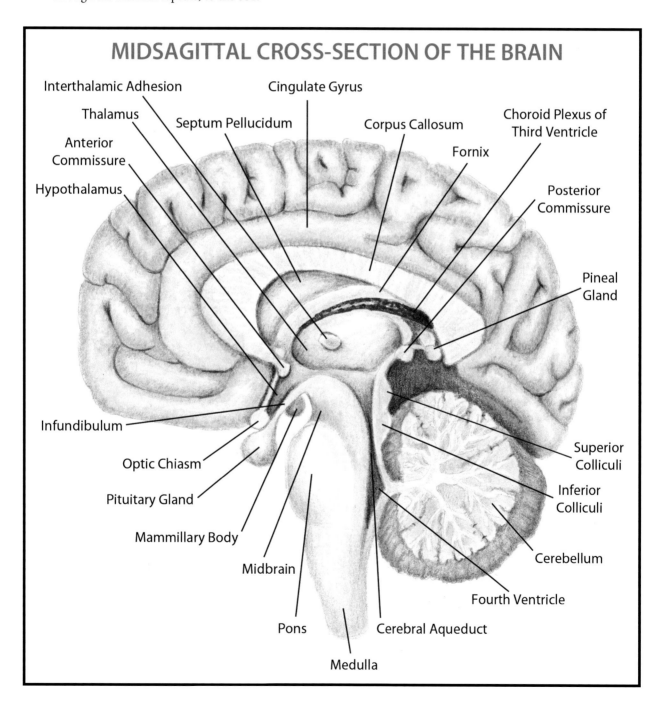

MIDSAGITTAL CROSS-SECTION OF THE BRAIN

Interthalamic Adhesion
Cingulate Gyrus
Thalamus
Septum Pellucidum
Corpus Callosum
Choroid Plexus of Third Ventricle
Anterior Commissure
Fornix
Hypothalamus
Posterior Commissure
Pineal Gland
Infundibulum
Superior Colliculi
Optic Chiasm
Inferior Colliculi
Pituitary Gland
Cerebellum
Mammillary Body
Midbrain
Fourth Ventricle
Pons
Cerebral Aqueduct
Medulla

Mammillary Bodies

- These structures form 2 protrusions that sit within the interpeduncular fossa on the anterior side of the midbrain.
- The mammillary bodies are nuclei groups that form attachments with the hypothalamus and fornix and may play a role in the processing of memory.[35]

Brainstem

- The brainstem is composed of 3 basic structures[36]:
  1. Midbrain
  2. Pons
  3. Medulla
- The brainstem controls vegetative functions:
  - Respiration
  - Cough and gag reflex
  - Pupillary response
  - Swallowing reflex

Midbrain

- The midbrain is the most rostral structure of the brainstem.
- It sits atop of the pons and is just inferior to the thalamus.
- The midbrain has a role in automatic reflexive behaviors dealing with vision, audition, motor control, alertness, temperature regulation, and sleep/wake patterns.[37-39]

External Structures of the Midbrain

Cerebral Peduncles

- Cerebral peduncles are large fiber bundles located on the anterior surface of the midbrain.
- They carry descending motor tracts from the cerebrum to the brainstem.[1-6]

Interpeduncular Fossa

- The interpeduncular fossa is the indentation between the pair of cerebral peduncles.
- The mammillary bodies sit within the interpeduncular fossa on the anterior aspect of the midbrain.[40]

Superior and Inferior Colliculi

- The superior and inferior colliculi sit on the posterior surface of the midbrain just beneath the posterior commissure.
- The superior colliculi are located just above the inferior colliculi.
- The superior colliculi are a pair of relay centers for vision. They communicate directly with the thalamic nuclei (lateral geniculate nuclei) that process visual stimuli. This pathway allows visual information to be processed at an unconscious level.[41]
- The inferior colliculi are a pair of relay centers for audition. They communicate directly with the thalamic nuclei (medial geniculate nuclei) that process auditory stimuli. This pathway allows auditory information to be processed at an unconscious level.[42]

Internal Structures of the Midbrain (seen on cross-section)

Cerebral Aqueduct (also called Aqueduct of Sylvius)

- The cerebral aqueduct is part of the ventricular system. It connects the third and fourth ventricles. Cerebrospinal fluid (CSF) flows through the cerebral aqueduct.[43]

Superior and Inferior Colliculi

- Superior and inferior colliculi can be seen on cross-section.[41,42]

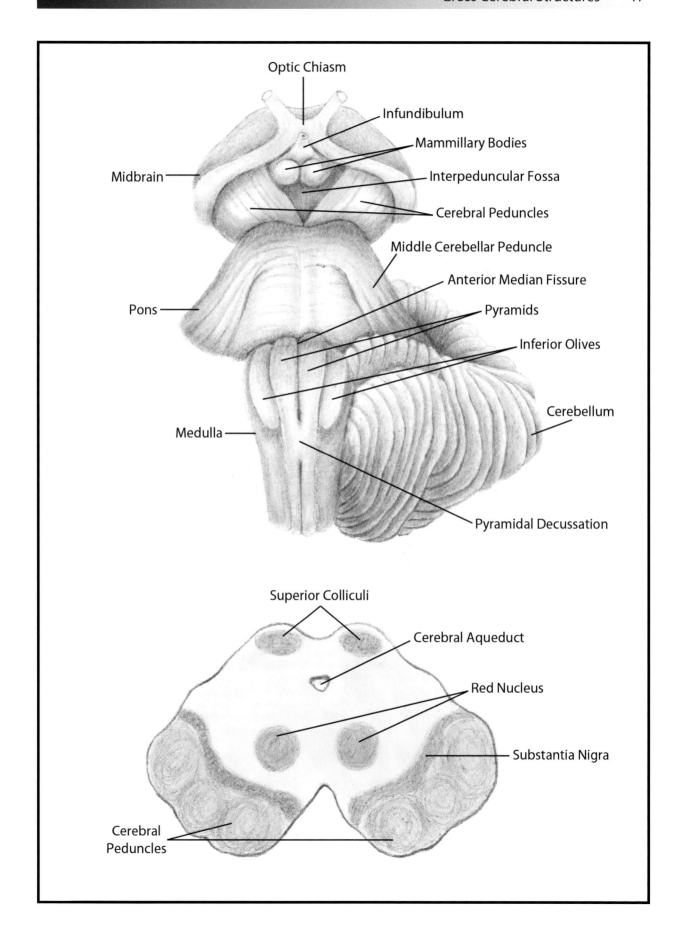

Cerebral Peduncles

- The cerebral peduncles have an inner and outer coat.[1-6]
- The outer coat consists of the crus cerebri.
- The inner coat consists of the red nucleus and the substantia nigra.

Tegmentum

- The substantia nigra and the red nucleus are collectively called the *tegmentum*.[44]

Tectum

- The superior and inferior colliculi are collectively called the *tectum*.[45]

PONS

- The pons is located just caudal to the midbrain and rostral to the medulla.
- The pons is a relay system among the spinal cord, cerebellum, and cerebrum.
- It largely mediates motor information on an unconscious level; for example, shifting weight to maintain balance and making fine motor adjustments in one's muscles to perform precise coordinated limb movement.[46,47]

External Structures of the Pons

Cerebellar Peduncles

- Cerebellar peduncles largely carry sensory information from the pons to the cerebellum about the body's position in space.
- Each cerebellar peduncle is paired; one on each side.
- There are 3 cerebellar peduncles on each side:
  1. *Middle cerebellar peduncle*
     - This peduncle carries sensory information about the body's position in space to the cerebellum.[48]
  2. *Inferior cerebellar peduncle*
     - This peduncle is located in the pons and medulla and carries sensory information about the body's position in space from the pons/medulla to the cerebellum.
     - The cerebellum then analyzes this sensory information and makes decisions about how to readjust the body for precision movement and balance.
     - The cerebellum then sends its decision to the thalamus via the superior cerebellar peduncles. The thalamus sends this motor information back down through the brainstem to the spinal cord and to the skeletal muscles.[49]
  3. *Superior cerebellar peduncle*
     - This peduncle is located in the pons and carries sensory information from the pons to the cerebellum.
     - It also carries sensorimotor information from the cerebellum to the thalamus.[50]

Internal Structures of the Pons

Fourth Ventricle

- The fourth ventricle is located in the posterior pons.
- It is a continuation of the cerebral aqueduct and leads into the central canal of the spinal cord.[51]

Corticospinal Tracts

- These are descending motor tracts that originate in M1 and descend through the internal capsule, thalamus, brainstem, and spinal cord.
- The corticospinal tracts are responsible for voluntary movement.[52]

Middle and Superior Cerebellar Peduncles

- These can be seen in a cross-section of the pons.
- These cerebellar peduncles carry sensory information from the pons to the cerebellum.[48,50]

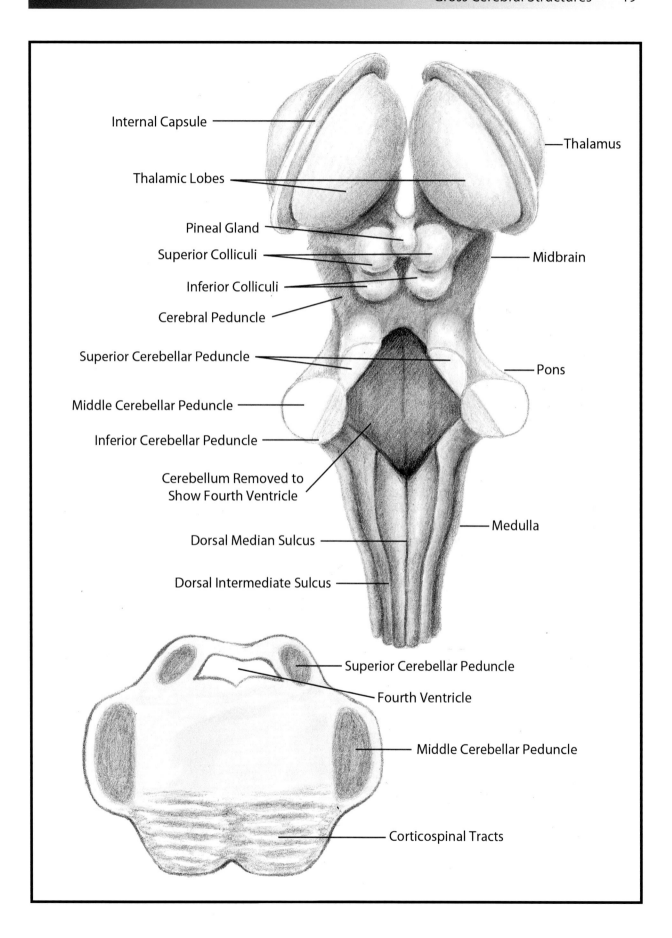

Internal Capsule

Thalamus

Thalamic Lobes

Pineal Gland

Superior Colliculi

Inferior Colliculi

Cerebral Peduncle

Midbrain

Superior Cerebellar Peduncle

Pons

Middle Cerebellar Peduncle

Inferior Cerebellar Peduncle

Cerebellum Removed to Show Fourth Ventricle

Medulla

Dorsal Median Sulcus

Dorsal Intermediate Sulcus

Superior Cerebellar Peduncle

Fourth Ventricle

Middle Cerebellar Peduncle

Corticospinal Tracts

MEDULLA

- The medulla is just caudal to the pons.
- Because the medulla is long, it is divided into the rostral and caudal medulla.
- The medulla carries descending motor messages from the cerebrum to the spinal cord.
- It also carries ascending sensory messages from the spinal cord to the cerebrum.
- Located within the medulla are ANS centers for blood pressure, heart rate, respiration, vasoconstriction and dilation, and the reflex functions of vomiting, coughing, sneezing, and swallowing.[53]

External Structures of the Medulla—Anterior Side

Anterior Median Fissure

- The anterior median fissure divides the medulla into equal right and left halves.
- This fissure continues all the way down the spinal cord.[54]

Pyramids

- The pyramids are 2 large structures that are divided by the anterior median fissure.
- They are motor tracts (the corticospinal tracts), or fiber bundles, that carry descending motor information from the cortex to the spinal cord.[54]

Pyramidal Decussation

- This is the crossing-over point where motor fibers from the left cortex cross to the right side of the spinal cord. Motor fibers from the right side of the cortex cross to the left side of the spinal cord.
- This is why the right cerebral hemisphere controls the left side of the body and the left cerebral hemisphere controls the right side of the body.[1-6,54]

Inferior Olives

- The olives are located just lateral to each pyramid.
- They are relay nuclei that carry ascending sensory information to the cerebellum. This sensory data pertain to the body's position in space.[1-6,54]

External Structures of the Medulla—Posterior Side

Dorsal Median Sulcus

- The dorsal median sulcus is the midline that divides the posterior medulla into equal left and right sides.[55]
- The dorsal median sulcus is not as well-defined as the anterior median fissure.

Dorsal Intermediate Sulcus

- These sulci are located just lateral to the dorsal median sulcus.[55]

Internal Structures of the Medulla (seen in cross-section)

Rostral Medulla

- Caudal end of the fourth ventricle
- Pyramids
- Inferior olivary nuclei
- Inferior cerebellar peduncles

Caudal Medulla

- Central canal (this is where the end of the fourth ventricle meets the spinal cord)
- Pyramids
- Fasciculus gracilis and cuneatus (these are ascending sensory tracts)
- Nucleus gracilis and cuneatus (these are where the nuclei or cell bodies of the fasciculus gracilis and cuneatus are located)

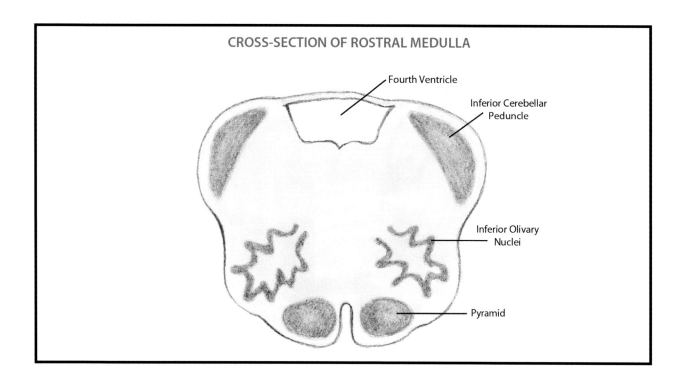

CROSS-SECTION OF ROSTRAL MEDULLA

Fourth Ventricle

Inferior Cerebellar Peduncle

Inferior Olivary Nuclei

Pyramid

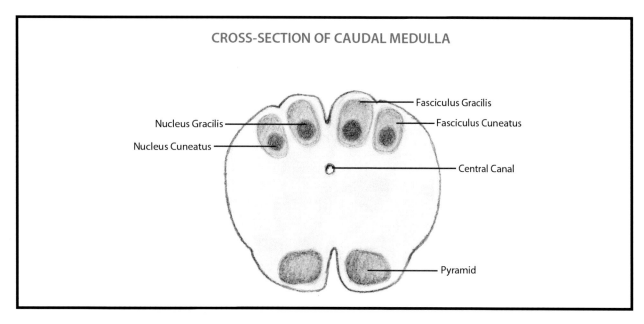

CROSS-SECTION OF CAUDAL MEDULLA

Fasciculus Gracilis

Nucleus Gracilis

Fasciculus Cuneatus

Nucleus Cuneatus

Central Canal

Pyramid

RETICULAR FORMATION

- The reticular formation is diffusely located in the brainstem and plays a role in screening information before it reaches the cortex. Important information critical to functional survival is amplified, while less important information is habituated or not readily noticed by the cortex.
- The reticular formation consists of 2 systems[56]:
  1. Reticular activating system (RAS)
  2. Reticular inhibiting system (RIS)

Reticular Activating System

- The RAS is the brainstem center that is involved in states of wakefulness and sets the general level of brain activation.
- It plays a role in alerting the cortex to attend to important sensory stimuli.
- The RAS is located in the rostral midbrain.[57]

Reticular Inhibiting System

- The RIS is the brainstem center that is involved in states of unconsciousness such as sleep, stupor, or coma.
- It plays a role in habituation or screening of unimportant information so that the cortex can concentrate on information critical to survival or goal-directed behavior.
- The RIS extends from the caudal midbrain to the caudal medulla.[58]

Columns

- The reticular formation is also divided into 3 columns[59]:
  1. *Raphe nuclei*: involved in the neurochemical synthesis of serotonin and mood regulation
  2. *Red nucleus*: involved in motor coordination
  3. *Reticular nucleus*: involved in respiratory exhalation

BASAL GANGLIA

- The basal ganglia form an unconscious motor system that operates on a subcortical level.
- They specifically mediate stereotypic or automatic motor patterns such as those involved in walking, riding a bike, and writing.[60]
- These are activities that are initially learned by using the cortex to think about how to perform such motor movements.
- Once learned, such motor patterns are stored subcortically and become integrated by the basal ganglia.
- Recent research suggests that the basal ganglia also appear to work collaboratively in certain cognitive and affective processes that require timing, such as the ability to appropriately time verbal contributions in group situations and the ability to delay impulses. Some theorists suggest that pathology of the basal ganglia may be involved in attention deficit hyperactivity disorder (ADHD) and autism spectrum disorder.[61]
- The basal ganglia consist of 3 primary structures[60,61]:
  1. Caudate nucleus
  2. Putamen
  3. Globus pallidus
- Three other structures that are considered to be part of the basal nuclei are the subthalamic nucleus of the diencephalon, the substantia nigra of the midbrain, and the nucleus accumbens of the basal forebrain.[60,61]
- The basal ganglia form clusters of neurons within the cerebrum. They are the only ganglia located directly in the CNS.

Caudate Nucleus

- The caudate is an arch-shaped structure that follows the arc of the fornix and lateral ventricles.
- The caudate has a head, body, and tail. The tail attaches to the amygdala of the limbic system.
- This structure is involved in the planning and execution of automatic movement patterns.
- It is also involved in the evaluation of that movement's appropriateness.
- The caudate has strong connections with the frontal lobe and interacts with it in motor planning.
- The caudate also plays a role in the inhibitory control of movement; it acts like a brake on certain motor activities.
- When the brake is not working—when the caudate is damaged—extraneous, purposeless movements appear. Examples include tics and tardive dyskinesias (tongue protrusions, facial grimacing, and lip smacking).[62]
- Tardive means that the disorder occurred after chronic use of certain drugs that affect the caudate nucleus.

Putamen and Globus Pallidus

- The putamen and globus pallidus are located just lateral to the internal capsule.
- These have excitatory and inhibitory properties. If the caudate nucleus and globus pallidus act like a brake to inhibit movement, the putamen serves as an activating mechanism.
- The basal ganglia's ability to achieve balance between inhibitory and excitatory movement is a key component in the precision and timed execution of specific behaviors and actions.[63,64]

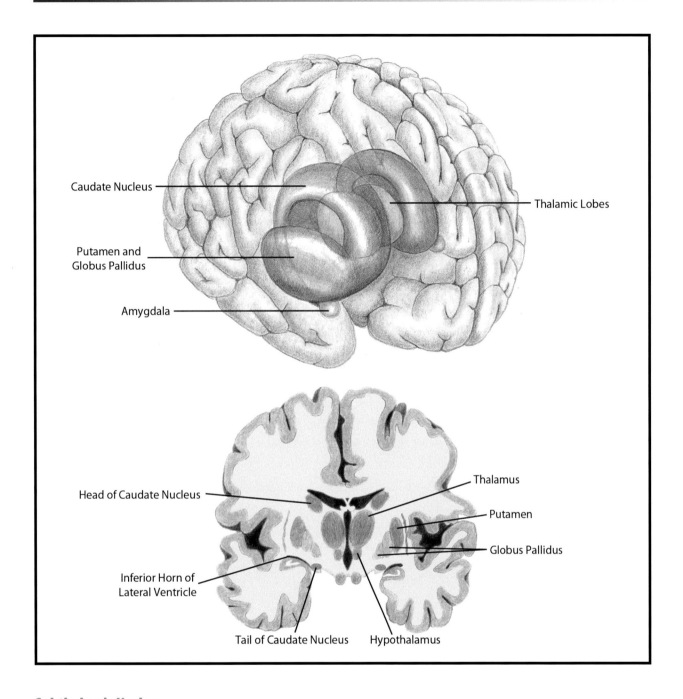

Caudate Nucleus

Thalamic Lobes

Putamen and
Globus Pallidus

Amygdala

Head of Caudate Nucleus

Thalamus

Putamen

Globus Pallidus

Inferior Horn of
Lateral Ventricle

Tail of Caudate Nucleus   Hypothalamus

Subthalamic Nucleus

- The subthalamic nucleus is a thalamic nuclei group located caudal to the thalamus.
- It contains cells that use dopamine and is a key structure connecting feedback and feedforward circuits of the thalamus and basal ganglia.
- In addition to motor control, the subthalamic nucleus is believed to play roles in the timing of cognitive decision making and the processing of emotional information.[65,66]

Substantia Nigra

- The substantia nigra is located in the midbrain.
- The red nucleus and the substantia nigra of the midbrain form the inner coat of the cerebral peduncles.
- The substantia nigra produces dopamine, a neurotransmitter that functions in movement and mood regulation.
- The axons of the substantia nigra form the nigrostriatal pathway. This pathway is referred to as a *dopaminergic pathway* supplying dopamine to the striatum.[67]

Nucleus Accumbens

- The nucleus accumbens is a region of the basal forebrain that is just rostral to the preoptic area of the hypothalamus.
- Together with the olfactory tubercle, this region forms the ventral striatum of the basal ganglia.
- It is believed that the nucleus accumbens has a role in the cognitive processing of behaviors involved in reward and addiction.[68]

Pathology of the Basal Ganglia

- The basal ganglia have been implicated in disorders involving the inability to appropriately time one's social expression and participation. For example, some researchers have suggested that ADHD, which involves difficulty timing one's verbalizations and movements, difficulty delaying urges and actions, and responding impulsively, may be related to pathology of the basal ganglia.[69]
- Deterioration of the basal ganglia has been identified as a key component in Parkinson disease. When dopamine neurons degenerate, automated movements that are controlled by the basal ganglia (such as walking or reacting to a sudden fall) become inhibited.[70]

Extrapyramidal System

- The basal ganglia are considered to be an extrapyramidal system, or *motor system*, that does not use the pyramids to send motor messages to the skeletal muscles.[71]

Corpus Striatum

- *Corpus striatum* is a collective name for the caudate, putamen, and globus pallidus.[60,61]

Neostriatum

- *Neostriatum* is a collective name for the caudate and putamen.[60,61]

Lenticular Nucleus

- *Lenticular nucleus* is a collective name for the globus pallidus and putamen.[60,61]

Paleostriatum

- *Paleostriatum* is another name for the globus pallidus because of its striped appearance.[60,61]

Claustrum

- The claustrum is not considered to be part of the basal ganglia, although it is a group of nuclei located just lateral to the extreme capsule and just medial to the insula.
- Its function is not well understood but may relate to segregated attention of sensory input.[72]

CEREBELLUM

- *Cerebellum* means "little brain," and in many ways, it is like a brain unto itself.
- The cerebellum has 2 hemispheres that are connected by a vermis, much like the corpus callosum connects the cerebral hemispheres.
- It has a cerebellar cortex, with an outer coat of gray matter and an inner core of white matter.
- The cerebellum has 3 lobes.
- The traditional view of the cerebellum holds that it is a sensorimotor system that oversees proprioception (or the unconscious awareness of the body's position in space). In this view, the cerebellum is a sensory and motor system that receives sensory information from joint and muscle receptors concerning the body's position. The cerebellum uses this sensory information to make decisions about how to adjust the body for the coordinated, precision control of movement and balance. These decisions are made on an unconscious level; the messages never reach the cortex for conscious awareness.[73]
- More recent research suggests that the cerebellum has a role in a wider range of functions including attention shifting, practice-related learning, spatial organization, and memory. The cerebellum appears to work collaboratively with cortically based cognitive functions to predict and prepare functional responses to environmental demands.[73,74]
- An additional function of the cerebellum is the regulation of speech. The cerebellum is largely responsible for the timing and fluidity of speech.[73]

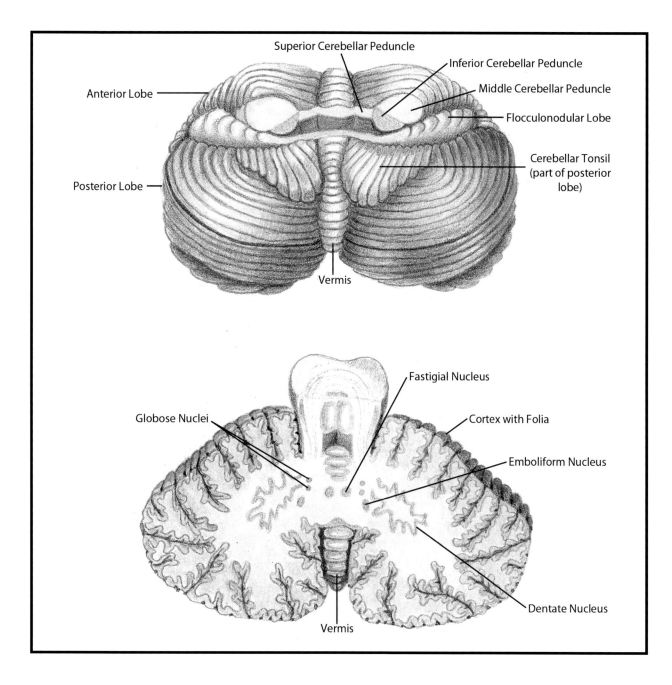

External Structures of the Cerebellum

- The cerebellum has 2 hemispheres; each hemisphere has 3 lobes.

Flocculonodular Lobe

- The flocculonodular lobe is also called the *archicerebellum* (ie, ancient brain) because it used to be considered the oldest part of the cerebellum (in phylogenetic terms).
- It is believed to have developed in organisms without limbs.
- It plays a role in trunk control, postural reflexes, and balance.[75]

Anterior Lobe

- The anterior lobe is also called the *paleocerebellum* (ie, old brain).
- It is often large in size in organisms with limbs.
- It functions in extremity control, postural adjustments, and stereotypic movement patterns.[76]

Posterior Lobe

- The posterior lobe is also called the *neocerebellum* (ie, new brain).
- It is commonly large in size in organisms having a cortex.
- It plays a role in motor planning (praxis) and the precise timing and coordination of multiple muscle groups.
- Some researchers have found evidence that the coordination of cognitive functions may take place in this lobe.[77]

Lateral vs Intermediate Zones

- Functionally, the cerebellum can also be organized into lateral and intermediate zones.
- The lateral zone is believed to have a large role in motor planning.
- The intermediate zone is believed to function in posture and trunk and limb movements.[78]

Three Primary Fissures

- *Primary fissure*: separates the anterior and posterior lobes
- *Posterolateral fissure*: divides the flocculonodular and posterior lobes
- *Horizontal fissure*: divides the posterior lobe in half[74,75,78]

Cerebellar Peduncles

- The peduncles are composed of axons or fibers that travel between the cerebellum and the brainstem (superior and middle cerebellar peduncles travel through the pons; inferior cerebellar peduncle travels through the medulla).
- They are located in the anterior lobe of the cerebellum.[79]

Vermis

- The vermis is a midline structure that has a role in the integration of information used by the right and left cerebellar hemispheres.
- Some have also suggested that the vermis has a role in emotion and the timing of appropriate affective responses.[76]

Internal Structures of the Cerebellum

Cortex with Folia

- The outer covering of the cerebellum is lined with gray matter that has many folds, called *folia*.[74,75,78]

White and Gray Matter

- The interior of the cerebellum consists of a central mass of white matter surrounded by gray matter.
- There are also some smaller masses of gray matter within the central white core. These are the cerebellar nuclei.[80]

Four Pairs of Nuclei

- There are 4 pairs of nuclei, 1 in each hemisphere[81]:
  1. Dentate nuclei (looks similar to the inferior olivary nuclei of the medulla)
  2. Globose nuclei
  3. Emboliform nuclei
  4. Fastigial nuclei

Vermis

- The vermis can also be seen in the interior of the cerebellum.
- As noted previously, evidence is growing that the vermis has a role in emotional processing and the timing of appropriate affective responses.[82]

Pathology of the Cerebellum

- The most evident pathologies of the cerebellum take the form of motor incoordination, decreased proprioception, ataxia, and dysarthric speech.[83]
- A growing body of research, however, suggests that damage to the cerebellum may also result in impaired cognitive functions and a decreased ability to shift attention and respond appropriately to social situations.[73,74]
- Several studies have shown that the most consistent site of neural abnormality in people with autism spectrum disorder is the cerebellum.[84]

- Autopsy and neuroimaging reports have also indicated the presence of cerebellar abnormality in a variety of conditions including ADHD, autism spectrum disorder, unipolar depression, bipolar disorder, and schizophrenia.[85]
- Cognitive and behavioral problems associated with cerebellar pathology include distractibility, hyperactivity, impulsiveness, disinhibition, obsessive behaviors, lowered emotional intelligence, and difficulty with abstraction and planning.[84]

Cerebellar Cognitive Affective Syndrome (CCAS; also called Schmahmann Syndrome)

- CCAS results from damage to or disease of the cerebellum and is a constellation of affective and cognitive problems.[86]
- Signs and symptoms include the following:
  - Disinhibition, blunted affect, impulsivity
  - Obsessive behaviors
  - Problems with planning and anticipating consequences
  - Problems in working memory and abstraction
  - Emotional regulation dysfunction
  - Perseveration
  - Distractibility and inattention
- The cognitive and affective problems of CCAS suggest that the cerebellum has a robust role in cognitive and affective functions that we are only beginning to understand.

LIMBIC SYSTEM

- Phylogenetically, the limbic system is considered to be a very old part of the brain. It is located deep within the core of the brain.
- The limbic system appears to be the source of our raw emotions before they are modulated by the frontal lobes.
- The limbic system is also a formation and retrieval system for long-term memories, particularly memories that have a strong emotional component.
- Although the limbic system used to be considered a separate, distinct neural region, primarily functioning in emotion, it is now understood to be a system highly connected with many brain areas and having an array of functions including emotion, behavior, memory generation and retrieval, and olfaction.[87]

Cingulate Gyrus

- The cingulate gyrus is the most medial and deepest gyrus in the frontal and parietal lobes and is located directly above the corpus callosum.
- The cingulate gyrus has vast connections to the other structures within the brain's emotional limbic system and plays a role in decision making in response to sensory data.[88]

Parahippocampal Gyrus

- The parahippocampal gyrus is the most medial and deepest gyrus in the temporal lobes.
- This gyrus folds back on itself at its anterior end to become the uncus.
- It relays information between the hippocampus and other cerebral areas, particularly the frontal lobes.
- The gyrus functions when we compare a present event to an event stored in long-term memory in order to decide how to handle a present situation.[89]

Uncus

- The uncus is the bulb-like, anterior end of the parahippocampal gyrus.[90]

Fornix

- The fornix bodies are a pair of arch-shaped fibers that begin in the uncus and wrap around to the mammillary bodies.
- The fornix is a relay system for messages generated by the limbic system.[91]

Amygdala

- The amygdalae are an almond-shaped group of nuclei located in each anterior temporal lobe.

- These bihemispheric structures have neural connections to the prefrontal cortex, occipitofrontal cortex, caudate nucleus, hippocampus, ventral tegmental area, nucleus accumbens, hypothalamus, thalamus, and anterior cingulate.
- The amygdalae play a primary role in the mediation of fear, anger, and anxiety.[92]
- They also play a role in the perception of social cues and the generation of feelings of empathy.
- The amygdalae have an additional role in the memory formation of emotionally arousing events.[93]
- The size of the amygdalae have been found to be significantly smaller in some people with autism who have difficulty perceiving and interpreting social cues. A significant number of children with autism also have abnormally densely packed neurons in the amygdala, suggesting a deficiency of dendrites. The neuronal branches connecting neurons appear to be diminished.[94]
- Patients with amygdala damage or pathology may not be able to interpret emotionally laden social cues. For example, they may not recognize the expression of fear on another's face or interpret someone's verbal tone as indicative of irritation.
- Researchers have found that in the normal human brain, a significantly greater number of neural pathways run from the amygdalae to the cortex than from the cortex to the amygdalae. This suggests that the amygdalae may, in part, be responsible for the generation of anxiety and worry. These structures alerts the cortex that a condition of crisis exists.
- Because far fewer pathways run from the cortex to the amygdalae, it is likely that the amygdalae are better at generating anxiety than the cortex is at calming one's worries.[95]
- The amygdalae are also a critical component of the brain reward system (see Section 29), a group of neuroanatomical structures, chemicals, and pathways that are responsible for the processes of addiction and relapse as well as the experience of pleasure and aversion.[96]
- Pathology of the amygdala may be linked to social phobia and social anxiety, autism spectrum disorder, addiction, obsessive-compulsive disorder, and post-traumatic stress disorder.

Olfactory Bulb and Tract

- The olfactory bulb and tract are also known as *cranial nerve* 1.
- The olfactory tract connects to limbic system structures directly through its pathway to the hippocampus. This connection accounts for the deep association between specific odors and long-term memories that hold emotional significance.[97]

Hippocampus

- The hippocampus is located within the parahippocampal gyrus.
- In a coronal section, the hippocampus looks like a seahorse (in Latin, *hippocampus* means "seahorse").
- It is one of the major storehouses in the brain for long-term memory, particularly for memories that are traumatic or emotionally laden.[98]
- In psychoanalytic terms, the hippocampus has been proposed as the storehouse of repressed memories that are gated by the processes of the amygdala.
- There is evidence that the hippocampus also functions in the spatial memory needed for navigating familiar terrains and routes.[99]
- Research has shown that neurogenesis—or the cell birth and maturation of neurons—occurs in the hippocampus throughout life. This may account for the clinical finding that long-term memory is often spared in brain trauma, while short-term memory commonly becomes impaired. Long-term memory is believed to be a function of the hippocampus, while short-term memory occurs largely in the frontal lobes. Neurogenesis in the hippocampus may help to maintain long-term memory despite brain damage that impairs other cognitive functions.[100]
- There has also been evidence that patients with depression or post-traumatic stress disorder have reduced hippocampal volume and cell proliferation; in other words, a reduction in hippocampal neurogenesis. Animal models have shown that chronic stress reduces cell proliferation in the hippocampus. Researchers have found that several classes of antidepressant drugs actually enhance hippocampal neurogenesis—a finding that may, in part, account for antidepressant drug effectiveness.[101]
- Hippocampal damage has been identified in Alzheimer disease and likely results in the common signs of memory loss and disorientation associated with this disease.[102]

LIMBIC SYSTEM

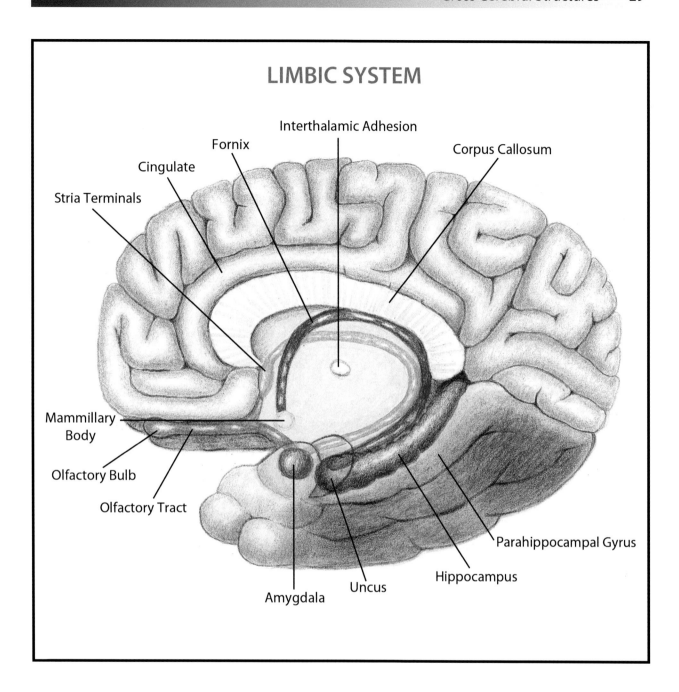

REFERENCES

1. Haines DE. *Neuroanatomy in Clinical Context: An Atlas of Structures, Sections, and Systems.* 9th ed. Philadelphia, PA: Wolters Kluwer, Lippincott, Williams, and Wilkins; 2014.

2. Notle J. *The Human Brain: An Introduction to Its Functional Anatomy.* 6th ed. St. Louis, MO: Mosby; 2008.

3. Woolsey TA, Hanaway J, Gado MH. *The Brain Atlas: A Visual Guide to the Human Central Nervous System.* 3rd ed. New York, NY: Wiley; 2007.

4. Hendelman W. *Atlas of Functional Neuroanatomy.* 3rd ed. Boca Raton, FL: CRC Press; 2015.

5. England M, Wakeley J. *Color Atlas of the Brain and Spinal Cord.* 2nd ed. St. Louis, MO: Mosby; 2005.

6. Felten DL, Shetty A. *Netter's Atlas of Neuroscience.* 2nd ed. Philadelphia, PA: Saunders; 2010.

7. Davatzikos C, Bryan RN. Morphometric analysis of cortical sulci using parametric ribbons: a study of the central sulcus. *J Comput Assist Tomogr.* 2002;(2):298-307.

8. Sun B, Ge H, Tang Y, et al. Asymmetries of the central sulcus in young adults: effects of gender, age and sulcal pattern. *Int J Dev Neurosci.* 2015;44:65-74. doi:10.1016/j.ijdevneu.2015.06.003.

9. Radoš M, Nikić I, Radoš M, Kostović I, Hof PR, Šimić G. Functional reorganization of the primary motor cortex in a patient with a large arteriovenous malformation involving the precentral gyrus. *Transl Neurosci.* 2013;4(2):269-272. doi:10.2478/s13380-013-0122-5.

10. Kato H, Izumiyama M. Impaired motor control due to proprioceptive sensory loss in a patient with cerebral infarction localized to the postcentral gyrus. *J Rehabil Med.* 2015;47(2):187-190. doi:10.2340/16501977-1900.

11. Tanriover N, Rhoton AL Jr, Kawashima M, Ulm AJ, Yasuda A. Microsurgical anatomy of the insula and the Sylvian fissure. *J Neurosurg.* 2004;100(5):891-922.

12. Stuss DT. Functions of the frontal lobes: relation to executive functions. *J Int Neuropsychol Soc.* 2011;17(05):759-765. doi:10.1017/S1355617711000695.

13. Bruner E, Iriki A. Extending mind, visuospatial integration, and the evolution of the parietal lobes in the human genus [published online ahead of print May 2015]. *Quat Int.* doi:10.1016/j.quaint.2015.05.019.

14. Simmons W, Martin A. The anterior temporal lobes and the functional architecture of semantic memory. *J Int Neuropsychol Soc.* 2009;15(05):645-649. doi:10.1017/S1355617709990348.

15. van Lamsweerde A, Johnson J. The role of the occipital cortex in capacity limits and precision of visual working memory. *J Vision.* 2015;15(12):661-661. doi:10.1167/15.12.661.

16. Gasquoine PG. Contributions of the insula to cognition and emotion. *Neuropsychol Rev.* 2014;24(2):77-87. doi:10.1007/s11065-014-9246-9.

17. MacNeilage PF, Rogers LJ, Vallortigara G. Origins of the left and right brain. *Sci Am.* 2009;301(1):60-67. doi:10.1038/scientificamerican0709-60.

18. Pinel P, Dehaene S. Beyond hemispheric dominance: brain regions underlying the joint lateralization of language and arithmetic to the left hemisphere. *J Cog Neurosci.* 2010;22(1):48-66. doi:10.1162/jocn.2009.21184.

19. Martinez-Ferre A, Martinez S. Molecular regionalization of the diencephalon. *Front Neurosci.* 2012;6:73. doi:10.3389/fnins.2012.00073.

20. Constantinople CM, Bruno RM. Deep cortical layers are activated directly by thalamus. *Science.* 2013;340(6140):1591-1594. doi:10.1126/science.1236425.

21. Saper CB, Lowell BB. The hypothalamus. *Curr Biol.* 2014;24(23):R1111-R1116. doi:10.1016/j.cub.2014.10.023.

22. Guilding C, Hughes ATL, Piggins HD. Circadian oscillators in the epithalamus. *Neuroscience.* 2010;169(4):1630-1639. doi:10.1016/j.neuroscience.2010.06.015.

23. Turner DA. Re-engineering the subthalamus. *World Neurosurg.* 2013;80(5):476-478. doi:10.1016/j.wneu.2012.05.014.

24. Perez-Castro C, Renner U, Haedo MR, Stalla GK, Arzt E. Cellular and molecular specificity of pituitary gland physiology. *Physiol Rev.* 2012;92(1):1-38. doi:10.1152/physrev.00003.2011.

25. Tsutsumi S, Hori M, Ono H, Tabuchi T, Aoki S, Yasumoto Y. The infundibular recess passes through the entire pituitary stalk [published online ahead of print April 18, 2015]. *Clin Neuroradiol.* 2015:1-5. doi:10.1007/s00062-015-0391-1.

26. Borjigin J, Zhang LS, Calinescu AA. Circadian regulation of pineal gland rhythmicity. *Mol Cell Endocrinol.* 2012;349(1):13-19. doi:10.1016/j.mce.2011.07.009.

27. Liu Y, Dawant BM. Automatic detection of the anterior and posterior commissures on MRI scans using regression forests. *Engineering in Medicine and Biology Society (EMBC), 2014 36th Annual International Conference of the IEEE,* 1505-1508. doi:10.1109/EMBC.2014.6943887.

28. Peltier J, Verclytte S, Delmaire C, Pruvo JP, Havet E, Le Gars D. Microsurgical anatomy of the anterior commissure: Correlations with diffusion tensor imaging fiber tracking and clinical relevance. *Neurosurgery.* 2011;69:ons241-247. doi:10.1227/NEU.0b013e31821bc822.

29. Cheng S, Tan K, Bilston LE. The effects of the interthalamic adhesion position on cerebrospinal fluid dynamics in the cerebral ventricles. *J Biomech*. 2010;43(3):579-582. doi:10.1016/j.neuroimage.2010.01.110.

30. Sen F, Ulubay H, Ozeksi P, Sargon MF, Tascioglu AB. Morphometric measurements of the thalamus and interthalamic adhesion by MR imaging. *Neuroanatomy*. 2005;4:10-12.

31. Raybaud C. The corpus callosum, the other great forebrain commissures, and the septum pellucidum: anatomy, development, and malformation. *Neuroradiology*. 2010;52(6):447-477. doi:10.1007/s00234-010-0696-3.

32. Luders E, Toga AW, Thompson PM. Why size matters: differences in brain volume account for apparent sex differences in callosal anatomy: the sexual dimorphism of the corpus callosum. *Neuroimage*. 2014;84:820-824. doi:10.1016/j.neuroimage.2013.09.040.

33. Petros TJ, Rebsam A, Mason CA. Retinal axon growth at the optic chiasm: to cross or not to cross. *Ann Rev Neurosci*. 2008;31:295-315. doi:10.1146/annurev.neuro.31.060407.125609.

34. Sullivan EV, Zahr NM, Rohlfing T, Pfefferbaum A. Fiber tracking functionally distinct components of the internal capsule. *Neuropsychologia*. 2010;48(14):4155-4163. doi:10.1016/j.neuropsychologia.2010.10.023.

35. Tagliamonte M, Sestieri C, Romani GL, Gallucci M, Caulo M. MRI anatomical variants of mammillary bodies. *Brain Struct Funct*. 2015;220(1):85-90. doi:10.1007/s00429-013-0639-y.

36. Itoi K, Sugimoto N. The brainstem noradrenergic systems in stress, anxiety and depression. *J Neuroendocrinol*. 2010;22(5):355-361. doi:10.1111/j.1365-2826.2010.01988.x.

37. Chaudhury D, Walsh JJ, Friedman AK, et al. Rapid regulation of depression-related behaviours by control of midbrain dopamine neurons. *Nature*. 2013;493(7433):532-536. doi:10.1038/nature11713.

38. Limbrick-Oldfield EH, Brooks JC, Wise RJ, et al. Identification and characterisation of midbrain nuclei using optimised functional magnetic resonance imaging. *NeuroImage*. 2012;59(2):1230-1238. doi:10.1016/j.neuroimage.2011.08.016.

39. D'Ardenne K, Eshel N, Luka J, Lenartowicz A, Nystrom LE, Cohen JD. Role of prefrontal cortex and the midbrain dopamine system in working memory updating. *Proc Natl Acad Sci USA*. 2012;109(49):19900-19909. doi:10.1073/pnas.1116727109.

40. Oyama K, Prevedello DM, Ditzel Filho LF, et al. Anatomic comparison of the endonasal and transpetrosal approaches for interpeduncular fossa access. *Neurosurg Focus*. 2014;37(4):E12. doi:10.3171/2014.7.FOCUS14329.

41. Fuchs I, Ansorge U. Unconscious cueing via the superior colliculi: evidence from searching for onset and color targets. *Brain Sci*. 2012;2(1):33-60. doi:10.3390/brainsci2010033.

42. Malmierca MS, Young ED. Inferior colliculus microcircuits. *Front Neural Circuits*. 2014;8:113. doi:10.3389/fncir.2014.00113.

43. Abbey P, Singh P, Khandelwal N, Mukherjee KK. Shunt surgery effects on cerebrospinal fluid flow across the aqueduct of Sylvius in patients with communicating hydrocephalus. *J Clin Neurosci*. 2009;16(4):514-518. doi:10.1016/j.jocn.2008.05.009.

44. Lodge DJ, Grace AA. The laterodorsal tegmentum is essential for burst firing of ventral tegmental area dopamine neurons. *Proc Natl Acad Sci U S A*. 2006;103(13):5167-5172. doi:10.1073/pnas.0510715103.

45. Nikolaou N, Lowe AS, Walker AS, et al. Parametric functional maps of visual inputs to the tectum. *Neuron*. 2012;76(2):317-324. doi:10.1523/JNEUROSCI.4990-12.2013.

46. Fuller PM, Saper CB, Lu J. The pontine REM switch: past and present. *J Physiol*. 2007;584(3):735-741. doi:10.1113/jphysiol.2007.140160.

47. Casanova E, Lazzari RE, Lotta S, Mazzucchi A. Locked-in syndrome: improvement in the prognosis after an early intensive multidisciplinary rehabilitation. *Arch Phys Med Rehabil*. 2003;84(6):862-867. doi:10.1016/S0003-9993(03)00008-X.

48. Uchino A, Sawada A, Takase Y, Kudo S. Symmetrical lesions of the middle cerebellar peduncle: MR imaging and differential diagnosis. *Magn Reson Med Sci*. 2004;3(3):133-140. doi:10.2463/mrms.3.133.

49. Lawton MT, Quinones-Hinojosa A, Jun P. The supratonsillar approach to the inferior cerebellar peduncle: anatomy, surgical technique, and clinical application to cavernous malformations. *Neurosurgery*. 2006;59(4):ONS-244. doi:10.1227/01.NEU.0000232767.16809.68.

50. Lea J, Lechner C, Halmagyi GM, Welgampola MS. Not so benign positional vertigo: paroxysmal downbeat nystagmus from a superior cerebellar peduncle neoplasm. *Otol Neurotology*. 2014;35(6):e204-e205. doi:10.1097/MAO.0000000000000359.

51. Sugimoto T, Uranishi R, Yamada T. Gradually progressive symptoms of normal pressure hydrocephalus caused by an arachnoid cyst in the fourth ventricle: a case report. *World Neurosurg*. 2016;85:364.e19-22. doi:10.1016/j.wneu.2015.08.061.

52. Freund P, Weiskopf N, Ashburner J, et al. MRI investigation of the sensorimotor cortex and the corticospinal tract after acute spinal cord injury: a prospective longitudinal study. *Lancet Neurol*. 2013;12(9):873-881. doi:10.1016/S1474-4422(13)70146-7.

53. Kumagai H, Oshima N, Matsuura T, et al. Importance of rostral ventrolateral medulla neurons in determining efferent sympathetic nerve activity and blood pressure. *Hypertens Res*. 2012;35(2):132-141. doi:10.1038/hr.2011.208.

54. Bican O, Minagar A, Pruitt AA. The spinal cord: a review of functional neuroanatomy. *Neurol Clin*. 2013;31(1):1-18. doi:10.1016/j.ncl.2012.09.009.

55. Jacquesson T, Streichenberger N, Sindou M, Mertens P, Simon E. What is the dorsal median sulcus of the spinal cord? Interest for surgical approach of intramedullary tumors. *Surg Radiol Anat.* 2014;36(4):345-351. doi:10.1007/s00276-013-1194-1.

56. Jang SH, Kwon HG. The ascending reticular activating system from pontine reticular formation to the hypothalamus in the human brain: a diffusion tensor imaging study. *Neurosci Lett.* 2015;590:58-61. doi:10.1016/j.neulet.2015.01.071.

57. Jang SH, Do Lee H. Ascending reticular activating system recovery in a patient with brain injury. *Neurology.* 2015;84(19):1997-1999. doi:10.1212/ WNL. 0000000000001563.

58. Vanini G, Nemanis K, Baghdoyan HA, Lydic R. GABAergic transmission in rat pontine reticular formation regulates the induction phase of anesthesia and modulates hyperalgesia caused by sleep deprivation. *Eur J Neurosci.* 2014;40(1): 2264-2273. doi:10.1111/ejn.12571.

59. Commons KG. Two major network domains in the dorsal raphe nucleus. *J Compar Neurol.* 2015;523(10):1488-1504. doi:10.1002/cne.23748.

60. Nelson AB, Kreitzer AC. Reassessing models of basal ganglia function and dysfunction. *Ann Rev Neurosci.* 2014;37:117. doi:10.1146/annurev-neuro-071013-013916.

61. Leisman G, Braun-Benjamin O, Melillo R. Cognitive-motor interactions of the basal ganglia in development. *Front Syst Neurosci.* 2014;8:16. doi:10.3389/fnsys.2014.00016.

62. Kotz SA, Anwander A, Axer H, Knösche TR. Beyond cytoarchitectonics: the internal and external connectivity structure of the caudate nucleus. *PLoS ONE.* 2013;8(7): e70141. doi:10.1371/journal.pone.0070141.

63. Vicente AF, Bermudez MA, del Carmen Romero M, Perez R, Gonzalez F. Putamen neurons process both sensory and motor information during a complex task. *Brain Res.* 2012;1466:70-81. doi:10.1016/j.brainres.2012.05.037.

64. Arimura N, Nakayama Y, Yamagata T, Tanji J, Hoshi, E. Involvement of the globus pallidus in behavioral goal determination and action specification. *J Neurosci.* 2013;33(34):13639-13653. doi:10.1523/JNEUROSCI.1620-13.2013.

65. Buot A, Welter ML, Karachi C, et al. Processing of emotional information in the human subthalamic nucleus. *J Neurol Neurosurg Psychiatry.* 2013;84(12):1331-1339. doi:10.1136/jnnp-2011-302158.

66. Cavanagh JF, Wiecki TV, Cohen MX, et al. Subthalamic nucleus stimulation reverses mediofrontal influence over decision threshold. *Nat Neurosci.* 2011;14(11):1462-1467. doi:10.1038/nn.2925.

67. Antal M, Beneduce BM, Regehr WG. The substantia nigra conveys target-dependent excitatory and inhibitory outputs from the basal ganglia to the thalamus. *J Neurosci.* 2014;34(23):8032-8042. doi:10.1523/JNEUROSCI.0236-14.2014.

68. Stuber GD, Sparta DR, Stamatakis AM, et al. Excitatory transmission from the amygdala to nucleus accumbens facilitates reward seeking. *Nature.* 2011;475(7356):377-380. doi:10.1038/nature10194.

69. Shaw P, De Rossi P, Watson B, et al. Mapping the development of the basal ganglia in children with attention-deficit/hyperactivity disorder. *J Am Acad Child Adolesc Psychiatry.* 2014;53(7):780-789. doi:10.1016/j.jaac.2014.05.003.

70. Rolinski M, Griffanti L, Szewczyk-Krolikowski K, et al. Aberrant functional connectivity within the basal ganglia of patients with Parkinson's disease. *Neuroimage Clin.* 2015;8:126-132. doi:10.1016/j.nicl.2015.04.003.

71. Zhang HY, Tang H, Chen WX, et al. Mapping the functional connectivity of the substantia nigra, red nucleus and dentate nucleus: a network analysis hypothesis associated with the extrapyramidal system. *Neurosci Lett.* 2015;606:36-41. doi:10.1016/j.neulet.2015.08.029.

72. Goll Y, Atlan G, Citri A. Attention: the claustrum. *Trends Neurosci.* 2015;38(8):486-495. doi:10.1016/j.tins.2015.05.006.

73. Stoodley CJ. The cerebellum and cognition: evidence from functional imaging studies. *Cerebellum.* 2012;11(2):352-365. doi:10.1007/s12311-011-0260-7.

74. Stoodley CJ, Valera EM, Schmahmann JD. (2012). Functional topography of the cerebellum for motor and cognitive tasks: an fMRI study. *Neuroimage.* 2012;59(2):1560-1570. doi:10.1016/j.neuroimage.2011.08.065.

75. Roostaei T, Nazeri A, Sahraian MA, Minagar A. The human cerebellum: a review of physiologic neuroanatomy. *Neurol Clin.* 2014;32(4):859-869. doi:10.1016/j.ncl.2014.07.013.

76. Cerebelar V, Variaciones T. Cerebellar vermis: topography and variations. *Int J Morphol.* 2010;28(2):439-443.

77. Schlerf JE, Verstynen TD, Ivry RB, Spencer RM. Evidence of a novel somatopic map in the human neocerebellum during complex actions. *J Neurophysiol.* 2010;103(6):3330-3336. doi:10.1152/jn.01117.2009.

78. Grimaldi G, Manto M. Topography of cerebellar deficits in humans. *Cerebellum.* 2012;11(2):336-351. doi:10.1007/s12311-011-0247-4.

79. Kataoka H, Izumi T, Kinoshita S, Kawahara M, Sugie K, Ueno S. Infarction limited to both middle cerebellar peduncles. *J Neuroimaging.* 2011;21(2):e171-e172. doi:10.1111/j.1552-6569.2010.00503.x.

80. Cavanagh J, Krishnadas R, Batty GD, et al. Socioeconomic status and the cerebellar grey matter volume. Data from a well-characterised population sample. *Cerebellum.* 2013;12(6):882-891. doi:10.1007/s12311-013-0497-4.

81. Diedrichsen J, Maderwald S, Küper M., et al. Imaging the deep cerebellar nuclei: a probabilistic atlas and normalization procedure. *Neuroimage.* 2011;54(3):1786-1794. doi:10.1016/j.neuroimage.2010.10.035.

82. Baumann O, Mattingley JB. Functional topography of primary emotion processing in the human cerebellum. *Neuroimage.* 2012;61(4):805-811. doi:10.1016/j.neuroimage.2012.03.044.

83. Miyai I, Ito M, Hattori N, et al. Cerebellar ataxia rehabilitation trial in degenerative cerebellar diseases. *Neurorehabil Neural Repair.* 2012;26(5):515-522. doi:10.1177/1545968311425918.

84. Fatemi SH, Aldinger KA, Ashwood P. Consensus paper: pathological role of the cerebellum in autism. *Cerebellum.* 2012;11(3):777-807. doi:10.1007/s12311-012-0355-9.

85. Stoodley CJ. The cerebellum and neurodevelopmental disorders. *Cerebellum.* 2016;15(1):34-37. doi:10.1007/s12311-015-0715-3.

86. Wolf U, Rapoport MJ, Schweizer TA. Evaluating the affective component of the cerebellar cognitive affective syndrome. *J Neuropsychiatry.* 2014;21(3):245-253.

87. Rolls ET. Limbic systems for emotion and for memory, but no single limbic system. *Cortex.* 2015;62:119-157. doi:10.1016/j.cortex.2013.12.005.

88. Merkley TL, Larson MJ, Bigler ED, Good DA, Perlstein WM. Structural and functional changes of the cinguålate gyrus following traumatic brain injury: relation to attention and executive skills. *J Int Neuropsychol Soc.* 2013;19(08):899-910. doi:10.1017/S135561771300074X.

89. Ward AM, Schultz AP, Huijbers W, et al. The parahippocampal gyrus links the default mode cortical network with the medial temporal lobe memory system. *Hum Brain Mapp.* 2014;35(3):1061-1073. doi:10.1002/hbm.22234.

90. Poppenk J, Evensmoen HR, Moscovitch M, Nadel L. Long-axis specialization of the human hippocampus. *Trends Cogn Sci.* 2013;17(5):230-240. doi:10.1016/j.tics.2013.03.005.

91. Mielke MM, Okonkwo OC, Oishi K, et al. Fornix integrity and hippocampal volume predict memory decline and progression to Alzheimer's disease. *Alzheimers Dement.* 2012;8(2):105-113. doi:10.1016/j.jalz.2011.05.2416.

92. Li H, Penzo MA, Taniguchi H, Kopec CD, Huang ZJ, Li B. Experience-dependent modification of a central amygdala fear circuit. *Nat Neurosci.* 2013;16(3):332-339. doi:10.1038/nn.3322.

93. Goerlich-Dobre KS, Lamm C, Pripfl J, Habel U, Votinov M. The left amygdala: a shared substrate of alexithymia and empathy. *NeuroImage.* 2015;122:20-32. doi:10.1016/j.neuroimage.2015.08.014.

94. Bellani M, Calderoni S, Muratori F, Brambilla P. Brain anatomy of autism spectrum disorders II. Focus on amygdala. *Epidemiol Psychiatr Sci.* 2013;22(04):309-312. doi:10.1017/S2045796013000346.

95. Tye KM, Prakash R, Kim SY, et al. Amygdala circuitry mediating reversible and bidirectional control of anxiety. *Nature.* 2011;471(7338):358-362. doi:10.1038/nature09820.

96. Pauli WM, Hazy TE, O'Reilly RC. Expectancy, ambiguity, and behavioral flexibility: separable and complementary roles of the orbital frontal cortex and amygdala in processing reward expectancies. *J Cogn Neurosci.* 2012;24(2):351-366. doi:10.1162/jocn_a_00155.

97. Czerniawska E, Zegardło E, Wojciechowski J. Memories evoked by odors stimulating the olfactory nerve versus odors stimulating both the olfactory and trigeminal nerves: possible qualitative differences? *Percept Mot Skills.* 2013;117(1): 248-256. doi:10.2466/24.27.PMS.117x15z5.

98. Edelson M, Sharot T, Dolan RJ, Dudai Y. Following the crowd: brain substrates of long-term memory conformity. *Science.* 2011;333(6038):108-111. doi:10.1126/science.1203557.

99. Jadhav SP, Kemere C, German PW, Frank LM. Awake hippocampal sharp-wave ripples support spatial memory. *Science.* 2012;336(6087):1454-1458. doi:10.1126/science.1217230.

100. Spalding KL, Bergmann O, Alkass K. Dynamics of hippocampal neurogenesis in adult humans. *Cell.* 2013;153(6): 1219-1227. doi:10.1016/j.cell.2013.05.002.

101. Mahar I, Bambico FR, Mechawar N, Nobrega JN. Stress, serotonin, and hippocampal neurogenesis in relation to depression and antidepressant effects. *Neurosci Biobehav Rev.* 2014;38:173-192. doi:10.1016/j.neubiorev.2013.11.009.

102. Fjell AM, McEvoy L, Holland D, Dale AM, Walhovd KB. What is normal in normal aging? Effects of aging, amyloid and Alzheimer's disease on the cerebral cortex and the hippocampus. *Prog Neurobiol.* 2014;117:20-40. doi:10.1016/j.pneurobio.2014.02.004.

CLINICAL TEST QUESTIONS

Sections 1 to 3

1. Five days after a stroke, Mr. Peters cannot move his right arm and leg and lists to the right when seated in his wheelchair. In which hemisphere did Mr. Peters experience a stroke?
    a. left hemisphere
    b. right hemisphere

2. After his motorcycle accident 1 year ago, Jim's personality and behavior have changed significantly. He now has severe short-term memory problems and is disorganized, foul-mouthed, and impulsive. Jim can neither foresee the consequences of his actions nor does he possess insight into his behaviors. Damage of which cerebral lobe would largely be responsible for these problems?
    a. occipital
    b. temporal
    c. frontal
    d. parietal

3. After his brain injury, Jack has difficulty regulating his temperature, has experienced acne due to hormonal imbalances, and is unable to assume a normal sleep-wake cycle. Which neurological structure is primarily thought to be responsible for these functions?
    a. hypothalamus
    b. thalamus
    c. cerebellum
    d. brainstem

4. After a gunshot wound to the head, Jose has been in a vegetative state. Although he shows no response to verbal commands, his cough and gag reflex, swallowing reflex, and pupillary response all remain intact. Which neurological structure is responsible for these reflexive functions?
    a. thalamus
    b. brainstem
    c. frontal lobe
    d. basal ganglia

5. From the time Francis was a young child, he displayed tics and uncontrollable movements (eg, tongue protrusion and neck snapping). Although these dyskinesias have improved somewhat as he has aged, they still remain to a moderate extent as an adult. Which neurological structure is believed to be responsible for this movement disorder?
    a. occipital lobe
    b. brainstem
    c. hippocampus
    d. basal ganglia

6. Mr. Jones has been diagnosed with Parkinson disease and displays the festinating gait, intention tremors, and masked face associated with this disease. Which neurological structure is believed to be responsible for these symptoms and is often the target of drug and surgical treatment?
    a. hippocampus
    b. brainstem
    c. basal ganglia
    d. thalamus

7. Alice has been experiencing decreased proprioception; she has difficulty understanding the location of her limbs in space and in relation to each other. She walks with great clumsiness or motor incoordination and ataxia. Magnetic resonance imaging has most likely detected a tumor in which neurological structure?

    a. cerebellum

    b. hypothalamus

    c. cerebral peduncles

    d. parietal lobe

8. Josh, a 7 year old in elementary school, has difficulty interpreting others' emotions through their facial expressions, verbal tone, and body language. He also has difficulty generating age-appropriate feelings of empathy for his classmates. Josh has been given a diagnosis of autism spectrum disorder (ASD) by his pediatrician. Researchers have targeted which one of the below neurological structures as dysfunctional in ASD?

    a. medial longitudinal fissure

    b. amygdala

    c. pyramidal decussation

    d. anterior median fissure

9. When Mrs. Anderson walked into the hospital to visit her newly born grandson, the scents and odors of the hospital setting reminded her of the time when, 5 years ago, her husband was a hospital patient after experiencing cardiac arrest. Which 2 structures are primarily responsible for long-term memory storage of emotionally laden events associated with a distinct odor?

    a. hippocampus and optic chiasm

    b. reticular formation and optic chiasm

    c. reticular formation and olfactory bulb and tract

    d. hippocampus and olfactory bulb and tract

10. After a stroke, Ms. Rodriguez displays aphasia, a language disorder in which she has difficulty speaking and interpreting others' words. Language disorders such as aphasia commonly occur in which hemisphere?

    a. left

    b. right

Answers

1. a
2. c
3. a
4. b
5. d
6. c
7. a
8. b
9. d
10. a

Ventricular System

Ventricular System

- In embryonic development, the brain begins as a flat plate that fuses into a tube.
- The space within the tube becomes the ventricular system.
- The walls of the tube become the brain; the ventricles are the hollow spaces in the brain that contain cerebrospinal fluid (CSF).[1]

There Are Four Ventricles in the Brain

- One pair of lateral ventricles (one in each hemisphere)
- One third ventricle
- One fourth ventricle[2]

Two Lateral Ventricles

- There is one lateral ventricle in each hemisphere.
- The lateral ventricles are divided by the septum pellucidum, a thin partition covering the medial wall of each lateral ventricle.
- Each lateral ventricle has 3 horns[3]:
    1. *Anterior horn*: projects into the frontal lobe
    2. *Inferior horn*: projects into the temporal lobe
    3. *Posterior horn*: projects into the occipital lobe

One Third Ventricle

- The third ventricle is surrounded by the diencephalon.
- The thalamic lobes form the walls of the third ventricle.
- The hypothalamic lobes form the floor of the third ventricle.[4]

One Fourth Ventricle

- The fourth ventricle is located within the pons, rostral medulla, and the cerebellum.[5]

Choroid Plexus

- The choroid plexus is made up of the vascular structures in the brain that protrude into the ventricles and produce CSF.
- All of the ventricles contain choroid plexus, but the lateral ventricles contain the most.[6]

Cerebral Aqueduct (also called *Aqueduct of Sylvius*)

- The cerebral aqueduct is a narrow channel that descends through the midbrain.
- It connects the third and fourth ventricles and is a common site of blockage.[7]

Gutman SA. *Quick Reference Neuroscience for Rehabilitation Professionals:
The Essential Neurologic Principles Underlying Rehabilitation Practice,
Third Edition* (pp 38-43).
© 2017 Taylor & Francis Group.

VENTRICULAR SYSTEM

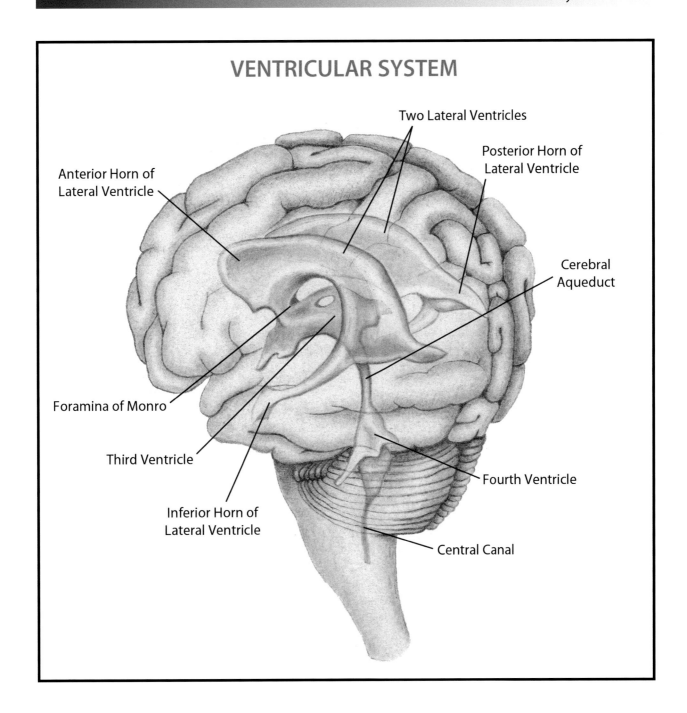

Two Lateral Ventricles

Posterior Horn of
Lateral Ventricle

Anterior Horn of
Lateral Ventricle

Cerebral
Aqueduct

Foramina of Monro

Fourth Ventricle

Third Ventricle

Inferior Horn of
Lateral Ventricle

Central Canal

Central Canal
- The central canal begins in the caudal medulla and descends all the way down the spinal cord.
- This canal connects the ventricular system with the spinal cord and contains CSF.[8]

Foramina of Monro
- There are 2 foramina of Monro, 1 in each hemisphere.
- These foramina are small channels that connect the lateral ventricles with the third ventricle.[9]

Foramen of Magendie (also called *Median Aperture*)
- There is only one foramen of Magendie, which is an opening in the fourth ventricle (in the rostral medulla).
- The foramen of Magendie opens to the subarachnoid space below the cerebellum. This space is located above the brain and beneath the skull.

- The subarachnoid space is the space between the arachnoid membrane and the pia mater.
- This foramen is also a potential site of CSF blockage.[10]

Foramina of Luschka (also called *Lateral Apertures*)

- There are 2 foramina of Luschka. These are openings in the fourth ventricle (in the pons) through which CSF can exit to the subarachnoid space.
- The foramina are potential sites of CSF blockage.[11]

CEREBROSPINAL FLUID

- CSF is a clear, colorless fluid that bathes and nourishes the brain and spinal cord.[12]

Arachnoid Villi

- CSF is reabsorbed in the arachnoid villi and returns to blood circulation through the venous sinuses.
- The arachnoid villi are projections of the arachnoid mater into the dura mater.[13]

Cerebrospinal Fluid Pressure

- CSF maintains a constant circulatory pressure.
- The formation of CSF is independent of the pressure.
- This is important with regard to hydrocephalus (a buildup of CSF pressure and fluid).
- Even if CSF pressure increases, CSF continues to be produced.
- There is no neurologic mechanism that detects too much CSF and regulates its pressure and production.[14]

Composition of Cerebrospinal Fluid

- CSF composition and rate of flow are used for diagnostic purposes to identify disease processes.
- Example: Spinal tap (or lumbar puncture) is a procedure in which the spinal cavity is punctured with a needle to extract CSF for diagnostic purposes.[14]

Flow of Cerebrospinal Fluid

- The CSF is produced in the choroid plexus; travels through the ventricles, subarachnoid space, and spinal cord; and then returns to the circulatory system.[15]

Function of the Cerebrospinal Fluid

- One function of CSF is protection of the brain; the fluid acts as a shock absorber.
- Another function is the exchange of nutrients and waste; CSF plays a role in the transfer of substances between the blood and the nervous tissue.
- CSF helps in diagnosis and is examined for its rate of pressure and fluid composition.
- CSF also has a role in the transport of some hormones throughout the central nervous system.[14]

HYDROCEPHALUS

- Hydrocephalus is an abnormal accumulation of pressure and fluid that results in compression of neural tissue and enlargement of the ventricles.
- This condition causes intracranial pressure and progressive enlargement of the head in childhood if not corrected. If onset occurs in adulthood, the condition can be lethal if not addressed.[16]

Noncommunicating Hydrocephalus

- Noncommunicating hydrocephalus occurs when blockage in the ventricular system prevents the CSF from reaching the arachnoid villi for reabsorption.
- This condition occurs from obstruction of the foramina or cerebral aqueduct.
- The most commonly obstructed site is the cerebral aqueduct.[17]

Communicating Hydrocephalus

- Communicating hydrocephalus results from impaired reabsorption of CSF that does not occur from blockage of the foramina.

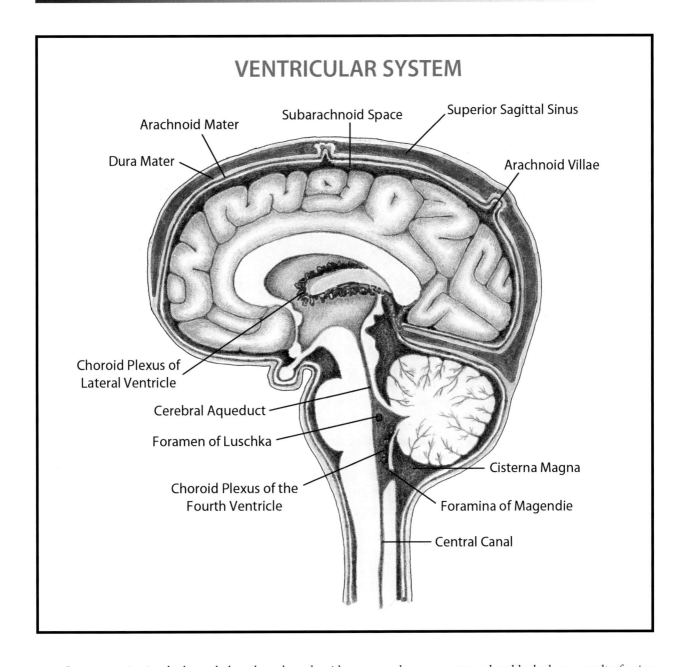

VENTRICULAR SYSTEM

- In communicating hydrocephalus, the subarachnoid space can become narrowed or blocked as a result of prior bleeding or meningitis.
- In normal pressure hydrocephalus, a form of communicating hydrocephalus often occurring in the elderly, the CSF flow spaces become enlarged without an accompanying increase in intracranial pressure. This condition can result in dementia, incontinence, and gait abnormalities.[18]

Congenital Hydrocephalus in Infants

Etiology

- Blockage (particularly in the foramina of Luschka and Magendie)
- Excessive production of CSF for unknown reasons
- Meningitis, causing adhesions and resultant blockages in the subarachnoid space
- Tumors of the choroid plexus, causing excessive CSF production
- Hemorrhage or inflammation; the ependyma (the lining of the ventricles) is especially sensitive to viral infections during embryonic development.[19,20]

Common Sites of Blockage
- Cerebral aqueduct
- Foramen of Luschka
- Foramen of Magendie[19,20]

Pathological Effects
- The infant's skull expands to accommodate the increased fluid. The cranial sutures separate.
- Head expansion and bulging of the fontanels
- Compression of neural tissue
- Because the skull can expand, increased intracranial pressure is usually not present; intelligence is often spared.[19,20]

Treatment
- If hydrocephalus was caused by a blockage, then treatment requires a shunt, or tube, that bypasses the blockage.
- If there is excessive production of CSF, treatment requires a shunt usually placed from the fourth ventricle to the abdomen to drain the excess CSF.
- If diagnosed, hydrocephalus can be successfully treated in utero.[21]

Adult Onset Hydrocephalus

Etiology
- Tumors
- Meningitis
- Hemorrhage and inflammation
- Unknown causes[22]

Pathological Effects
- Enlarged ventricles and rapid atrophy of neural tissue; there is no place for the fluid to go.
- Increased intracranial pressure
- Headache and vomiting
- Cognitive deterioration
- This condition is life-threatening unless treatment occurs quickly.[23]

Treatment
- Treatment for an adult usually involves surgical shunt placement (to the abdomen) to drain the excess fluid.
- In noncommunicating hydrocephalus, surgical shunt placement is attempted to bypass the blockage.
- In communicating hydrocephalus, attempts to clear the arachnoid villi of exudate are made first. If this is unsuccessful, surgical shunting is often indicated.[23]

Normal Pressure Hydrocephalus

- A form of hydrocephalus that develops in adulthood, usually in the fifth, sixth, or seventh decade.
- This occurs because the arachnoid villi cannot absorb the CSF. The CSF pressure remains normal.
- It is characterized by the following[23]:
  - Unsteady gait
  - Progressive dementia
  - Urinary incontinence
- Treatment usually involves surgical shunt placement.

REFERENCES

1. Lowery LA, Sive H. Totally tubular: the mystery behind function and origin of the brain ventricular system. *Bioessays.* 2009;31(4):446-458. doi:10.1002/bies.200800207.

2. Haines DE. *Neuroanatomy in Clinical Context: An Atlas of Structures, Sections, and Systems.* 9th ed. Philadephia, PA: Wolters Kluwer, Lippincott, Williams, and Wilkins; 2014.

3. Zhu DC, Xenos M, Linninger AA, Penn RD. Dynamics of lateral ventricle and cerebrospinal fluid in normal and hydrocephalic brains. *J Magn Reson Imaging.* 2006;24(4):756-770. doi:10.1002/jmri.20679.

4. Kurtcuoglu V, Soellinger M, Summers P, et al. Computational investigation of subject-specific cerebrospinal fluid flow in the third ventricle and aqueduct of Sylvius. *J Biomech.* 2007;40(6):1235-1245. doi:10.1016/j.jbiomech.2006.05.031.

5. Longatti P, Fiorindi A, Feletti A, Baratto V. Endoscopic opening of the foramen of Magendie using transaqueductal navigation for membrane obstruction of the fourth ventricle outlets: technical note. *J Neurosurg.* 2006;105(6):924-927.

6. Wolburg H, Paulus W. Choroid plexus: Biology and pathology. *Acta Neuropathol.* 2010;119(1):75-88. doi:10.1007/s00401-009-0627-8.

7. Longatti P, Fiorindi A, Perin A, Martinuzzi A. Endoscopic anatomy of the cerebral aqueduct. *Neurosurgery.* 2007;61(3):1-7. doi:10.1227/01.neu.0000289705.64931.0c.

8. Woolsey TA, Hanaway J, Gado MH. *The Brain Atlas: A Visual Guide to the Human Central Nervous System.* 3rd ed. New York, NY: Wiley; 2007.

9. Tubbs RS, Oakes P, Maran IS, Salib C, Loukas, M. The foramen of Monro: a review of its anatomy, history, pathology, and surgery. *Childs Nerv Syst.* 2014;30(10):1645-1649. doi:10.1007/s00381-014-2512-6.

10. Ciołkowski M, Sharifi M, Tarka S, Ciszek B. Median aperture of the fourth ventricle revisited. *Folia Morphol.* 2011;70(2):84-90.

11. Takami H, Shin M, Kuroiwa M, Isoo A, Takahashi K, Saito N. Hydrocephalus associated with cystic dilation of the foramina of Magendie and Luschka: case report. *J Neurosurg Pediatr.* 2010;5(4):415-418.

12. Engelhardt B, Sorokin L. The blood-brain and the blood-cerebrospinal fluid barriers: function and dysfunction. *Sem Immunopathol.* 2009;31(4):497-511. doi:10.1007/s00281-009-0177-0.

13. Ohnishi YI, Iwatsuki K, Morii E, et al. Histopathological study of spinal meningioma originating from the arachnoid villi. *Brain Tumor Pathol.* 2011;28(1):77-81. doi:10.1007/s10014-010-0003-3.

14. Sakka L, Coll G, Chazal J. Anatomy and physiology of cerebrospinal fluid. *Eur Ann Otorhinolaryngol Head Neck Dis.* 2011;128(6):309-316. doi:10.1016/j.anorl.2011.03.002

15. Bunck AC, Kröger JR, Jüttner A, et al. Magnetic resonance 4D flow characteristics of cerebrospinal fluid at the craniocervical junction and the cervical spinal canal. *Eur Radiol.* 2011;21(8):1788-1796. doi:10.1007/s00330-011-2105-7.

16. Lorenzo AV, Page LK, Watters GV. Relationship between cerebrospinal fluid formation, absorption and pressure in human hydrocephalus. *Brain.* 2015;93(4):679-692. doi.org/10.1093/brain/93.4.679.

17. Sæhle T, Eide PK. Association between ventricular volume measures and pulsatile and static intracranial pressure scores in non-communicating hydrocephalus. *J Neurol Sci.* 2015;350(1):33-39. doi:10.1016/j.jns.2015.02.003.

18. Abbey P, Singh P, Khandelwal N, Mukherjee KK. Shunt surgery effects on cerebrospinal fluid flow across the aqueduct of Sylvius in patients with communicating hydrocephalus. *J Clin Neurosci.* 2009;16(4):514-518. doi:10.1016/j.jocn.2008.05.009.

19. Munch TN, Rasmussen MLH, Wohlfahrt J, Juhler M, Melbye M. Risk factors for congenital hydrocephalus: a nationwide, register-based, cohort study. *J Neurol Neurosurg Psychiatry.* 2014;85(11):1253-1259. doi:10.1136/jnnp-2013-306941.

20. Tully HM, Dobyns WB. Infantile hydrocephalus: a review of epidemiology, classification and causes. *Eur J Med Genet.* 2014;57(8):359-368. doi:10.1016/j.ejmg.2014.06.002.

21. Jernigan SC, Berry JG, Graham DA, Goumnerova L. The comparative effectiveness of ventricular shunt placement versus endoscopic third ventriculostomy for initial treatment of hydrocephalus in infants. *J Neurosurg Pediatrics.* 2014;13(3):295-300. doi:10.3171/2013.11.PEDS13138.

22. Kasanmoentalib ES, Brouwer MC, van der Ende A, van de Beek D. Hydrocephalus in adults with community-acquired bacterial meningitis. *Neurology.* 2010;75(10):918-923. doi:10.1212/ WNL.0b013e3181f11e10.

23. Siraj S. An overview of normal pressure hydrocephalus and its importance: how much do we really know? *J Am Med Dir Assoc.* 2011;12(1):19-21. doi:10.1016/j.jamda.2010.05.005.

The Cranium

SKULL

- The skull is the bony framework of the head and supports, anchors, and protects the brain.
- It is composed of 14 bones of the face, 28 adult teeth, and 8 cranial bones.[1-3]

Cranium

- The cranium is the portion of the skull that encloses the brain.
- It consists of 8 separate fused bones: frontal bone, occipital bone, sphenoid bone, ethmoid bone, 2 temporal bones, and 2 parietal bones.[1-3]

Suture Lines

- The suture lines are junctions between the skull bones. These are areas where the bones have fused.
- The cranial sutures begin to fuse at 2 months and are complete at 18 months.
- There are 3 suture lines: coronal, sagittal, and lambdoid.[1-4]

Coronal Suture

- This suture runs along the coronal plane and connects the frontal bone with the parietal bones.[5]

Sagittal Suture

- This suture runs along the midsagittal plane and connects the 2 parietal bones.[5]

Lambdoid Suture

- This suture connects the 2 parietal bones to the occipital bone.[5]

Fontanels

- The fontanels are nonossified spaces, or soft spots, located between the cranial bones of a fetus and newborn.
- These allow the skull to expand to accommodate the growing brain.[6]
  - Anterior fontanel
  - Posterior fontanel
  - Sphenoid fontanel
  - Mastoid fontanel

Gutman SA. *Quick Reference Neuroscience for Rehabilitation Professionals: The Essential Neurologic Principles Underlying Rehabilitation Practice, Third Edition* (pp 44-47).
© 2017 Taylor & Francis Group.

Floor of the Cranial Cavity

- The undersurface of the brain sits within the floor of the cranial cavity.
- The cranial cavity holds the anterior–inferior aspect of the frontal lobes, the inferior aspect of the temporal lobes, and the inferior aspect of the cerebellum.[1-3]

Fossa

- The undersurface of the brain sits in 3 cranial sections, or fossae[1-3,7]:
    1. *Anterior cranial fossa*: primarily supports the frontal lobes
    2. *Middle cranial fossa*: supports the anterior-inferior temporal lobes and the diencephalon
    3. *Posterior cranial fossa*: supports the cerebellum

Sharp Edges of the Fossa

- The fossae are problematic in brain injuries caused by motor vehicle accidents (MVA).
- Sharp edges of each fossa can shear brain tissue and vessels, causing brain damage.[8]

Foramina

- The foramina are openings in the skull for the passage of blood vessels and nerves.[9]

Foramen Magnum

- The foramen magnum is the largest foramen in the skull.
- It is the opening through which the brainstem connects with the spinal cord and is located in the occipital bone.[10]

Function of the Cranial Bones

- The cranial bones provide protection for the brain.[1-3]

Skull Fractures

- One of the weakest cranial sutures is at the pterion, a site that joins the frontal, parietal, temporal, and sphenoid bones.
- The pterion often fractures upon strong impact, causing penetration of bone fragments entering the brain; cerebral arteries are easily ruptured as a result.[11]
- Frontal and parietal bone fractures are often seen as a result of MVAs.[12]

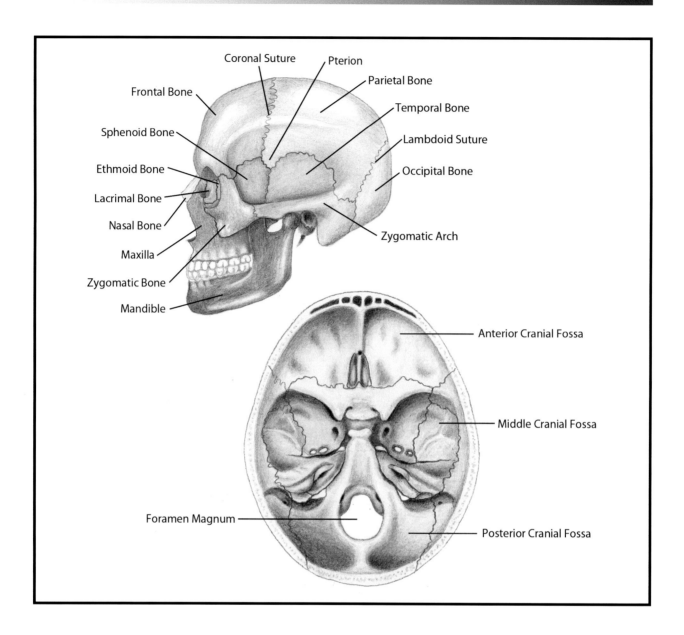

REFERENCES

1. Marieb EN, Wilhelm PB, Mallatt JB. *Human Anatomy.* 7th ed. New York, NY: Pearson; 2013.

2. Martini FH, Timmons MJ, Tallitsch RB. *Human Anatomy.* 8th ed. New York, NY: Pearson; 2014.

3. Hansen JT. *Netter's Clinical Anatomy.* 3rd ed. Philadelphia, PA: Elsevier Saunders; 2014.

4. Sanchez T, Stewart D, Walvick M, Swischuk L. Skull fracture vs. accessory sutures: how can we tell the difference? *Emerg Radiol.* 2010;17(5):413-418. doi:10.1007/s10140-010-0877-8.

5. Slater BJ, Lenton KA, Kwan MD, Gupta DM, Wan DC, Longaker MT. Cranial sutures: a brief review. *Plast Reconstr Surg.* 2008;121(4):170e-178e. doi:10.1097/01.prs.0000304441.99483.97.

6. Pindrik J, Ye X, Ji BG, Pendleton C, Ahn ES. (2014). Anterior fontanelle closure and size in full-term children based on head computed tomography. *Clin Pediatr.* 2014;53(12):1149-57. doi:10.1177/0009922814538492.

7. Lieberman DE, McBratney BM, Krovitz G. The evolution and development of cranial form in Homo sapiens. *Proc Natl Acad Sci U S A.* 2002;99(3):1134-1139. doi:10.1073/pnas.022440799.

8. Bigler ED. Anterior and middle cranial fossa in traumatic brain injury: relevant neuroanatomy and neuropathology in the study of neuropsychological outcome. *Neuropsychology.* 2007;21(5):515. doi:10.1037/0894-4105.21.5.515.

9. Berge JK, Bergman RA. Variations in size and in symmetry of foramina of the human skull. *Clin Anat.* 2001;14(6): 406-413. doi:10.1002/ca.1075.

10. Rhoton AL Jr. The foramen magnum. *Neurosurgery.* 2000;47(3):S155-S193.

11. Hussain Saheb S, Haseena S, Prasanna LC. Unusual Wormian bones at Pterion—three case reports. *J Biomed Sci Res.* 2010;2(2);116-118.

12. Mulligan RP, Mahabir RC. The prevalence of cervical spine injury, head injury, or both with isolated and multiple cranio-maxillofacial fractures. *Plast Reconstr Surg.* 2010;126(5):1647-1651. doi:10.1097/PRS.0b013e3181ef90e4.

The Meninges

LOCATION

- The meninges are located between the skull and brain, and they cover the spinal cord. They form a seal around the central nervous system (CNS).
- There are 3 layers of meninges: dura mater, arachnoid mater, and pia mater.
- The following are the layers of structures as they are positioned between the skull and brain[1]:
  - Skull
  - Epidural space
  - Dura mater
  - Subdural space
  - Arachnoid mater
  - Subarachnoid space
  - Pia mater
  - Brain

DURA MATER

- The dura mater is the outermost meningeal layer.
- It is a very tough and thick membrane that is attached to the inner surface of the cranium.[1]
- The dura has 2 projections that extend into the brain:
  1. *Falx cerebri*: extends into the medial longitudinal fissure[2]
  2. *Tentorium*: the horizontal shelf of dura that sits between the occipital lobe and the cerebellum[3]
- The falx cerebri and tentorium decrease linear and rotary forces on the brain.

Dural Sinuses

- The dural sinuses function as large veins and are located above the frontal and parietal lobes.
- The sinuses act like a circulatory system, allowing cerebral veins to empty into them.
- The cerebral veins also receive cerebrospinal fluid (CSF) from the subarachnoid space via the arachnoid villi.
- These fluids are then returned to their general circulatory systems.[4]

Gutman SA. *Quick Reference Neuroscience for Rehabilitation Professionals: The Essential Neurologic Principles Underlying Rehabilitation Practice, Third Edition* (pp 48-51).
© 2017 Taylor & Francis Group.

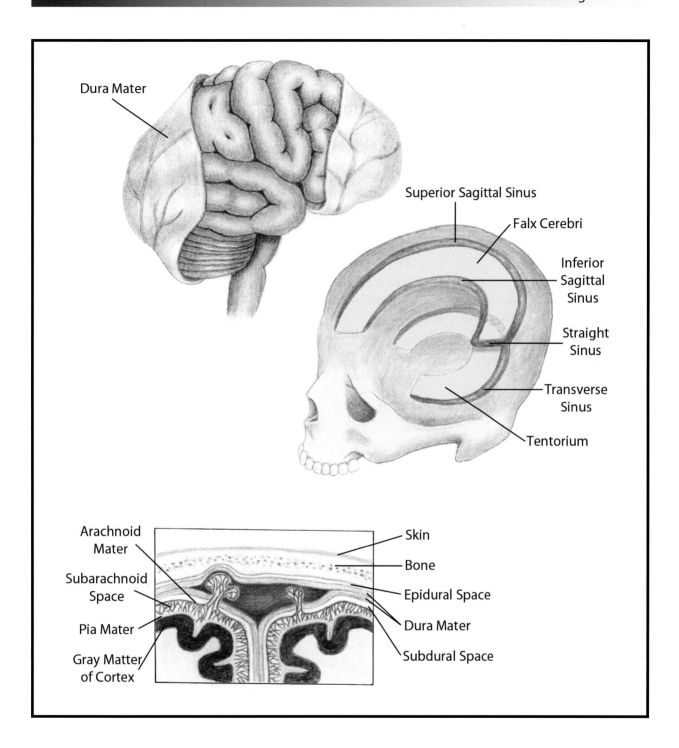

Dura Mater

Superior Sagittal Sinus

Falx Cerebri

Inferior Sagittal Sinus

Straight Sinus

Transverse Sinus

Tentorium

Arachnoid Mater

Skin

Bone

Subarachnoid Space

Epidural Space

Pia Mater

Dura Mater

Gray Matter of Cortex

Subdural Space

Blood Supply of the Dura

- The blood supply of the dura comes from the middle meningeal artery.
- This artery often ruptures during head injury, resulting in hemorrhages in the subdural space, or *subdural hematomas.*
- Subdural hematomas can also result from a cerebrovascular accident, or *stroke.*
- Hemorrhages in the subdural space cause increased cranial pressure that compresses neural tissue, a condition that is fatal if not treated promptly.[5]

Dural Neuronal Innervation

- The dura mater is innervated by the nervous system and can experience physical sensation.
- The brain is unable to detect pain, having no pain receptors of its own.
- Some headaches are caused by the constriction of meningeal membranes.[6]

ARACHNOID MATER

- The arachnoid mater is the middle meningeal layer and is located just below the subdural space.
- The arachnoid looks like a spider web (*arachnoid* means "spider" in Greek).
- It protects the brain and acts as a seal around the CNS.[7]

Subarachnoid Space

- Beneath the arachnoid is the subarachnoid space, which holds the CSF.[8]

Cisterns

- The cisterns are openings or large spaces in the subarachnoid space.[9]

Cisterna Magna (also called the *Cerebellar Medullary Cistern*)

- The cisterna magna is the largest subarachnoid cistern and is located between the cerebellum and the medulla.
- It is often used as a shunt placement in hydrocephalus.[10]

PIA MATER

- The pia mater is the deepest meningeal layer and is located directly on the *gyri* and sulci of the brain and on the spinal cord.
- There are 2 subdivisions of the pia mater: the cranial pia mater and the spinal pia mater.[11]

Cranial Pia Mater

- The cranial pia is anchored to the brain by glial cells.[12,13]

Spinal Pia Mater

- The spinal pia mater encloses the spinal cord and attaches to the dura mater through 21 pairs of denticulate ligaments.
- These ligaments anchor the spinal cord and provide stability to it.[14]

BLOOD-BRAIN BARRIER

- The blood-brain barrier is a highly effective bulwark that consists of the meninges, protective glial cells, and capillary beds of the brain.
- The blood-brain barrier occurs along all neural capillaries and consists of tight junctions between endothelial cells that are responsible for the exchange of nutrients between the CNS and the vascular system. The barrier acts as a wall that controls which molecules in the bloodstream will be able to enter the CNS.
- Oxygen, sugars, and amino acids are allowed entrance, while most other compounds are not.
- This protective mechanism ensures that the brain will not be exposed to toxins that could impair its function. However, because of the efficiency of the blood-brain barrier, approximately 98% of therapeutic drugs cannot access the brain. Pharmaceuticals cannot presently reach brain regions that are implicated in such diseases as meningitis, rabies, tumors, Alzheimer disease, Parkinson disease, and multiple sclerosis.[15]

REFERENCES

1. Mack J, Squier W, Eastman JT. Anatomy and development of the meninges: implications for subdural collections and CSF circulation. *Pediatr Radiol.* 2009;39(3):200-210. doi:10.1007/s00247-008-1084-6.

2. Erdogan S, Zorludemir S, Erman T, et al. Chondromas of the falx cerebri and dural convexity: report of two cases and review of the literature. *J Neuro-Oncol.* 2006;80(1):21-25. doi:10.1007/s11060-005-9082-0.

3. Kurucz P, Baksa G, Patonay L, Hopf NJ. Endoscopic anatomical study of the arachnoid architecture on the base of the skull. Part II: level of the tentorium, posterior fossa and the craniovertebral junction. *Innovative Neurosurgery.* 2013;1(2): 91-108. doi:10.1515/ins-2013-0008.

4. Davidson JR, Mack J, Gutnikova A, Varatharaj A, Darby S, Squier W. Developmental changes in human dural innervation. *Childs Nerv Syst.* 2012;28(5):665-671. doi:10.1007/s00381-012-1727-7.

5. Jussen D, Wiener E, Vajkoczy P, Horn P. Traumatic middle meningeal artery pseudoaneurysms. *Neuroradiology.* 2012;54(10):1133-1136. doi:10.1007/s00234-011-1003-7.

6. Kemp WJ, Tubbs RS, Cohen-Gadol AA. The innervation of the cranial dura mater: neurosurgical case correlates and a review of the literature. *World Neurosurg.* 2012;78(5):505-510. doi:10.1016/j.wneu.2011.10.045.

7. Adeeb N, Deep A, Griessenauer CJ, et al. The intracranial arachnoid mater. *Childs Nerv Syst.* 2013;29(1):17-33. doi:10.1007/s00381-012-1910-x.

8. Gupta S, Soellinger M, Boesiger P, Poulikakos D, Kurtcuoglu V. Three-dimensional computational modeling of subject-specific cerebrospinal fluid flow in the subarachnoid space. *J Biomech Eng.* 2009;131(2):021010. doi:10.1115/1.3005171.

9. Inoue K, Seker A, Osawa S, Alencastro LF, Matsushima T, Rhoton AL Jr. Microsurgical and endoscopic anatomy of the supratentorial arachnoidal membranes and cisterns. *Neurosurgery.* 2009;65(4):644-665. doi:10.1227/01. NEU.0000351774.81674.32.

10. Whitney N, Sun H, Pollock JM, Ross DA. The human foramen magnum—normal anatomy of the cisterna magna in adults. *Neuroradiology.* 2013;55(11):1333-1339. doi:10.1007/s00234-013-1269-z.

11. Ozawa H, Matsumoto T, Ohashi T, Sato M, Kokubun S. Mechanical properties and function of the spinal pia mater. *J Neurosurg Spine.* 2004;1(1):122-127.

12. Aimedieu P, Grebe R. Tensile strength of cranial pia mater: preliminary results. *J Neurosurg.* 2004;100(1):111-114.

13. Adeeb N, Mortazavi MM, Deep A, et al. The pia mater: a comprehensive review of literature. *Childs Nerv Syst.* 2013;29(10):1803-1810. doi:10.1007/s00381-013-2044-5.

14. Nam MH, Baek M, Lim J, et al. Discovery of a novel fibrous tissue in the spinal pia mater by polarized light microscopy. *Connect Tissue Res.* 2014;55(2):147-155. doi:10.3109/03008207.2013.879864.

15. Lawther BK, Kumar S, Krovvidi H. Blood-brain barrier. *Cont Ed Anaesth Crit Care Pain.* 2011;11(4):128-132. doi:10.1093/bjaceaccp/mkr018.

Spinal Cord Anatomy

SPINAL CORD ANATOMY

Boundaries of the Spinal Cord

- Boundaries of the spinal cord (SC) extend from the foramen magnum to the conus medullaris.
- The conus medullaris is the end of the SC at the L1-L2 vertebral area.[1,2] The SC then becomes the cauda equina (this means "horse's tail").[3]
- The cauda equina are spinal nerves that have not yet exited the vertebral column.

Enlargements of the Spinal Cord

- The SC has an hourglass shape. Enlargements of the SC occur in the cervical and lumbar sections.
- The cervical enlargement is due to the brachial plexus, a network of spinal nerves from C5 to T1 that extend from the cervical vertebrae to the upper extremities.[4]
- When the spinal nerves of the brachial plexus enter the SC (and synapse with SC tracts), they account for the large area of white matter in the cervical SC.
- The lumbar enlargement is due to the lumbar plexus, a network of spinal nerves from L1 to S3 that extend from the lumbar vertebrae to the lower extremities.[5]
- When the spinal nerves of the lumbar plexus enter the SC (and synapse with SC tracts), they account for the large area of white matter in the lumbar SC.

Anterior Median Fissure

- The anterior median fissure continues from the anterior aspect of the medulla to the end of the SC.[6,7]

Dorsal Median Sulcus

- The dorsal median sulcus continues from the posterior aspect of the medulla to the end of the SC.[6-8]

Dorsal Intermediate Sulcus

- The dorsal intermediate sulcus continues from the posterior aspect of the medulla and extends only throughout the thoracic levels of the SC.
- This sulcus separates 2 ascending sensory pathways: the fasciculus gracilis and cuneatus of the dorsal columns.[6,7]

Central Canal

- The central canal contains cerebrospinal fluid (CSF).[6,7,9]

SPINAL CORD ANATOMY: PNS VS CNS

Spinal Nerves

- The spinal nerves are located in the peripheral nervous system (PNS).
- The spinal nerves consist of (a) ascending sensory pathways and (b) descending motor pathways.
- Ascending sensory spinal nerves extend from a sensory receptor to the dorsal rootlets.
- Descending motor spinal nerves extend from the ventral horn of the SC to skeletal muscles.
- There are 31 pairs of spinal nerves: 8 cervical, 12 thoracic, 5 lumbar, 5 sacral, and 1 coccygeal.[10]

Gutman SA. *Quick Reference Neuroscience for Rehabilitation Professionals: The Essential Neurologic Principles Underlying Rehabilitation Practice, Third Edition* (pp 52-67).
© 2017 Taylor & Francis Group.

Dorsal Root Ganglion

- The dorsal root ganglion contains the cell bodies of sensory nerves that are part of the somatic PNS.
- Each sensory nerve has its own dorsal root ganglion.
- The dorsal root emerges from the dorsal ganglia.[11]

Dorsal Root and Rootlets

- The dorsal roots are ascending spinal nerves that carry sensory data from the sensory receptors (in the PNS) to the dorsal horn of the SC.
- Dorsal roots are axon bundles that emerge from a spinal nerve.
- The dorsal root leads into the dorsal rootlets, which are thin string-like axons that emerge from the dorsal root and synapse in the dorsal horn of the SC.
- The dorsal root and rootlets are considered to be within the PNS.[6,7,10]

Dorsal Horn

- The dorsal horn is considered to be part of the central nervous system (CNS).
- The dorsal horn contains the cell bodies of many of the sensory SC tracts.
- In the dorsal horn, the dorsal rootlets (of the PNS) may synapse on interneurons. These interneurons then synapse with SC tracts, or the rootlets may synapse directly on the cell bodies of the SC tracts.
- When the spinal nerves have synapsed with an SC tract, the SC tract ascends through the SC and brainstem and travels to the cortex.[6,7,10,12]

Ventral Horn, Root, and Rootlets

- Descending motor SC tracts travel from the cerebrum down through the brainstem and SC.
- Motor SC tracts synapse with interneurons in the ventral horn.
- These interneurons then synapse with motor spinal nerves and exit the ventral horn through the ventral rootlets.
- The ventral rootlets merge into the ventral roots and extend to skeletal muscles.
- The ventral horn, rootlets, and root are all considered to be within the PNS.[6,7,10,13]

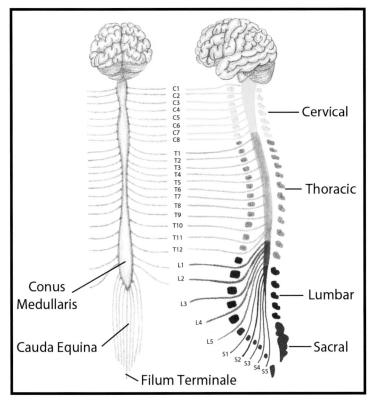

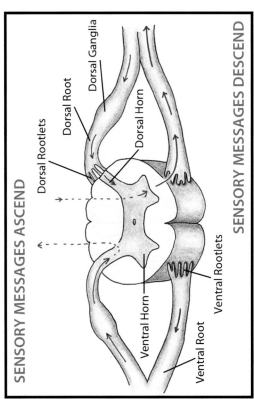

SPINAL NERVES AND THE DERMATOMES

Dermatome Distribution

- A dermatome is a skin segment that receives its innervation from one specific spinal nerve.
- Each spinal nerve is responsible for carrying messages about the sensation of a specific skin region to the primary somatosensory area.[14]

Referred Pain

- Referred pain occurs when a specific body region shares its spinal nerve innervation with a separate dermatomal skin segment.
- The pain experienced by the body part is misinterpreted by the cortex as pain coming from a separate dermatomal skin segment level.[15,16]
- Example: Referred pain in heart attack
- The spinal nerves that innervate the heart share interneurons that innervate the dermatomal level of the left arm (T1).
- When the heart experiences pain, the cortex misinterprets the origin of the pain as coming from the medial aspect of the left arm.

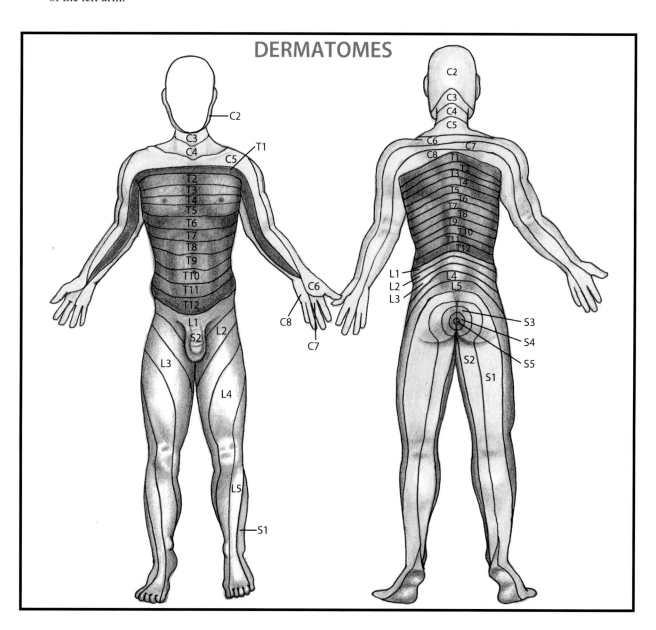

DERMATOMES

- This cortical misinterpretation occurs because the cortex does not have prior experience interpreting pain from the heart. The cortex relies on past experience when interpreting pain from a visceral source. Because it is uncommon for pain sensations to originate in the viscera, the cortex initially interprets the pain as coming from the left arm (T1 dermatome).
- As the pain increases, the cortex is able to correctly identify the source of the pain as the heart.

Clinical Use of the Dermatomal Distribution

- When a therapist performs a sensory evaluation and determines that a specific body region does not register sensation, the therapist is then able to identify the lesion level.
- For example, if a patient cannot perceive sensation on the dorsal forearm, the therapist is able to determine that there is some impairment at C6 level.

Transcutaneous Electrical Nerve Stimulation Unit

- The use of transcutaneous electrical nerve stimulation (TENS) is based on the dermatomal distribution.
- The therapist places the TENS unit on the identified dermatome region to stimulate nerve regeneration or to reduce pain in a peripheral nerve injury.
- There is limited evidence for nerve growth regeneration using TENS.[17]

SPINAL NERVES AND THE VERTEBRAL COLUMN

Relationship of the Spinal Cord to the Vertebral Column

Ontogenetic Development

- The SC is the same length as the vertebral column in utero.
- However, the vertebral column continues to grow after birth, while the SC does not.
- The adult SC ends at the L1-L2 vertebral region.
- The remainder of the spinal nerves (the cauda equina) must descend through the vertebral column to exit their intervertebral foramina.[18]

There Is One More Pair of Spinal Nerves Than There Are Vertebrae

- From C1 to C7, the spinal nerves exit above their corresponding vertebrae.
- There is a pair of C8 spinal nerves but no C8 vertebra.
- This means that the C8 spinal nerve must exit below C7 vertebra and above T1 vertebra.
- T1 spinal nerve exits below T1 vertebra and above T2 vertebra.
- From C8 down, the spinal nerves exit below their corresponding vertebrae.[6,7,10,19]

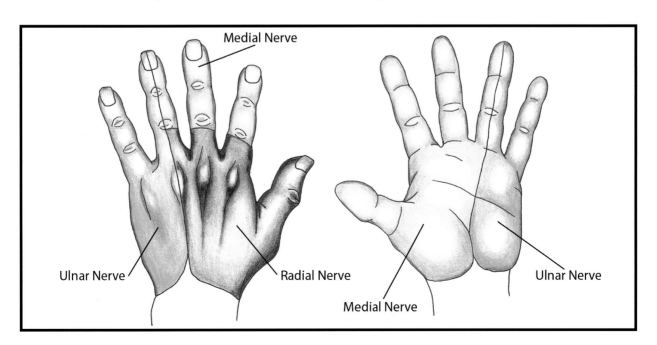

Intervertebral Discs

- The nucleus pulposus is a soft, pulpy, highly elastic tissue in the center of the intervertebral disc that functions as a shock absorber. With age, the nucleus pulposus loses water, begins to shrink, and cannot absorb pressure as well.[6,7,10,19,20]
- The annulus fibrosus is the more fibrous outer covering of the disc that consists of several layers of fibrocartilage. With age, the annulus fibrosis becomes weaker and can tear easily.[21]

Ruptured Disc

- The nucleus pulposus is the part of the disc most likely to rupture, or herniate.
- When the nucleus pulposus ruptures, it travels to the place of least resistance: the intervertebral foramina.
- Disc herniation can result in a pinched spinal nerve, because the nerves exit the vertebral column through the intervertebral foramina.[22]

Cervical Rupture

- Cervical nerves exit through the foramina above their corresponding vertebra.
- When a cervical disc has ruptured, or herniated, the nerve above the rupture will be impinged.[23]
- Example: A ruptured C5 disc will impinge the C5 spinal nerve.

Lumbar Rupture

- The lumbar and sacral nerves exit through the foramina below their corresponding vertebrae.
- Because the cauda equina forms the lumbar plexus, a ruptured lumbar or sacral disc will often impinge several spinal nerves.[24]
- An example is sciatica—pain that radiates down the leg due to a ruptured disc in the lumbar or sacral regions. A ruptured disc in the lumbosacral region will impinge several spinal nerves that innervate the lower extremities.

Cross-Sections of the Spinal Cord

Cervical Levels

- The cervical sections are large and oval in appearance.
- They consist of a large amount of white matter, which is made up of the axons of the sensory and motor tracts.
- At the cervical level, the descending motor tracts have not yet exited the SC, and most of the ascending sensory tracts have already entered the cord. This abundant presence of spinal cord tracts (axons) accounts for the large, oval appearance of the cervical SC sections.
- The amount of gray matter (nerve cell bodies) in the cervical sections is small.[6,7,10,19]

Thoracic Levels

- The thoracic levels are also oval-shaped but are smaller than the cervical levels.
- The thoracic sections have a lateral horn (also called an *intermediolateral horn*) which is part of the autonomic nervous system (ANS).
- The lateral horn is where the cell bodies for the sympathetic nervous system are located.[6,7,10,19]

Lumbar Levels

- The lumbar sections are large and round in shape.
- These sections have the largest amount of gray matter (cell bodies) because a great number of peripheral spinal nerves that carry sensory and motor messages from and to the lower extremities synapse with cell bodies in the lumbar SC levels.[6,7,10,19]
- Peripheral spinal nerves carrying sensory information from the lower extremities enter the lumbar SC sections and synapse on cell bodies in the dorsal horn.
- Peripheral spinal nerves carrying motor messages to the lower extremities synapse with cell bodies in the ventral horn and exit the cord to the lower extremities.

Sacral Levels

- The sacral sections appear similar to the lumbar sections but are much smaller.
- Most of the descending motor tracts have already exited the SC.
- Many of the ascending sensory tracts have not yet entered the SC.[6,7,10,19]

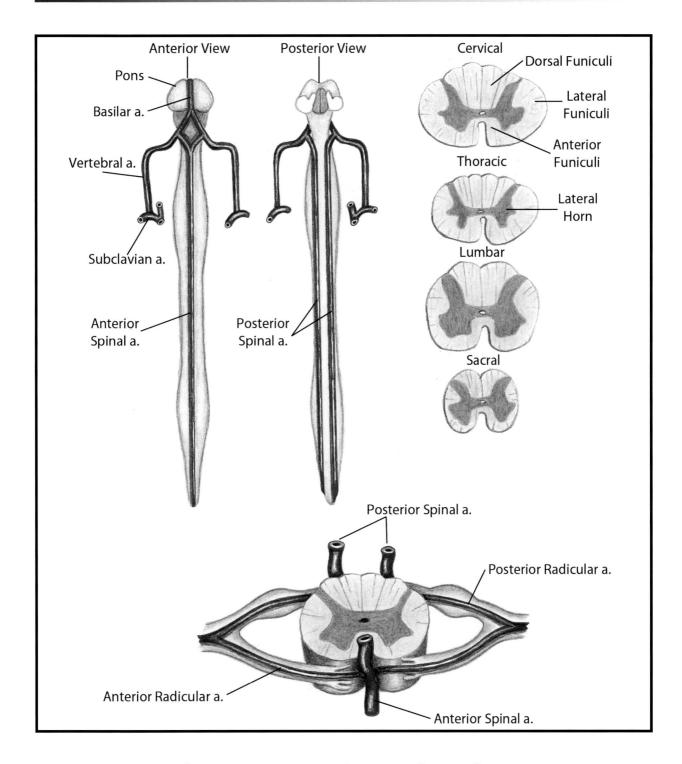

ORGANIZATION OF THE INTERNAL SPINAL CORD

White Matter

- White matter consists of myelinated axons.
- The white matter is divided into 3 pairs of funiculi[6,7,10,19]:
  1. Anterior
  2. Lateral
  3. Dorsal
- The SC tracts are located in the funiculi.

Gray Matter

- Gray matter contains the cell bodies of the sensory SC tracts (in the dorsal horn) and the cell bodies of the motor spinal nerves (in the ventral horn).
- The cell bodies for the motor spinal nerves (which innervate the skeletal muscles) are organized in a precise pattern in the ventral horn[6,7,10,19]:
  - ○ The cell bodies for the motor spinal nerves that innervate the proximal muscle groups are located in the medial ventral horn.
  - ○ The cell bodies for the motor spinal nerves that innervate the distal muscle groups are located in the lateral ventral horn.

BLOOD SUPPLY OF THE SPINAL CORD

- The blood supply of the SC comes from the vertebral arteries.
- The vertebral arteries are 2 branches that give rise to 1 anterior spinal artery and 2 posterior spinal arteries.

Anterior Spinal Artery (1)

- The vertebral artery traverses the medulla and sends off a branch called the *anterior spinal artery*.
- The anterior spinal artery descends down the medulla and the anterior aspect of the SC.
- The artery runs along the anterior median fissure and supplies the anterior aspect of the SC.[25,26]

Posterior Spinal Arteries (2)

- The vertebral artery also gives rise to 2 posterior spinal arteries.
- These descend down the dorsal intermediate sulci on the posterior aspect of the SC.
- These arteries supply the posterior aspect of the SC.[26]

Radicular Arteries

- The radicular arteries encircle the SC at all levels.
- The radicular arteries meet up with and supply the anterior spinal artery and the posterior spinal arteries.[26,27]

MENINGES OF THE SPINAL CORD

- The meninges of the SC are the same as those of the brain.
- Their function is to protect and anchor the SC.
- There are 3 layers of meninges[28]:
  1. Dura mater
  2. Arachnoid mater
  3. Pia mater

Dura Mater

- The dura is the most superficial and thickest membrane.[29]

Arachnoid Mater

- The arachnoid mater is the middle meningeal membrane.
- CSF bathes the SC in the subarachnoid space.[30]

Pia Mater

- The pia mater is the deepest and thinnest membrane.
- It adheres to the SC and sends off 2 projections: filum terminale and dentate ligaments.[31]

Filum Terminale (Projection of the Pia)

- The filum terminale is a slender median fibrous thread that attaches the conus medullaris to the coccyx.
- This thread-like structure anchors the end of the SC to the vertebral column.[32]

Denticulate Ligaments (Projections of the Pia)

- The denticulate ligaments are a series of 21 triangular bodies that anchor the SC.[33]

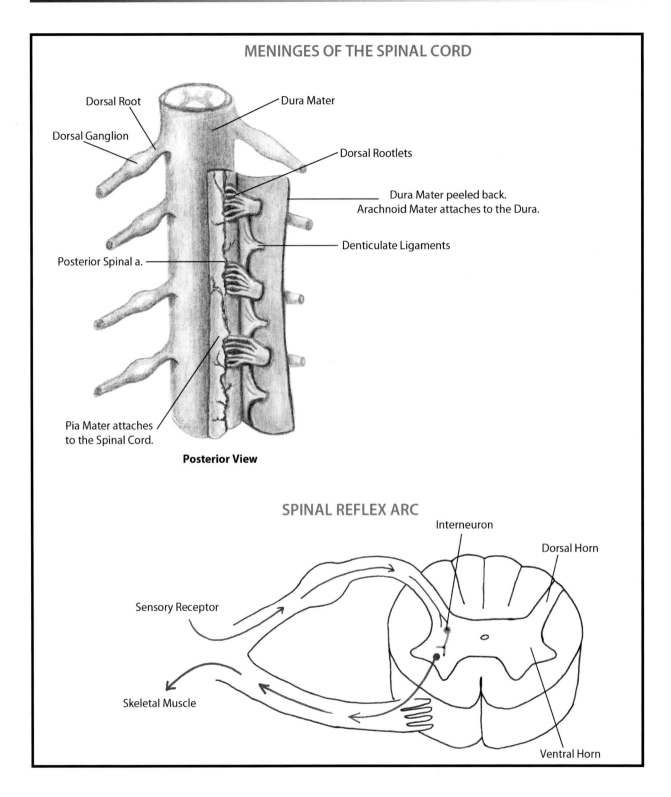

MENINGES OF THE SPINAL CORD

Dorsal Root

Dorsal Ganglion

Dura Mater

Dorsal Rootlets

Dura Mater peeled back.
Arachnoid Mater attaches to the Dura.

Denticulate Ligaments

Posterior Spinal a.

Pia Mater attaches
to the Spinal Cord.

Posterior View

SPINAL REFLEX ARC

Interneuron

Dorsal Horn

Sensory Receptor

Skeletal Muscle

Ventral Horn

SPINAL REFLEX ARC

- A spinal reflex arc is a reflex that is mediated solely at the SC level. There is no cortical involvement, no conscious decision making.
- Spinal reflexes allow sensory information to be processed and acted upon quickly, without cortical processing, although the cortex will be alerted to the processed reflex.[34]

Pathway of a Spinal Reflex Arc

- A sensory receptor in the PNS sends a message along an ascending sensory spinal nerve.
- The sensory spinal nerve travels to the dorsal horn where it synapses on an interneuron.
- The interneuron synapses on a motor cell body located in the ventral horn.
- The motor cell body in the ventral horn relays the message to a motor spinal nerve in the PNS.
- The message travels to a skeletal muscle group for action in response to the initial sensory message.[6,7,10]

DEEP TENDON REFLEXES

- A deep tendon reflex is a reflex arc in which a muscle contracts when its tendon is percussed.
- Such reflexes are also called *myotatic reflexes*, *monosynaptic reflexes*, and *muscle stretch reflexes*.
- Deep tendon reflexes work on the principle of the spinal reflex arc.
- Common deep tendon reflexes are those of the biceps, brachioradialis, triceps, patella, and Achilles tendons.
- In an upper motor neuron (UMN) injury, deep tendon reflexes become hyperreflexive.
- In a lower motor neuron (LMN) injury, deep tendon reflexes become hyporeflexive.[35]

WITHDRAWAL REFLEX

- The withdrawal reflex is a spinal reflex that works similarly to the spinal reflex arc.
- This reflex is a protective mechanism that allows reflexive withdrawal of a body part from physical danger while simultaneously adjusting posture to avoid imbalance. Quickly pulling one's hand from a hot stove is an example of a withdrawal reflex. The hand is pulled away from the stove before the cortex consciously perceives pain.
- The withdrawal reflex is polysynaptic; in other words, signals (to withdraw a limb) that enter one side of the SC will synapse with interneurons on the contralateral side of the cord. For example, if the right hand is withdrawn, the left limbs will also adjust to maintain balance.
- A painful stimulus to one side of the body will activate the flexors and inhibit the extensors on the ipsilateral side.
- Simultaneously, the flexors will be inhibited and the extensors activated on the contralateral side of the body.
- This allows for the quick withdrawal of the limb while maintaining balance.[6,7,10,36]

UPPER VS LOWER MOTOR NEURONS

- Motor neurons carry motor messages from different areas of the nervous system.
- Motor neurons are divided into 2 categories: UMN and LMN.

Upper Motor Neurons

- An UMN carries motor messages from the primary motor cortex to the following[37]:
  - The cranial nerve nuclei (located in the brainstem)
  - Interneurons in the ventral horn. An UMN travels up to the ventral horn and synapses with an interneuron that connects to a motor cell body located in the ventral horn.
- UMNs are considered to be part of the CNS.

Lower Motor Neurons

- A LMN carries motor messages from the motor cell bodies in the ventral horn to the skeletal muscles in the periphery.
- LMNs are considered to be part of the PNS.
- LMNs include the cranial nerves, spinal nerves, cauda equina, and ventral horn.[6,7,10]

Upper Motor Neuron Lesion

- In an UMN lesion, spasticity occurs below the lesion level.[37,38]
  - Spasticity occurs because the spinal reflex arcs below the lesion level remain intact.
  - The spinal reflex arcs operate without cortical modification.
  - Thus, increased muscle tone (or spasticity) occurs.

- In an UMN lesion, flaccidity occurs at the lesion level.[37,38]
  - ○ Flaccidity occurs because the spinal reflex arc at the lesion level is lost.
  - ○ Thus, nothing is innervating the muscles.
  - ○ The muscles (at the lesion level) lose all tone and become flaccid.
- In reality, this type of lesion involves both UMN and LMN damage. Because the motor cell bodies in the ventral horn are no longer innervated, this type of lesion is also considered a LMN lesion.

Lower Motor Neuron Lesion

- In a LMN lesion, flaccidity occurs at and below the lesion level.[38]
- Flaccidity occurs in all LMN lesions because a LMN does not involve any spinal reflex arcs.
- Because spinal reflex arcs are not part of LMN lesions, there is nothing that continues to innervate the muscles.

Congenital Anomalies of the Spinal Cord

Spina Bifida
- Spina bifida is a congenital disorder involving the incomplete closure of the neural tube during fetal development. A section of the SC does not unite in midline. Usually, the opening occurs in the low thoracic and lumbar sections of the SC.
- Meningocele
  - A meningocele is a form of spina bifida that occurs when the meninges and the CSF protrude through the opening of the vertebral column.
  - This results in compression of the SC and some nerve roots.
  - There is a visible cyst on the infant's back that is filled with CSF and neural tissue.
  - Possible problems may include lower extremity weakness or paralysis, incontinence, and orthopedic impairment (eg, club foot, scoliosis).[39]
- Meningomyelocele
  - This is a severe form of spina bifida that occurs when the meninges, SC, and spinal nerves all protrude through an opening in the vertebral column.
  - All motor and sensory information below the level of the cyst are lost.[40]

Arnold Chiari Malformation
- Arnold Chiari malformation involves displacement of the cerebellar vermis, brainstem, and fourth ventricle.
- The cerebellar tonsils are often displaced downward into the upper cervical canal.
- Arnold Chiari malformation is often associated with a meningomyelocele.
- Individuals with Arnold Chiari malformation may present with hydrocephalus and cerebellar and lower cranial nerve signs.[41]

SPINA BIFIDA

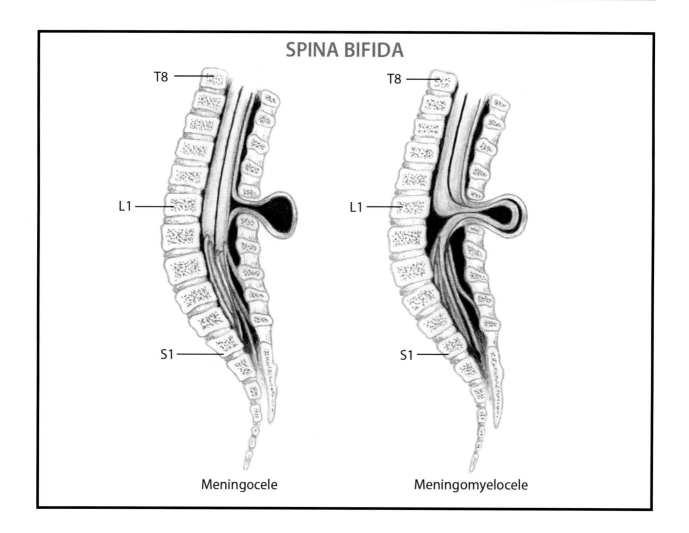

T8

L1

S1

Meningocele

T8

L1

S1

Meningomyelocele

REFERENCES

1. Harrop JS, Naroji S, Maltenfort MG, et al. Neurologic improvement after thoracic, thoracolumbar, and lumbar spinal cord (conus medullaris) injuries. *Spine.* 2011;36(1):21-25. doi:10.1097/BRS.0b013e3181fd6b36.

2. Podnar S. Epidemiology of cauda equina and conus medullaris lesions. *Muscle Nerve.* 2007;35(4):529-531. doi:10.1002/mus.20696.

3. Ogikubo O, Forsberg L, Hansson T. The relationship between the cross-sectional area of the cauda equina and the preoperative symptoms in central lumbar spinal stenosis. *Spine.* 2007;32(13):1423-1428. doi:10.1097/BRS.0b013e318060a5f5.

4. Johnson EO, Vekris M, Demesticha T, Soucacos PN. Neuroanatomy of the brachial plexus: normal and variant anatomy of its formation. *Surg Radiol Anat.* 2010;32(3):291-297. doi:10.1007/s00276-010-0646-0.

5. Matejčík V. Anatomical variations of lumbosacral plexus. *Surg Radiol Anat.* 2010;32(4):409-414. doi:10.1007/s00276-009-0546-3.

6. Haines DE. *Neuroanatomy in Clinical Context: An Atlas of Structures, Sections, and Systems.* 9th ed. Philadelphia, PA: Wolters Kluwer, Lippincott, Williams, and Wilkins; 2014.

7. England M, Wakley J. *Color Atlas of the Brain and Spinal Cord.* 2nd ed. St. Louis, MO: Mosby; 2005.

8. Jacquesson T, Streichenberger N, Sindou M, Mertens P, Simon E. What is the dorsal median sulcus of the spinal cord? Interest for surgical approach of intramedullary tumors. *Surg Radiol Anat.* 2014;36(4):345-351. doi:10.1007/s00276-013-1194-1.

9. Petit-Lacour MC, Lasjaunias P, Iffenecker C, et al. Visibility of the central canal on MRI. *Neuroradiology.* 2000;42(10):756-761. doi:10.1007/s002340000373.

10. Felten DL, Shetty A. *Netter's Atlas of Neuroscience.* 2nd ed. Philadelphia, PA: Saunders; 2010.

11. Sapunar D, Kostic S, Banozic A, Puljak L. Dorsal root ganglion—a potential new therapeutic target for neuropathic pain. *J Pain Res.* 2012;5:31-38. doi:10.2147/JPR.S26603.

12. Peirs C, Williams SPG, Zhao X, et al. Dorsal horn circuits for persistent mechanical pain. *Neuron.* 2015;87(4):797-812. doi:10.1016/j.neuron.2015.07.029.

13. Ruven C, Chan TK, Wu W. Spinal root avulsion: an excellent model for studying motoneuron degeneration and regeneration after severe axonal injury. *Neural Regen Res.* 2014;9(2):117-118. doi:10.4103/1673-5374.125338.

14. Haas S, Marovich L, Young C, Voissem P, Jablonski S, Thill S. Standardizing nursing assessments of dermatome levels of postoperative patients with spinal blocks, epidural analgesia. *J Perianesth Nurs.* 2015;30(4):e17-e18. doi:10.1016/j.jopan.2015.05.049.

15. Alonso-Blanco C, Fernández-de-las-Peñas C, Fernández-Mayoralas DM, de-la-Llave-Rincón AI, Pareja JA, Svensson P. Prevalence and anatomical localization of muscle referred pain from active trigger points in head and neck musculature in adults and children with chronic tension-type headache. *Pain Med.* 2011;12(10):1453-1463. doi:10.1111/j.1526-4637.2011.01204.x.

16. Graven-Nielsen T, Arendt-Nielsen L. Induction and assessment of muscle pain, referred pain, and muscular hyperalgesia. *Curr Pain Headache Rep.* 2003;7(6):443-451. doi:10.1007/s11916-003-0060-y.

17. Lynch PJ, McJunkin T, Eross E, Gooch S, Maloney J. Case report: successful epiradicular peripheral nerve stimulation of the C2 dorsal root ganglion for postherpetic neuralgia. *Neuromodulation.* 2011;14(1):58-61.

18. Jessell TM. Neuronal specification in the spinal cord: inductive signals and transcriptional codes. *Nat Rev Genet.* 2000;1(1):20-29. doi:10.1038/35049541.

19. Nolte J. *The Human Brain: An Introduction to Its Functional Anatomy.* 6th ed. St. Louis, MO: Mosby; 2008.

20. Walter BA, Purmessur D, Likhitpanichkul M, et al. Inflammatory kinetics and efficacy of anti-inflammatory treatments on human nucleus pulposus cells. *Spine.* 2015;40(13):955-963. doi:10.1097/BRS.0000000000000932.

21. Jin L, Liu Q, Scott P, et al. Annulus fibrosus cell characteristics are a potential source of intervertebral disc pathogenesis. *PLoS ONE.* 2014;9(5):e96519. doi:10.1371/journal.pone.0096519.

22. Kamper SJ, Ostelo RW, Rubinstein SM, et al. Minimally invasive surgery for lumbar disc herniation: a systematic review and meta-analysis. *Eur Spine J.* 2014;23(5):1021-1043. doi:10.1007/s00586-013-3161-2.

23. Wong JJ, Côté P, Quesnele JJ, Stern PJ, Mior SA. The course and prognostic factors of symptomatic cervical disc herniation with radiculopathy: a systematic review of the literature. *Spine J.* 2014;14(8):1781-1789. doi:10.1016/j.spinee.2014.02.032.

24. Lurie JD, Tosteson TD, Tosteson AN, et al. Surgical versus non-operative treatment for lumbar disc herniation: Eight-year results for the Spine Patient Outcomes Research Trial (SPORT). *Spine.* 2014;39(1):3-16. doi:10.1097/BRS.0000000000000088.

25. Biglioli P, Spirito R, Roberto M, et al. The anterior spinal artery: the main arterial supply of the human spinal cord—a preliminary anatomic study. *J Thorac Cardiovasc Surg.* 2000;119(2):376-379. doi:10.1016/S0022-5223(00)70194-2.

26. Martirosyan NL, Feuerstein JS, Theodore N, Cavalcanti DD, Spetzler RF, Preul MC. Blood supply and vascular reactivity of the spinal cord under normal and pathological conditions: a review. *J Neurosurg Spine.* 2011;15(3):238-251. doi:10.3171/2011.4.SPINE10543.

27. Simon JI, McAuliffe M, Smoger D. Location of radicular spinal arteries in the lumbar spine from analysis of CT angiograms of the abdomen and pelvis [published online ahead of print September 1, 2015]. *Pain Med.* doi:10.1111/pme.12891.

28. Decimo I, Fumagalli G, Berton V, Krampera M, Bifari F. Meninges: from protective membrane to stem cell niche. *Am J Stem Cells.* 2012;1(2):92-105.

29. Reina MI, Lopez A, Dittman M, De Andres JA. Ultrastructure of spinal dura mater. In: Reina MA, De Andres JA, Hadzic A, Prats-Galino A, Sala-Branch X, van Zundert AAJ, eds. *Atlas of Functional Anatomy for Regional Anesthesia and Pain Medicine.* New York, NY: Springer; 2015:411-434. doi:10.1007/978-3-319-09522-6_20.

30. Adeeb N, Deep A, Griessenauer CJ, et al. The intracranial arachnoid mater. *Childs Nerv Syst.* 2013;29(1):17-33. doi:10.1007/s00381-012-1910-x.

31. Machés F, Reina MA, Casasola ODL. Ultrastructure of spinal pia mater. In: Reina MA, De Andres JA, Hadzic A, Prats-Galino A, Sala-Branch X, van Zundert AAJ, eds. *Atlas of Functional Anatomy for Regional Anesthesia and Pain Medicine.* New York, NY: Springer; 2015:499-522. doi:10.1007/978-3-319-09522-6_25.

32. Fontes RB, Saad F, Soares MS, de Oliveira F, Pinto FC, Liberti EA. Ultrastructural study of the filum terminale and its elastic fibers. *Neurosurgery.* 2006;58(5):978-984. doi:10.1227/01.NEU.0000210224.54816.40.

33. Ceylan D, Tatarlı N, Abdullaev T, et al. The denticulate ligament: anatomical properties, functional and clinical significance. *Acta Neurochir.* 2012;154(7):1229-1234. doi:10.1007/s00701-012-1361-x.

34. Ghosh A, Haggard P. The spinal reflex cannot be perceptually separated from voluntary movements. *J Physiol.* 2014;592(1):141-152.

35. Chardon MK, Rymer WZ, Suresh NL. Quantifying the deep tendon reflex using varying tendon indentation depths: Applications to spasticity. *IEEE Transactions on Neural Systems and Rehabilitation Engineering.* 2014;22(2):280-289. doi:10.1109/TNSRE.2014.2299753.

36. Neziri AY, Andersen OK, Petersen-Felix S, et al. The nociceptive withdrawal reflex: normative values of thresholds and reflex receptive fields. *Eur J Pain.* 2010;14(2):134-141. doi:10.1016/j.ejpain.2009.04.010.

37. Ivanhoe CB, Reistetter TA. Spasticity: the misunderstood part of the upper motor neuron syndrome. *Am J Phys Med Rehabil.* 2004;83(10):S3-S9.

38. Barnes MP. An overview of the clinical management of spasticity. In: Barnes MP, Johnson GR, eds. *Upper Motor Neurone Syndrome and Spasticity: Clinical Management and Neurophysiology.* 2nd ed. Cambridge, United Kingdom: Cambridge University Press; 2008:1-9.

39. Paul P, Tiwari M, Kumar H. Anterior sacral meningocele presenting with purulent rectal discharge and altered mental status. *Neurol Clin Pract.* 2015;5(1):89-90.

40. Valenca MP, de Menezes TA, Calado AA, de Aguiar Cavalcanti G. Burden and quality of life among caregivers of children and adolescents with meningomyelocele: measuring the relationship to anxiety and depression. *Spinal Cord.* 2012;50(7):553-557. doi:10.1038/sc.2012.10.

41. Parfitt SE, Roth CK. Chiari malformation in pregnancy. *Nurs Womens Health.* 2015;19(2):177-181. doi: 10.1111/1751-486X.12189.

CLINICAL TEST QUESTIONS

Sections 4 to 7

1. A newborn infant has increased cranial expansion with accompanying cranial suture separation and neural tissue compression. This condition is called _____ and can result from _____.
   a. congenital hydrocephalus; foramina blockage, excessive production of CSF, choroid plexus tumors
   b. normal pressure hydrocephalus; reduced absorption of CSF by the arachnoid villae
   c. congenital hydrocephalus; reabsorption of CSF by the arachnoid villae
   d. normal pressure hydrocephalus; foramina blockage

2. Mr. Wilson has been diagnosed with normal pressure hydrocephalus. This form of hydrocephalus is caused by _____ and can result in _____.
   1. blockage of the foramen of Luschka
   2. impaired reabsorption of the CSF without foramina blockage
   3. fontanel bulging and increased cranial expansion
   4. dementia, incontinence, and gait abnormalities
   a. 1, 3
   b. 2, 4
   c. 1, 4
   d. 2, 3

3. Joshua has been admitted to the emergency room after a severe auto vehicle accident in which he was a passenger. He is diagnosed with increased intracranial pressure and neural tissue compression resulting from hemorrhage into the subdural space. Traumatic brain injuries often involve:
   a. blockage of the foramen of Magendie, resulting in hydrocephalus
   b. rupture of the middle meningeal artery, resulting in hemorrhage

4. Mrs. Greenly has been diagnosed with Parkinson disease. Her physician explains to the family that, while several pharmaceutical options are available, none are highly effective because such drugs cannot reach the brain. The neurological structure by which potentially toxic molecules are prevented from reaching the brain is called the:
   a. dura mater
   b. cerebral aqueduct
   c. blood-brain barrier
   d. arachnoid villae

5. After his spinal cord injury, Andrew has no sensation above his nipple line. It is likely that his injury occurred at which level of the spinal cord?
   a. C4-C2
   b. S1-L4
   c. S5-S1
   d. T3-T5

6. Mr. Amadi was rushed to the hospital after experiencing pain in his left jaw that radiated down his left arm. This type of pain is called _____ and occurs as a result of _____.
   1. neurogenic pain
   2. referred pain
   3. stimulation of a spinal nerve that innervates both a specific dermatome level and visceral organ
   4. stimulation of adjacent sensory and motor spinal nerves
   a. 1, 3
   b. 2, 4
   c. 1, 4
   d. 2, 3

7. Ms. Henderson has been diagnosed with a lumbar disc rupture at L4, causing impingement of the lumbosacral plexus. As a result, she has been experiencing severe pain in her back that radiates down her legs. This type of pain is called:

   a. sciatic pain or sciatica
   b. brachial plexus pain
   c. referred pain
   d. angina

8. Mr. Cho had a spinal cord injury that occurred at T6 1 year ago. He has spasticity in all muscle groups below T7. Mr. Cho's spinal cord injury is considered:

   a. a lower motor neuron injury
   b. an upper motor neuron injury

9. When playing high school football, Tyler sustained a peripheral nerve injury at the brachial plexus when he was hit by another player. As a result, he experienced a nerve root avulsion or severe tear. This injury is accompanied by numbness and weakness in Tyler's right arm and hand. This type of injury is considered:

   a. a lower motor neuron injury
   b. an upper motor neuron injury

10. Anna's infant was born with a congenital disorder in which the neural tube did not completely fuse and the spinal cord has not united. The meninges and CSF protrude through the vertebral column and a visible cyst is present on the infant's back filled with CSF and neural tissue. This disorder is called:

    a. Arnold Chiari malformation
    b. meningomyelocele
    c. meningocele

Answers

1. a
2. b
3. b
4. c
5. d
6. d
7. a
8. b
9. a
10. c

The Cranial Nerves

THE CRANIAL NERVES

Cranial Nerve Anatomy

- There are 12 pairs of cranial nerves (CN).
- The CNs are considered to be part of the peripheral nervous system (PNS).
- Their nuclei (cell bodies) are located in the brainstem.
- CN nuclei are considered to be part of the central nervous system (CNS).
- CNs begin exiting the brain at the midbrain level and lead all the way down the medulla.
- CNs use Roman numerals (however, Arabic numerals will be used in this text).[1-4]

List of Cranial Nerves

- Olfactory nerve
- Optic nerve
- Oculomotor nerve
- Trochlear nerve
- Trigeminal nerve
- Abducens nerve
- Facial nerve
- Vestibulocochlear nerve
- Glossopharyngeal nerve
- Vagus nerve
- Accessory nerve
- Hypoglossal nerve

Function

- CNs carry sensory and motor information to and from the following receptors of the head, face, and neck[1-4]:
    - Special sense receptors (for vision, audition, olfaction, gustation, and equilibrium)
    - Somatosensory receptors
    - Proprioceptors

Lesions

- Most CN lesions produce ipsilateral signs and symptoms.[1-4]

Gutman SA. *Quick Reference Neuroscience for Rehabilitation Professionals: The Essential Neurologic Principles Underlying Rehabilitation Practice, Third Edition* (pp 68-98). © 2017 Taylor & Francis Group.

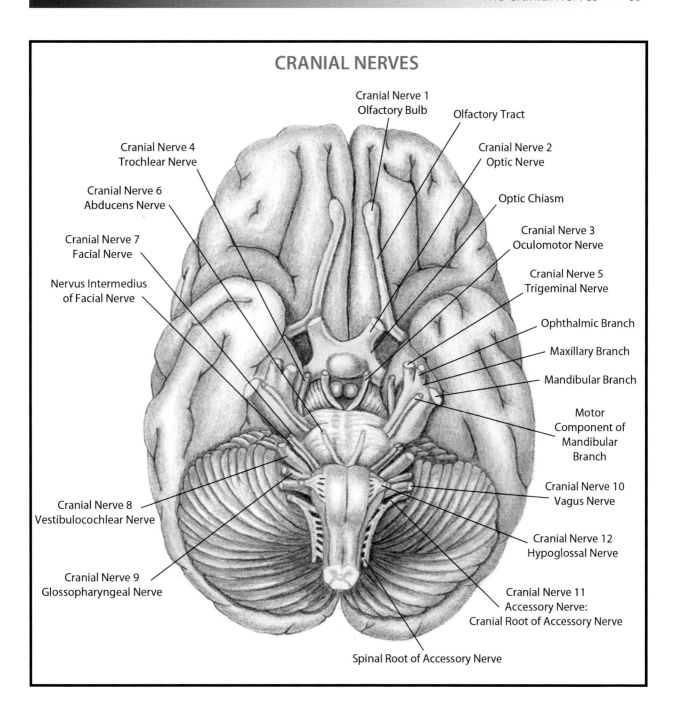

CRANIAL NERVES

CRANIAL NERVE 1: OLFACTORY NERVE

Carries
- Sensory information[1-5]

Nuclei Location
- Chemoreceptors in the nose[1-5]

Function
- Olfaction (smell)[1-5]

Pathway
- Chemoreceptors in the nose send olfactory messages to the inferior frontal lobes, where the olfactory bulb is located.
- The olfactory information then travels from the olfactory bulb down the olfactory cranial nerve to the hippocampal formation in the temporal lobe.
- The hippocampus is responsible for long-term storage of odor memories. This is why odors can elicit old memories with an efficiency far greater than any other sense.
- Olfactory messages are then sent to the hypothalamus, thalamus, and finally to the orbitofrontal cortex, where they are interpreted and eventually integrated with gustatory information.[1-5]

Lesion Symptoms
- If the lesion is unilateral (only occurs in one olfactory nerve)[5,6]:
  - There are no symptoms because the opposite olfactory nerve compensates for the lost sense of smell on one side.
- If the lesion is bilateral[5,6]:
  - The individual loses the sense of smell; this is called *anosmia*.
  - Often, anosmia occurs as a result of head injury.
  - There is also a lack of olfactory function.

Test
- Test one olfactory nerve at a time.
- Occlude vision.
- Block the patient's nostril on the side opposite to the side being tested.
- Present one odor at a time.
- Provide the patient with a verbal choice of specific odors if he or she has difficulty identifying the odors but can easily smell them, or if the patient has word-finding difficulties.[7]

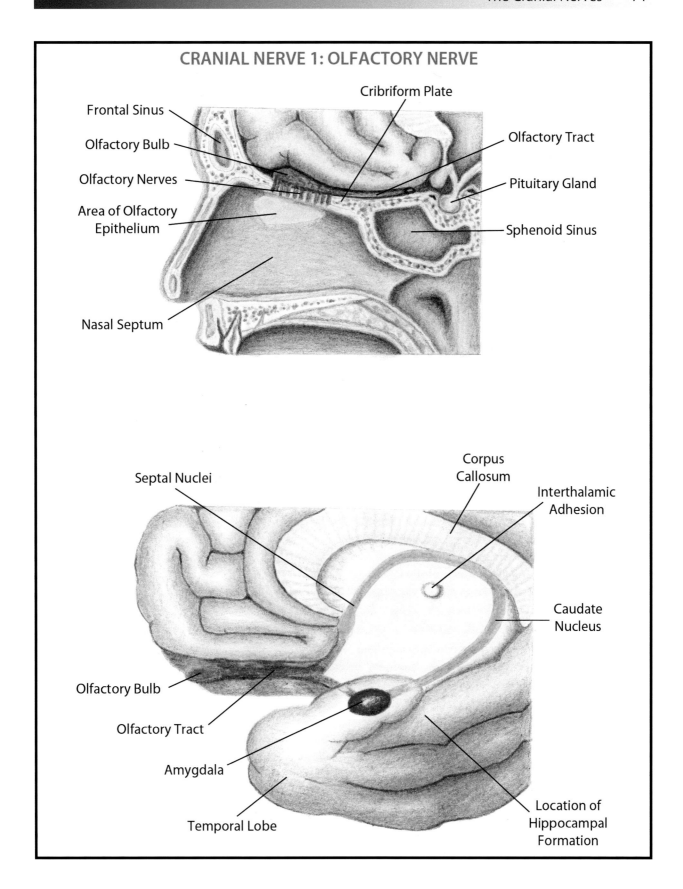

CRANIAL NERVE 1: OLFACTORY NERVE

CRANIAL NERVE 2: OPTIC NERVE

Carries

- Sensory information[1-4]

Nuclei Location

- Photoreceptors of the retina (rods and cones)[1-4]

Function

- Visual acuity (the accuracy of sight; not the interpretation of visual information).[1-4]
- Visual messages that travel from the thalamus to the superior colliculi (and back) are involved in the following:
  - Pupillary reflexes
  - Awareness of light and dark
  - Orientation of head and eye movements

Pathway

- The rods and cones of the retina send visual information down the optic nerves to the optic chiasm.
- The visual information then travels from the optic chiasm through the optic tracts.
- Visual information travels from the optic tracts to the lateral geniculate bodies of the thalamus.
- A branch carries visual messages from the lateral geniculate bodies of the thalamus to the superior colliculi of the midbrain (the information is then processed back through the thalamus). This pathway allows certain visual information to be detected on an unconscious level, even in the case of cortical blindness, when the person's brain cannot interpret visual data but the visual anatomy remains intact.
- Visual messages then travel to the occipital lobes for visual detection and interpretation.[1-4,8]

Lesion Symptoms

- A unilateral lesion (in only one optic nerve) produces ipsilateral blindness.[1-4,8]
- A bilateral lesion (in both optic nerves) produces bilateral blindness.

Test

- When testing optic nerve function, 3 kinds of data should be collected, or the examination is not complete[1-4,8]:
  1. Results from a visual acuity test (Snellen eye chart)
  2. Results from a visual field test
  3. Results from a funduscopic examination
- Generally, therapists perform visual acuity tests and visual field tests. Ophthalmologists perform funduscopic exams.

Visual Acuity Test (Snellen Eye Chart)

- Test one eye at a time. Then test both eyes together.
- If the patient normally wears corrective lenses, test the patient with glasses on.[8]

Visual Field Test

- Test one eye at a time. Occlude vision in the opposite eye.
- Ask the patient to look straight ahead and not move the head.
- The examiner moves a visual stimulus in the 4 visual quadrants: right, left, superior, and inferior.
- The visual stimulus is moved in each quadrant one at a time.
- The examiner holds the visual stimulus at the 90 degree position in each quadrant and gradually moves the stimulus directly in front of the patient at 0 degrees. The patient is asked to alert the examiner when the visual stimulus first enters the patient's visual range.
- Test vertical (superior and inferior) and temporal (right and left) peripheral vision.
- Normal vertical vision begins at 45 degrees.
- Normal temporal vision begins at 85 degrees.[8]

CRANIAL NERVE 2: OPTIC NERVE

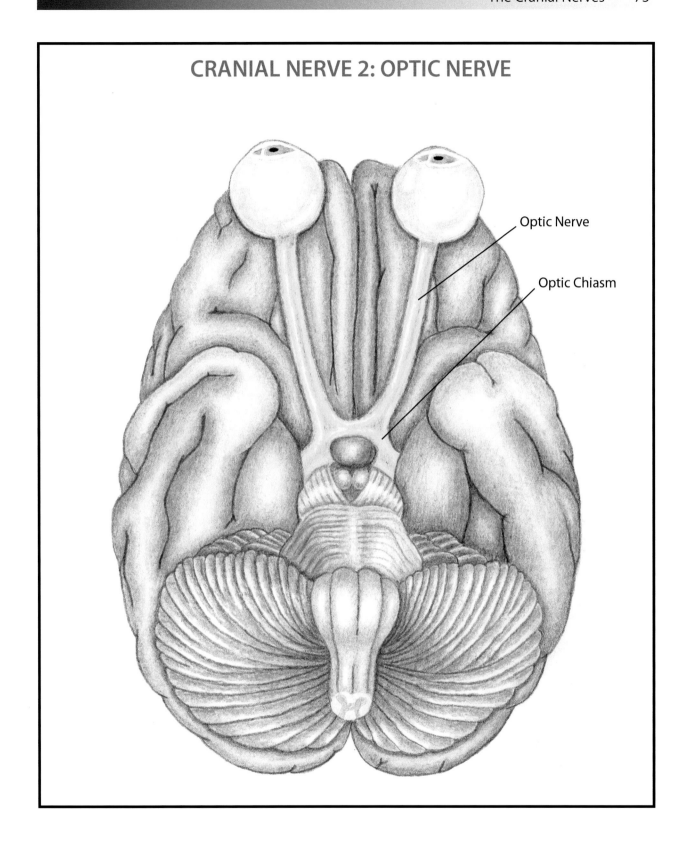

Optic Nerve

Optic Chiasm

CRANIAL NERVE 3: OCULOMOTOR NERVE

Carries

- Motor information[1-4]

Nuclei Location

- Midbrain at the level of the superior colliculi[1-4]

Function

- Extraocular eye movements.[1-4]
- CN 3 is responsible for eyeball movements up, down, medially, laterally, and downward deviation.
- The oculomotor nerve innervates the eye muscles that control these movements.
- The oculomotor nerve is considered to be one of the extraocular motor nerves, along with the trochlear and abducens nerves.
- The 3 extraocular motor nerves use the medial longitudinal fasciculus to communicate with each other and with the vestibular system.
- The medial longitudinal fasciculus is a brainstem tract that coordinates head and eye movements by providing bilateral connections among the vestibular nerve nuclei, extraocular nerve nuclei, and the accessory nerve nuclei in the brainstem.

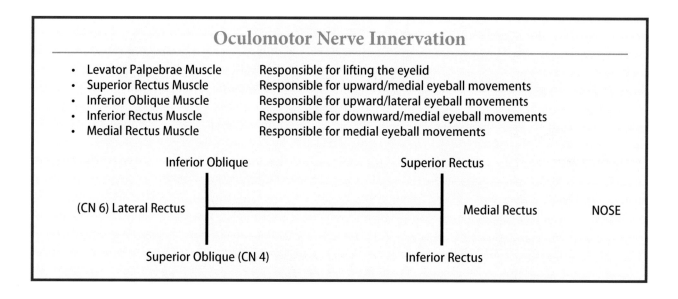

Oculomotor Nerve Innervation

- Levator Palpebrae Muscle — Responsible for lifting the eyelid
- Superior Rectus Muscle — Responsible for upward/medial eyeball movements
- Inferior Oblique Muscle — Responsible for upward/lateral eyeball movements
- Inferior Rectus Muscle — Responsible for downward/medial eyeball movements
- Medial Rectus Muscle — Responsible for medial eyeball movements

Inferior Oblique   Superior Rectus

(CN 6) Lateral Rectus   Medial Rectus   NOSE

Superior Oblique (CN 4)   Inferior Rectus

Oculomotor Nerve Reflexes

- Pupillary Reflex — Pupil of the eye constricts when light is shined into it.
- Accommodation — Lens of the eye adjusts to focus light on the retina.
- Convergence — Pupils move medially when viewing an object at close range.

CRANIAL NERVE 3: OCULOMOTOR NERVE

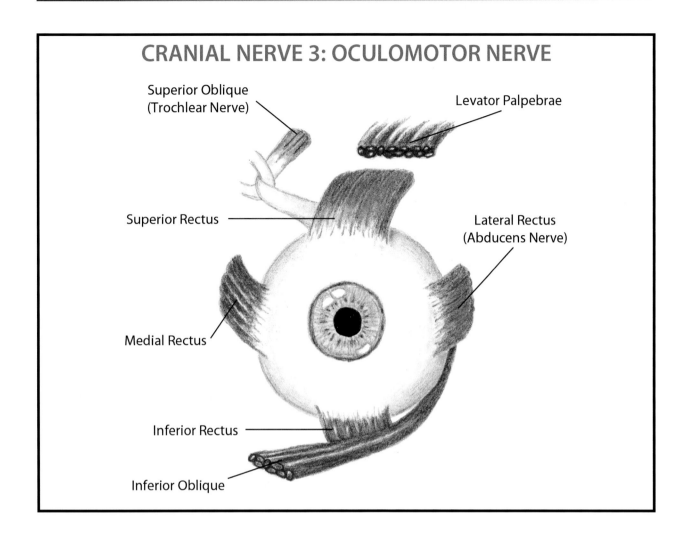

Superior Oblique
(Trochlear Nerve)

Levator Palpebrae

Superior Rectus

Lateral Rectus
(Abducens Nerve)

Medial Rectus

Inferior Rectus

Inferior Oblique

Lesion Symptoms

- Lateral strabismus (external strabismus or exotropia)[9]
- The eyeball deviates outward (or laterally) because the medial rectus is lost and the lateral rectus is working unopposed.
- This can cause diplopia, or *double vision.*

Ptosis

- Ptosis is the drooping of a body region; in this case, the ipsilateral eyelid droops.[9]

Nystagmus

- Nystagmus is involuntary back and forth movements of the eye in a quick, jerky, oscillating fashion when the eye moves laterally or medially to either the temporal or nasal extremes. Nystagmus can occur in the center of each visual field as well.
- Nystagmus can be normally elicited in an intact CNS using rotational or temperature stimulation of the semicircular canals.
- Pathological nystagmus is a sign of CNS abnormality and can occur with or without external stimulation.[9]

Test

- Therapists test the extraocular motor nerves simultaneously: the oculomotor, trochlear, and abducens nerves.[1-4,9]
- Test one eye at a time. Occlude the eye not being tested.
- Instruct the patient to maintain head in a fixed position while visually scanning a moving stimulus.
- The moving stimulus can be a colored pen cap.
- The therapist moves the visual stimulus in the shape of an H (see "Oculomotor Nerve Innervation" text box on p 74). This allows the therapist to determine if the eyeball muscles are functioning adequately (ie, if the extraocular muscles are adequately innervated by their extraocular motor CNs).
- Observe symmetry of pupil size.
- In a dimly lit area, shine a pen light at the bridge of the nose and observe for symmetrical corneal reflection. If corneal reflection is asymmetrical, strabismus is indicated.
- Shine the pen light into one eye at a time for a 2-second duration. Check for constriction of stimulated pupil.

SYMPTOMS OF OCULOMOTOR NERVE (CRANIAL NERVE 3) DAMAGE

Lateral Strabismus

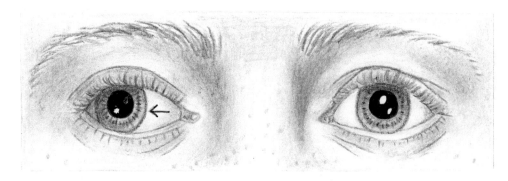

Ptosis

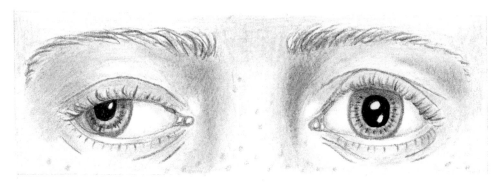

Nystagmus

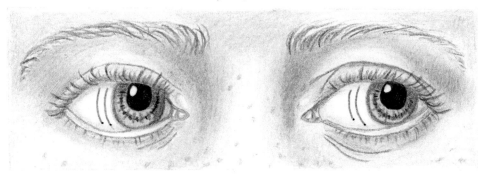

CRANIAL NERVE 4: TROCHLEAR NERVE

Carries

- Motor information[1-4]

Nuclei Location

- Midbrain at the level of the inferior colliculi[1-4]

Function

- Extraocular eye movements[1-4]
- Responsible for downward and lateral eyeball movements
- Considered to be one of the extraocular motor nerves

Innervates

- Superior oblique muscles[1-4]

Lesion Symptoms

- The patient will experience difficulty moving the eyeball down and laterally.[10]
- This occurs because the superior oblique muscle is lost. The medial rectus and the superior rectus muscles are working unopposed to pull the eyeball up and medially.
- This results in a subtle vertical, medial strabismus.
- The patient may display difficulty walking down steps.
- Vertical diplopia is often reported at both near and far distances.
- Nystagmus

Test

- Test the trochlear nerve function simultaneously with the oculomotor and abducens nerves (see Oculomotor Nerve Test section on p 76).[10]

SYMPTOMS OF TROCHLEAR NERVE DAMAGE (CN 4)

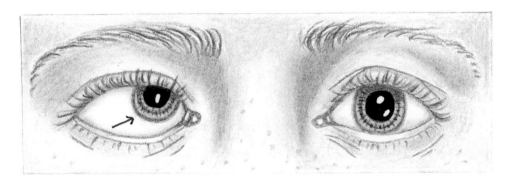

Vertical, Medial Strabismus

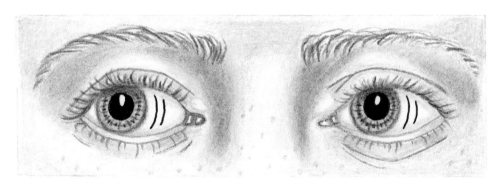

Nystagmus

CRANIAL NERVE 5: TRIGEMINAL NERVE

Carries
- Sensory and motor information[1-4]

Nuclei Location
- Mid pons[1-4]

Function

Sensory

- The sensory half of the trigeminal nerve mediates sensation of the face, head, cornea of the eye, and inner oral cavity (the ophthalmic, maxillary, and mandibular regions).
- Sensation includes pain, temperature, and discriminative touch.[1-4]

Motor

- The motor half of the trigeminal nerve innervates the jaw muscles that control chewing (or *mastication*).[1-4]

Lesion Symptoms

Sensory

- Damage to the sensory half of the trigeminal nerve causes ipsilateral loss of sensation to the head, face, and inner oral cavity.
- Trigeminal neuralgia occurs when half of the face loses sensation.[11]

Motor

- Damage to the motor half of the trigeminal nerve causes weakness in chewing (mastication).
- The jaw also deviates to the affected side.[11]

Test

Sensory Half of the Trigeminal Nerve

- Evaluate the patient's sensory abilities on the face, head, and inner oral cavity.
- Occlude vision.
- Use a cotton swab to stroke the inner oral cavity. Assess the intact side first. Then evaluate the involved side.
- Use a cotton swab to stroke the patient's forehead, cheek, jaw, and chin. Apply stimulus to the unaffected side first. Then proceed to the involved side.
- Touch the patient's cornea lightly with a cotton swab to check for corneal reflex; eyelid should close.[11]

Motor Half of the Trigeminal Nerve

- Occlude vision.
- Ask the patient to open his or her mouth. Check for deviation of the jaw to the affected side.
- Check for asymmetry of the size of the mouth opening; the patient will likely exhibit a decreased ability to open the mouth on the affected side.
- Ask the patient to move his or her jaw from side to side. Check for asymmetry of jaw movement.
- Instruct the patient to bite down on a tongue depressor. Ask the patient to resist attempts, made by the therapist, to pull the tongue depressor out. Check for asymmetry between right and left jaw strength.[11]

Trigeminal Neuralgia

- Trigeminal neuralgia involves sudden, excruciating pain of short duration along the second (maxillary region) and third (mandibular region) divisions of the trigeminal nerve.
- The etiology involves chronic compression of the trigeminal nerve as a result of a vessel position or tumor. This causes demyelination and impaired nerve signaling.
- Patients describe the pain of trigeminal neuralgia as sharp and shooting.
- Pain-free periods can be experienced between episodes, or a dull ache may continuously be felt in the affected region.
- Pharmacologic treatment includes antiseizure medications (eg, Tegretol [carbamazepine], Dilantin [phenytoin], or Neurontin [gabapentin]).
- Surgical intervention is attempted when drug therapy is unsuccessful. Such procedures involve surgical decompression of the trigeminal nerve.[12]

CRANIAL NERVE 5: TRIGEMINAL NERVE

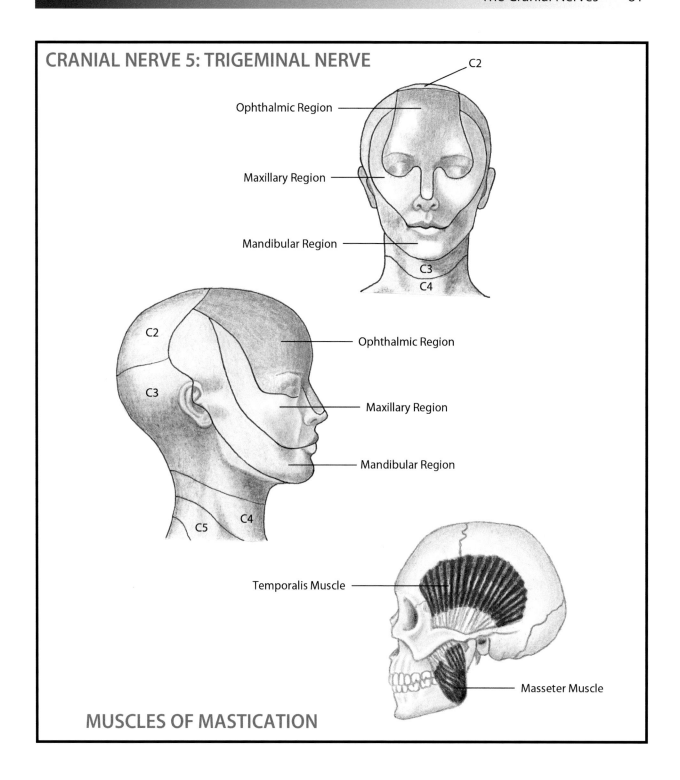

C2

Ophthalmic Region

Maxillary Region

Mandibular Region

C3

C4

C2

C3

Ophthalmic Region

Maxillary Region

Mandibular Region

C4

C5

Temporalis Muscle

Masseter Muscle

MUSCLES OF MASTICATION

Trigeminal Nerve Reflexes

Masseter Reflex
- When the masseter muscle is lightly tapped with a reflex hammer, the masseter contracts.

Corneal Reflex
- When the cornea is touched, the eyelids close.

CRANIAL NERVE 6: ABDUCENS NERVE

Carries

- Motor information[1-4]

Nuclei Location

- Low pons[1-4]

Function

- Extraocular eye movements[1-4]
- Responsible for lateral deviation of the eyeball (looking laterally)

Innervates

- Lateral rectus muscle[1-4]

Lesion Symptoms

Medial Strabismus (Internal Strabismus or Esotropia)

- Turning inward of the eyeball[13]
- This occurs because the lateral rectus muscle is lost. The medial rectus works unopposed to pull the eyeball medially.
- Can cause double vision or diplopia
- Nystagmus

Test

- The abducens nerve is simultaneously tested with the oculomotor and trochlear nerves (see Oculomotor Nerve Test section on p 76).[13]

SYMPTOMS OF ABDUCENS NERVE DAMAGE (CRANIAL NERVE 6)

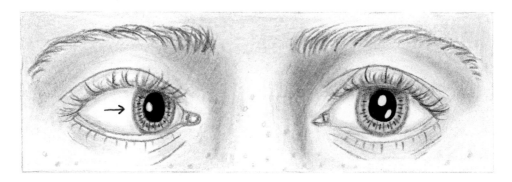

Medial Strabismus

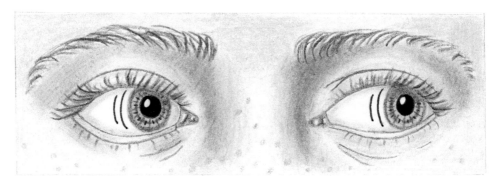

Nystagmus

CRANIAL NERVE 7: FACIAL NERVE

Carries

- Sensory and motor information[1-4]

Nuclei Location

- Mid to low pons[1-4]

Function

Sensory

- The sensory portion of the facial nerve comes off a separate branch of the facial nerve called the *nervous intermedius.*
- It innervates the taste receptors on the anterior tongue.[1-4]

Motor

- The motor portion of the facial nerve innervates the following[1-4]:
  - Muscles of facial expression
  - Muscles for eyelid closing
  - Stapedius muscle (controls the stapes of the middle ear)

Lesion Symptoms

- Decreased taste on the anterior of the tongue[14]
- Decreased corneal reflex

Test

Sensory Portion of the Facial Nerve

- Test the sense of taste on the anterior tongue.
- Occlude vision.
- Present sweet, salty, and sour solutions to the outer and lateral portions of the anterior tongue.
- Present each taste substance one at a time. Ask the patient to indicate if he or she can taste the substance and identify whether it is sweet, sour, or salty.[1-4,15]

Motor Portion of the Facial Nerve

- Test the strength and symmetry of facial muscles.
- Ask the patient to elevate eyebrows and forehead.
- The ability to wrinkle the forehead is used to distinguish an upper motor neuron (UMN) lesion from a lower motor neuron (LMN) lesion[1-4,15]:
  - In an UMN lesion, the muscles of the forehead will be spared (remain intact) even while the lower facial regions are not. This commonly occurs in cerebrovascular accident.
  - Bell palsy is a LMN disorder (the facial nerve has been lesioned). Both the forehead and the lower face are involved in the paralysis of facial muscles.
- Ask the patient to smile, frown, and pucker his or her lips. Check for asymmetry on the right and left sides of the face.
- Ask the patient to blow his or her cheeks up with air. Gently push on the cheeks while asking the patient to resist. Check for asymmetry of facial muscle strength.

Facial Nerve Reflex

- Corneal (or Blink Reflex)   When the cornea is touched, the eyelids close.[16]

Bell Palsy

- Occurs when the facial nerve swells and becomes compressed as it passes through the petrous temporal bone.
- The herpes simplex 1 virus is implicated in 60% to 70% of cases.
- Other viruses that may cause Bell palsy include cytomegalovirus, Epstein-Barr, rubella, and mumps.
- Trauma to the facial nerve may also play a role in some cases.
- Bell palsy is characterized by the following:
  - Drooping of the ipsilateral side of the face
  - Sagging eyebrow
  - Inability to close the affected eye completely
  - The mouth is drawn down toward the affected side
  - The ear on the affected side becomes hypersensitive to noise
- The acute phase is characterized by marked edema causing tension to the facial nerve.
- An inflammatory process begins; this induces edema with secondary vascular compromise.
- Inflammation and vascular compromise cause anoxia to the facial nerve.
- Anoxia then leads to vasodilation, transudation of fluid (oozing of fluid through the pores), and further pressure that confines the pathway of CN 7.
- Patients with diabetes are 4 times more likely to develop Bell palsy. It is also more common in the third trimester of pregnancy and in people who are immunocompromised (such as in AIDS).[17]

Hyperacusis in Bell Palsy (Increased Sensitivity to Sound)
- Because the facial nerve travels through the internal auditory meatus and later gives off branches to the stapedius muscle, patients with Bell palsy may have ipsilateral hyperacusis.[18]

CRANIAL NERVE 8: VESTIBULOCOCHLEAR NERVE

Carries

- Two sensory branches[1-4]

Nuclei Location

- Pons-medulla junction[1-4]

Function

Auditory Branch

- The auditory branch of the vestibulocochlear nerve transmits sensory impulses that result from the vibrations of the fluid in the cochlea.
- The function of the auditory branch is audition (hearing).[1-4]

Vestibular Branch

- The vestibular branch receives sensory stimulation from the semicircular canals of the inner ear.
- It is concerned with balance and the sensations of vertigo (dizziness).
- The functions of the vestibular branch are balance, equilibrium, and the position of the head in space.[1-4]

Pathway

Auditory Branch

- The auditory branch of the vestibulocochlear nerve runs from the hair cells (or receptors) of the organ of Corti (in the inner ear) to the vestibular nucleus in the brainstem.[1-4]

Vestibular Branch

- The vestibular branch runs from the semicircular canals, utricles, and saccules (of the inner ear) to the vestibular nuclei in the brainstem.
- The semicircular canals, utricles, and saccules detect changes in head position.[1-4]

Lesion Symptoms

Auditory Branch Lesions

- Deafness or tinnitus[19,20]

Vestibular Branch Lesions

- Nystagmus (due to connections to the extraocular motor nerve nuclei)
- Vertigo
- Decreased balance
- Decreased protective responses
- Changes in extensor tone (because the vestibulospinal tract is responsible for mediating extensor tone)[19,20]

Test

Auditory Branch of the Vestibulocochlear Nerve

- An audiologist must first distinguish between 2 possible types of hearing impairment[21]:
  - *Sensorineural*: involves the inner ear, vestibulocochlear nerve, and brain
  - *Conductive*: involves the outer ear and middle ear structures

Vestibular Branch of the Vestibulocochlear Nerve

- Test for nystagmus.[22]
- The patient should assume a seated position.
- Have the patient track a moving object (at a distance of 15 inches) in an H and X pattern.
- Check for nystagmus both within and at end ranges of visual fields.
- Test balance and the presence of protective responses (Romberg test).
- Have the patient stand with his or her eyes open, then closed.
  - Check for increased sway and loss of balance.
  - Gently displace patient's balance. Check for protective responses.
  - Test for the presence of extensor tone in the lower extremities.

Vestibular Neuritis

- Vestibular neuritis is characterized by an acute onset of vertigo, nausea, vomiting, disequilibrium, and nystagmus.
- Improvement usually occurs within 1 to 2 weeks; however, some patients develop recurrent episodes.
- A large percentage of patients report having had an upper respiratory tract infection 1 to 2 weeks prior to the onset of symptoms. This suggests a viral origin.
- In some patients, vestibular neuritis can recur over months or years. There is no way to determine whether a first attack will be followed by repeated occurrences.
- Drug treatment may involve anticholinergic drugs (eg, scopolamine, atropine), monoaminergic drugs (eg, amphetamine, ephedrine), and antihistamines (eg, Antivert [meclizine], Marezine [cyclizine], Dramamine [dimenhydrinate], and Phenergan [promethazine]).
- Vestibular rehabilitation usually involves balance training and habituation exercises that can retrain the brain's response to motion-induced vertigo.[23]

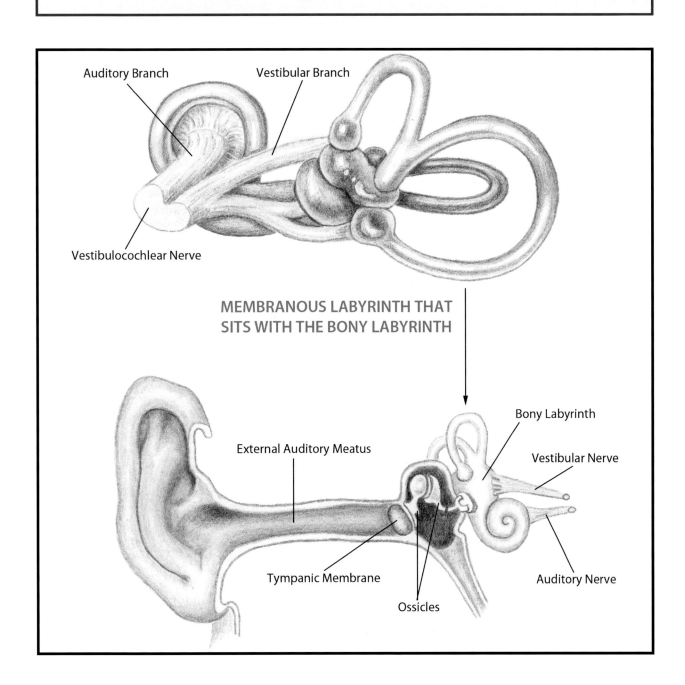

Auditory Branch

Vestibular Branch

Vestibulocochlear Nerve

MEMBRANOUS LABYRINTH THAT
SITS WITH THE BONY LABYRINTH

Bony Labyrinth

Vestibular Nerve

External Auditory Meatus

Tympanic Membrane

Ossicles

Auditory Nerve

CRANIAL NERVE 9: GLOSSOPHARYNGEAL NERVE

Carries

- Sensory and motor information[1-4]

Nuclei Location

- Nucleus ambiguous in the medulla[1-4]

Function

Sensory

- Taste on the posterior aspect of the tongue[1-4]

Motor

- Swallowing[1-4]

Lesion Symptoms

Sensory

- Loss of taste sensation on posterior aspect of tongue (loss of bitter taste modality)[24]

Motor

- Loss of the gag and swallowing reflexes
- Dysphagia: difficulty swallowing, leading to choking or food aspiration[25]

Test

- Because they mediate similar functions, the glossopharyngeal and vagus nerves are tested simultaneously.

Sensory

- Use the same testing procedures described for the sensory half of the facial nerve, except apply the procedure to the posterior aspect of the tongue (where bitter tastes are detected).
- Ask the patient to chew on a lemon rind to determine whether bitter tastes can be detected.[1-4]

Motor

- Attempt to elicit the gag reflex by swiping a tongue depressor or cotton swab at the back of the throat.
- Observe the patient's ability to swallow different consistencies of food.
- Present different consistencies of food one at a time (eg, solid foods, pureed foods, thick liquids, thin liquids).
- Ask the patient to consume each presented food type. Check for food aspiration, coughing, throat clearing, or a wet vocal quality (indicating that the food is pocketing in the larynx).
- If aspiration precautions have been indicated previously, modify this procedure accordingly.[1-4]

Glossopharyngeal Nerve Reflexes

Gag Reflex
- Touching the pharynx elicits contraction of the pharyngeal muscles.

Swallowing Reflex
- Food touching the pharynx elicits movement of the soft palate and contraction of the pharyngeal muscles.

CRANIAL NERVE 10: VAGUS NERVE

Carries
- Sensory and motor information[1-4]

Nuclei Location
- Dorsal vagal nuclei in the medulla
- Nucleus ambiguous in the medulla[1-4]

Function

Visceral Branches (to Hollow Organs)
- Visceral branches carry sensory and motor information. Sensory carries taste information from the palate and epiglottis.
- Motor carries parasympathetic information to and from the heart, pulmonary system, esophagus, and the gastro-intestinal tract.[1-4]

Skeletal Muscle Branches
- Skeletal muscle branches carry motor information to the muscles of the larynx, pharynx, and upper esophagus.
- These muscles are responsible for swallowing and speaking.[1-4]

Lesion Symptoms

Visceral Branch Lesions
- Transient tachycardia (irregular rapid heart beat)
- Dyspnea (difficulty breathing)[26,27]

Bilateral Visceral Branch Lesions
- Asphyxia (suffocation)[27]

Skeletal Muscle Branch Lesions
- Dysphonia (hoarse voice)[28]
- Dysphagia (difficulty swallowing)[29]
- Dysarthria (difficulty articulating words clearly; slurring words)[30]

Test
- The glossopharyngeal and vagus nerves are tested simultaneously. See testing procedures under Glossopharyngeal Nerve section (p 88).
- Observe the patient's ability to speak clearly without slurring words.
- Check for decreased phonal volume and hoarse voice.[27]

Vagus Nerve Reflexes

Gag Reflex
- Touching the pharynx elicits contraction of the pharyngeal muscles.

Swallowing Reflex
- Food touching the pharynx elicits movement of the soft palate and contraction of the pharyngeal muscles.

CRANIAL NERVE 11: ACCESSORY NERVE

Carries

- Motor information[1-4]

Accessory Nerve Has Two Roots

Cranial Nerve Root

- Emerges from the nucleus ambiguous and joins the vagus nerve
- Innervates the intrinsic muscles of the larynx[1-4]

Spinal Nerve Root

- Emerges from the ventral horn of the upper cervical spinal cord
- Innervates the sternocleidomastoid (SCM) and upper trapezius muscles[1-4]

Nucleus Location

Cranial Nerve Root

- Medulla[1-4]

Spinal Nerve Root

- C1-C5 spinal cord levels in the ventral horn[1-4]

Function

Cranial Nerve Root

- Controls elevation of the larynx during swallowing[1-4]

Spinal Nerve Root

- Innervation of the SCM muscle allows for the following[1-4]:
  - Head rotation to contralateral side
  - Head flexion/extension
- Innervation of the upper trapezius muscle allows for the following[1-4]:
  - Shoulder elevation and shoulder flexion above 90 degrees
- The accessory and vagus nerves are the only CNs that innervate organs and glands below the neck.

Lesion Symptoms

Cranial Nerve Root Lesions

- Dysphagia secondary to decreased laryngeal elevation[29]

Spinal Nerve Root Lesions

- Weakness rotating the head to the contralateral side (because the ipsilateral SCM muscle that is affected functions to rotate the head to the opposite side)
- Weakness flexing the head laterally and forward (SCM)
- Weakness extending the head (SCM)
- Weakness elevating the shoulder (shrugging the shoulder) on the ipsilateral side (upper trapezius muscle)
- Weakness flexing the arm above 90 degrees (upper trapezius muscle) on the ipsilateral side[31]

Test

Cranial Nerve Root

- Place index and middle fingers over the patient's Adam's apple (laryngeal muscles).
- Ask the patient to swallow.
- Check for normal rise and fall of the larynx.
- Check for presence of dysphagia using procedures described in the Glossopharyngeal Nerve section (p 88).[27]

Spinal Nerve Root

- Test SCM muscle as follows[27]:
    - Ask the patient to flex his or her head laterally and forward, and rotate the head to the opposite side (on both the involved and uninvolved sides). Instruct the patient to resist attempts to prevent the desired movement.
    - Compare both sides of the body to observe symmetry of movement and strength.
    - Check for atrophy in involved SCM muscles.
- Test upper trapezius muscles as follows[27]:
    - Ask the patient to shrug both shoulders toward his or her ears. Instruct the patient to resist attempts to depress the elevated shoulders.
    - Check for symmetry in shoulder movement and strength.
    - Check for atrophy of involved upper trapezius muscles.

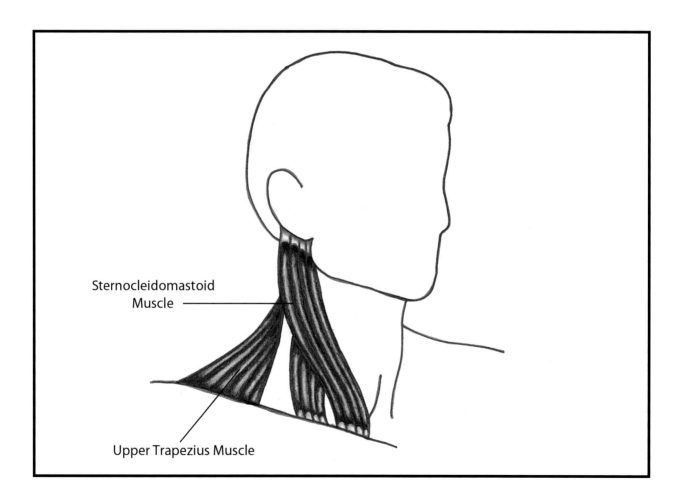

CRANIAL NERVE 12: HYPOGLOSSAL NERVE

Carries

- Motor information[1-4]

Nuclei Location

- Medulla[1-4]

Function

- Innervates the muscles of the tongue. The hypoglossal cranial nerve is responsible for tongue movement.[1-4]

Lesion Symptoms

- Dysarthria secondary to impaired tongue musculature; inability to produce required movements for sound and word formation[30]
- Ipsilateral deviation of the tongue[27]
- Dysphagia (because the tongue muscles are needed to manipulate food into a bolus in the mouth and propel bolus to the pharynx)[29]
- Ipsilateral atrophy and paralysis of tongue[27]

Test

- Ask the patient to protrude his or her tongue.
- Note whether the tongue deviates to the lesion side.
- Note whether there is unilateral or bilateral atrophy of the tongue muscles.
- Check for tongue tremors or involuntary tongue movements.
- Ask the patient to move his or her tongue from side to side.
- Check for asymmetry in movement and weakness.
- Ask the patient to push his or her tongue against both cheeks.
- Ask the patient to resist attempts to depress the cheek as the patient pushes the cheek outward.
- Note whether there is asymmetry in tongue strength.[27]

THE STAGES OF SWALLOWING:
CRANIAL NERVES THAT MEDIATE THE FUNCTION OF SWALLOWING

Three Stages of Swallowing

- Oral
- Pharyngeal/laryngeal
- Esophageal

Cranial Nerves Involved in Swallowing

- CN 5   Trigeminal nerve
- CN 7   Facial nerve
- CN 9   Glossopharyngeal nerve
- CN 10   Vagus nerve
- CN 11   Accessory nerve
- CN 12   Hypoglossal nerve

Stages of Swallowing

Stage	Function	CN
Oral	1. Food is brought into the mouth; the lips close.	CN 7
	2. Jaw, cheek, and tongue movements manipulate food into a bolus.	CN 5, 7, 12
	3. Tongue moves bolus to pharynx.	CN 12
	4. Larynx closes.	CN 10
	5. Swallow reflex is triggered.	CN 9
Pharyngeal/ Laryngeal	1. Food moves into pharynx.	CN 9
	2. Soft palate rises to block food from entering the nasal cavity.	CN 10
	3. Epiglottis covers trachea to prevent food from entering the lungs.	CN 10
	4. Pharynx rises and falls during swallowing.	CN 11
	5. Peristalsis moves food to the esophageal entrance, the sphincter opens, and food moves into the esophagus.	CN 10
Esophageal	Peristalsis moves food into the stomach.	CN 10

REFERENCES

1. Nowinski WL, Thaung TSL, Chua BC, et al. Three-dimensional stereotactic atlas of the adult human skull correlated with the brain, cranial nerves, and intracranial vasculature. *J Neurosci Methods.* 2015;246:65-74. doi:10.1016/j.jneumeth.2015.02.012.

2. Wilson-Pauwels L, Stewart PA, Akesson EJ, Spacey SD. *Cranial Nerves: Function and Dysfunction.* 3rd ed. Shelton, CT: People's Medical; 2010.

3. Damodaran O, Rizk E, Rodriguez J, Lee G. Cranial nerve assessment: a concise guide to clinical examination. *Clin Anat.* 2014;27(1):25-30. doi:10.1002/ca.22336.

4. Binder DK, Sonne C, Fischbein NJ. *Cranial Nerves: Anatomy, Pathology, Imaging.* New York, NY: Theime Medical; 2010.

5. Abolmaali N, Gudziol V, Hummel T. Pathology of the olfactory nerve. *Neuroimaging Clin N Am.* 2008;18(2):233-242. doi:10.1016/j.nic.2007.10.002.

6. Coello AF, Canals AG, Gonzalez JM, Martín JJA. Cranial nerve injury after minor head trauma: clinical article. *J Neurosurg.* 2010;113(3):547-555. doi:10.3171/2010.6.JNS091620.

7. Nordin S, Brämerson A. Complaints of olfactory disorders: epidemiology, assessment and clinical implications. *Curr Opin Allerg Clin Immunol.* 2008;8(1):10-15. doi:10.1097/ACI.0b013e3282f3f473.

8. Allen KF, Gaier ED, Wiggs JL. Genetics of primary inherited disorders of the optic nerve: clinical applications. *Cold Spring Harb Perspect Med.* 2015;5(7):a017277. doi:10.1101/cshperspect.a017277.

9. Sadagopan KA, Wasserman BN Managing the patient with oculomotor nerve palsy. *Curr Opin Ophthalmol.* 2013;24(5):438-447. doi:10.1097/ICU.0b013e3283645a9b.

10. Engel JM. Treatment and diagnosis of congenital fourth nerve palsies: an update. *Curr Opin Ophthalmol.* 2015;26(5):353-356. doi:10.1097/ICU.0000000000000179.

11. Heir GM, Nasri-Heir C, Thomas D, et al. Complex regional pain syndrome following trigeminal nerve injury: report of 2 cases. *Oral Surg Oral Med Oral Pathol Oral Radiol.* 2012;114(6):733-739. doi:10.1016/j.oooo.2012.06.001.

12. Zakrzewska JM, Linskey ME. Trigeminal neuralgia. *BMJ.* 2014;348:474. doi:10.1136/bmj.g474.

13. Quoc EB, Milleret C. Origins of strabismus and loss of binocular vision. *Front Integr Neurosci.* 2014;8:71. doi:10.3389/fnint.2014.00071.

14. Baricich A, Cabrio C, Paggio R, Cisari C, Aluffi P. Peripheral facial nerve palsy: how effective is rehabilitation? *Otol Neurotol.* 2012;33(7):1118-1126. doi:10.1097/MAO.0b013e318264270e.

15. Hohman MH, Hadlock TA. Etiology, diagnosis, and management of facial palsy: 2000 patients at a facial nerve center. *Laryngoscope.* 2014;124(7):E283-E293. doi:10.1002/lary.24542.

16. Pearce JMS. Observations on the blink reflex. *Eur Neurol.* 2008;59(3-4):221-223. doi:10.1159/000114053.

17. Patel DK, Levin KH. Bell palsy: clinical examination and management. *Cleve Clin J Med.* 2015;82(7):419-426.

18. Gilchrist JM. Seventh cranial neuropathy. *Sem Neurol.* 2009;29(1):5-13. doi:10.1055/s-0028-1124018.

19. Borghei-Razavi H, Darvish O, Schick U. Disabling vertigo and tinnitus caused by intrameatal compression of the anterior inferior cerebellar artery on the vestibulocochlear nerve: a case report, surgical considerations, and review of the literature. *J Neurol Surg Rep.* 2014;75(1):e47-e51. doi:10.1055/s-0033-1359299.

20. De Foer B, Kenis C, Van Melkebeke D, et al. Pathology of the vestibulocochlear nerve. *Eur J Radiol.* 2010;74(2):349-358. doi:10.1016/j.ejrad.2009.06.033.

21. Vermiglio AJ, Soli SD, Freed DJ, Fisher LM. The relationship between high-frequency pure-tone hearing loss, hearing in noise test (HINT) thresholds, and the articulation index. *J Am Acad Audiol.* 2012;23(10):779-788. doi:10.3766/jaaa.23.10.4.

22. Dumas G, Karkas A, Perrin P, Chahine K, Schmerber S. High-frequency skull vibration-induced nystagmus test in partial vestibular lesions. *Otol Neurotol.* 2011;32(8):1291-1301. doi:10.1097/MAO.0b013e31822f0b6b.

23. Roberts H, McGuigan S, Infeld B, Sultana R, Gerraty R. A video-oculographic study of acute vestibular neuritis. *J Clin Neurosci.* 2014;21(11):2035. doi:10.1016/j.jocn.2014.06.020.

24. Bartoshuk LM, Snyder DJ, Grushka M, Berger AM, Duffy VB, Kveton JF. Taste damage: previously unsuspected consequences. *Chem Senses.* 2005;30(Suppl 1):i218-i219. doi:10.1093/chemse/bjh192.

25. Steele CM, Miller AJ. Sensory input pathways and mechanisms in swallowing: a review. *Dysphagia.* 2010;25(4):323-333. doi:10.1007/s00455-010-9301-5.

26. Burki NK, Lee LY. Mechanisms of dyspnea. *CHEST Journal.* 2010;138(5):1196-1201. doi:10.1378/chest.10-0534.

27. Damodaran O, Rizk E, Rodriguez J, Lee G. Cranial nerve assessment: a concise guide to clinical examination. *Clin Anat.* 2014;27(1):25-30. doi:10.1002/ca.22336.

28. Cohen SM, Kim J, Roy N, Asche C, Courey M. Prevalence and causes of dysphonia in a large treatment-seeking population. *Laryngoscope*. 2012;122(2):343-348. doi:10.1002/lary.22426.

29. Umay EK, Unlu E, Saylam GK, Cakci A, Korkmaz H. Evaluation of dysphagia in early stroke patients by bedside, endoscopic, and electrophysiological methods. *Dysphagia*. 2013;28(3):395-403. doi:10.1007/s00455-013-9447-z.

30. Jordan LC, Hillis AE. Disorders of speech and language: aphasia, apraxia and dysarthria. *Curr Opin Neurol*. 2006;19(6): 580-585. doi:10.1097/WCO.0b013e3280109260.

31. Umeda M, Shigeta T, Takahashi H, et al. Shoulder mobility after spinal accessory nerve–sparing modified radical neck dissection in oral cancer patients. *Oral Surg Oral Med Oral Pathol Oral Radiol Endodontol*. 2010;109(6):820-824. doi:10.1016/j.tripleo.2009.11.027.

CLINICAL TEST QUESTIONS

Section 8

1. After sustaining a traumatic brain injury, Jayden lost his sense of smell and taste. Loss of these 2 senses likely resulted from damage to which cranial nerves?
     1. olfactory nerve (CN 1)
     2. facial nerve (CN 7)
     3. glossopharyngeal nerve (CN 9)
     4. vagus nerve (CN 10)
     5. hypoglossal nerve (CN 12)
   a. 1, 2
   b. 1, 2, 3
   c. 1, 2, 3, 4
   d. 1, 2, 3, 4, 5

2. Loss of smell is clinically termed:
   a. anomia
   b. anosmia
   c. agnosia
   d. aphasia

3. Which cranial nerves are being assessed when a therapist tests extraocular eye movements?
   a. optic nerve (CN 2), oculomotor nerve (CN 3), trochlear nerve (CN 4)
   b. optic nerve (CN 2), oculomotor nerve (CN 3), abducens nerve (CN 6)
   c. oculomotor nerve (CN 3), trochlear nerve (CN 4), trigeminal nerve (CN 5)
   d. oculomotor nerve (CN 3), trochlear nerve (CN 4), abducens nerve (CN 6)

4. Mary has a lateral strabismus (or external deviation) in her left eye accompanied by eyelid ptosis (drooping), and binocular nystagmus. Her therapist suspects involvement of which cranial nerve?
   a. optic nerve (CN 2)
   b. oculomotor nerve (CN 3)
   c. trochlear nerve (CN 4)
   d. abducens nerve (CN 6)

5. Ms. Chen is seeing her occupational therapist because she is experiencing loss of sensation to her head, face, and inner oral cavity on her left side. Her jaw is deviating to the left side and she is having difficulty chewing on that side. Her therapist suspects involvement of which cranial nerve?
   a. facial nerve (CN 7)
   b. abducens nerve (CN 6)
   c. trigeminal nerve (CN 5)
   d. glossopharyngeal nerve (CN 9)

6. Mr. Murakami presents with drooping of his right face, right eyelid ptosis, inability to completely close his right eyelid, and mouth deviation to the right. Additionally, he reports that he has become hypersensitive to noise in his right ear. This condition is called _____ and results from damage to cranial nerve _____.
   a. Bell palsy; CN 7 facial nerve
   b. Trigeminal neuralgia; CN 5 trigeminal nerve
   c. Bell palsy; CN 5 trigeminal nerve
   d. Trigeminal neuralgia; CN 8 vestibulocochlear nerve

7. After a viral infection of the upper respiratory tract, Ms. Schumacher began to experience vertigo, nausea, balance problems, and nystagmus. Her physician diagnosed _____, which is caused by damage to the _____.
   a. trigeminal neuraligia; CN 5 trigeminal nerve
   b. vestibular neuritis; CN 8 vestibulocochlear nerve
   c. vestibular neuritis; CN 10 vagus nerve
   d. Bell palsy; CN 7 facial nerve

8. After a head injury resulting from a fall, Mrs. Mazziotta has lost both the gag and swallowing reflexes. She is also experiencing dysphonia (hoarse voice), dysphagia (difficulty swallowing), and dysarthria (difficulty speaking clearly). These symptoms likely result from damage to which 2 cranial nerves?
   a. CN 11 accessory nerve, CN 12 hypoglossal nerve
   b. CN 9 glossopharyngeal nerve, CN 12 hypoglossal nerve
   c. CN 10 vagus nerve, CN 8 vestibulocochlear nerve
   d. CN 9 glossopharyngeal nerve, CN 10 vagus nerve

9. Howard presents with weakness rotating his head to the right, weakness flexing his head laterally and forward, weakness elevating his left shoulder, and weakness flexing his left arm above 90 degrees. His physician suspects involvement of which cranial nerve?
   a. CN 12 hypoglossal nerve
   b. CN 11 accessory nerve
   c. CN 10 vagus nerve
   d. CN 9 glossopharyngeal nerve

10. Emilia is experiencing tongue deviation to the right, atrophy and paralysis of the tongue, and dysphagia secondary to impaired tongue musculature. Her therapist immediately suspects impairment to which cranial nerve?
    a. CN 9 glossopharyngeal
    b. CN 11 accessory nerve
    c. CN 12 hypoglossal nerve
    d. CN 7 facial nerve

Answers

1. c
2. b
3. d
4. b
5. c
6. a
7. b
8. d
9. b
10. c

Sensory Receptors

- A sensory receptor is a specialized nerve cell that is designed to respond to a specific sensory stimulus (eg, touch, pressure, pain, temperature, light, sound, position in space).
- Normally, sensory receptors only accept molecules that have a complimentary receptor site organization. Exceptions occur in states of pathology.

THREE TYPES OF SENSORY RECEPTORS

Exteroceptors

- Exteroceptors are sensory receptors that are adapted for the reception of stimuli from the external world (outside the body).
- Example: visual, auditory, tactile, olfactory, and gustatory receptors[1]

Interoceptors

- Interoceptors receive sensory information from inside the body (eg, from the viscera, hollow organs, and glands).
- Interoceptors detect internal body sensations, such as stomach pain, pinched spinal nerves, or inflammatory processes in the deep layers of the skin.[2]

Proprioceptors

- Proprioceptors are sensory receptors located in the muscles, tendons, and joints of the body and in the utricles, saccules, and semicircular canals of the inner ear (ie, the labyrinths of the inner ear).
- These detect body position and movement.[3]

DEVELOPMENTAL CLASSIFICATION OF SENSORY RECEPTORS

Protopathic

- The protopathic sensory system is considered to be old phylogenetically.
- Protopathic receptors are adapted to identify gross bodily sensation rather than specific regions of sensation. Thus, protopathic receptors cannot precisely locate the origin of pain.
- Protopathic receptors detect crude touch and dull pain rather than discriminative touch and sharp pain.
- Evolutionary function: enables the organism to detect possible (but not imminent) danger in the environment.[4]

Epicritic

- With regard to phylogeny of the species, the epicritic sensory system is considered to have developed more recently than the protopathic system.
- Epicritic receptors can detect sensation with precision, accuracy, and acuteness. Discriminative touch, sharp pain, exact joint position, and the exact localization of a stimulus are within the functions of the epicritic system.
- Evolutionary function: allows the organism to explore the environment with precise detail, thus allowing the ability to detect imminent danger.[5]

Gutman SA. *Quick Reference Neuroscience for Rehabilitation Professionals: The Essential Neurologic Principles Underlying Rehabilitation Practice, Third Edition* (pp 100-105).

Children With Sensory Processing Problems

- The epicritic and protopathic sensory systems may not function optimally in children with sensory processing disorders.

A Child With a Dominant Protopathic Sensory System

- This child may not be able to receive adequate sensory stimulation from the environment, or the sensory data that enter the central nervous system (CNS) are experienced by the child as if they had been dulled. It would be as if the child received all sensory data filtered through gloves, earmuffs, and a heavy winter coat that decreased the child's direct sensory stimulation from the environment.
- Some children who display self-stimulation behaviors (eg, rocking, biting oneself, humming continuously) may have a dominant protopathic system. They may seek a great deal of sensory stimulation in an attempt to compensate for their inability to receive adequate sensory stimulation from the environment.
- Such sensory stimulation is necessary for the development of the CNS.

A Child With a Dominant Epicritic Sensory System

- These children may be hypersensitive to sensation from the environment. Some sensations that may be innocuous to others may be experienced as painful or intolerable to children with heightened epicritic systems.
- Tactile defensiveness is a condition in which certain normal sensations are experienced as highly noxious, such as the feel of water hitting the skin during bathing and showering or the feel of clothing labels rubbing against one's neck. Children with hypersensitive epicritic sensors may refuse to take showers and baths or may insist on wearing shorts in the winter because they cannot tolerate the feel of clothing against their skin.
- Children with hypersensitive proprioceptors may be unable to tolerate movement caused by gravitational displacement. Gravitational insecurity is a condition in which children experience gravitationally induced movement as frightening. For example, such children may be abnormally fearful of using playground equipment such as a swing, sliding board, seesaw, or jungle gym. While such playground games commonly provide exhilarating sensory stimulation to many children, those with gravitational insecurity may experience these sensations as frightening.[6]

SENSORY RECEPTORS CLASSIFIED BY ANATOMICAL LOCATION

Cutaneous Receptors

- Cutaneous receptors respond to pain, temperature, pressure, vibration, and discriminative touch.
- They are found in the superficial and deep layers of skin.
- Cutaneous receptors are also classified as exteroceptors (which receive stimuli from external sources) or interoceptors (eg, receiving stimuli from internal sources, such as an inflammatory process in the deep layers of the skin).[7]

Muscle, Tendon, and Joint Receptors (Proprioceptors)

- These sensory receptors are located in the muscles, tendons, and joints of the body.
- They detect muscle length, muscle tension, joint position, deep muscular and joint pain, and tendonitis.
- These sensory receptors are also classified as proprioceptors.[8]

Visceral Receptors

- Visceral receptors respond to pressure and pain from the internal organs.
- They are also considered to be interoceptors.[9]

Special Sense Receptors

Visual Receptors

- The visual receptors are the rods and cones of the retina. In addition to being called *special sense receptors*, they are considered exteroceptors because they respond to light stimuli from the external environment.[10]

Olfactory Receptors

- The olfactory receptors are the hair cells located in the mucous lining of the nasal canal. They are considered exteroceptors because they respond to scent and odor stimuli from the external environment.[11]

Auditory Receptors

- The auditory receptors are the hair cells of the cochlea. They are considered exteroceptors because they respond to sound stimuli from the external environment.[12]

Gustatory Receptors

- The gustatory receptors are the taste buds on the tongue. They are considered exteroceptors because they respond to taste stimuli from the external environment.[13]

Equilibrium

- Receptors for equilibrium are the semicircular canals, utricles, and saccules of the inner ear. These are also considered proprioceptors because they provide information about the head's position in relation to the body.[14]

SENSORY RECEPTORS CLASSIFIED BY STRUCTURAL DESIGN

Mechanoreceptors

- Mechanoreceptors are sensory receptors that are stimulated in response to mechanical pressure or deformation.
- Examples of mechanoreceptors are the hair cells of the labyrinth system, some receptors of the skin, and stretch receptors of the skeletal muscles.
- Mechanoreceptors detect touch, pressure, vibration, proprioception, equilibrium, and audition.[15]
- There are various types of mechanoreceptors:
  - Pacinian corpuscles (detect rapid vibration)
  - Meissner corpuscles (detect light touch and texture change)
  - Merkel discs (detect sustained pressure)
  - Ruffini endings (detect pressure and tension in deep skin layers and fascia)
  - Free nerve endings (detect touch, pressure, and stretch)
  - Baroreceptors (detect stretch of blood vessels)
  - Ligamentous receptors (detect ligament stretch and proprioception)

Thermoreceptors

- Thermoreceptors are sensory receptors that are stimulated in response to changes in temperature.
- Separate sensory receptors are believed to detect hot and cold sensation.
- Although thermoreceptors are located all over an organism's external and internal body, it is believed that the highest density of cold receptors are found in the facial skin, tongue, bladder, and cornea.
- Specialized pain receptors (nociceptors) that can detect changes in harmful temperatures (such as heat that can burn skin) have been identified.[16]

Chemoreceptors

- Chemoreceptors, or *chemosensors*, are sensory receptors that detect chemical stimuli from the environment.
- There are 2 primary categories of chemoreceptors: direct and distance.[17]
    1. Direct chemoreceptors become stimulated in response to immediate contact with a chemical from the environment. For example, the taste buds of the gustatory system respond when they are directly stimulated by food or liquid molecules on the tongue.
    2. Distance chemoreceptors become stimulated in response to molecules in a gaseous form (eg, the scent of freshly baked cookies) that emerge from the direct odorant (the actual cookies). For example, the olfactory receptors respond when they become stimulated by gaseous chemicals that contact the cilia in the mucosal lining of the nasal canal.

Photoreceptors

- Photoreceptors are highly specialized types of sensory receptors located on the retina that detect light from the environment.
- There are 2 primary forms of photoreceptors: rods and cones.[10]
    1. Rods allow vision in nighttime lighting and are responsible for black and white vision. Rods are primarily located in the periphery of the retina.
    2. Cones function in daytime and are responsible for color vision. The majority of cones are located in the fovea, the central region of the eye.
- We lose our color vision in very dim or dark lighting because only the rods are activated in low light levels.

RECEPTOR FIELDS

- A receptor field is a body area that contains specific types of sensory receptor cells.
- When stimulated, the receptors on a specific receptor field become activated.

Location of Small and Large Receptor Fields

Small Receptor Fields

- Small receptor fields are located on body areas with the greatest sensitivity, such as the lips, hands, face, and soles of the feet.[18,19]

Large Receptor Fields

- Large receptor fields are located on body regions with less discriminative sensitivity, such as the legs, abdomen, arms, and back.[18,19]

Function of Small vs Large Receptor Fields

Small Receptor Fields

- Small receptor fields function in fine discrimination and are necessary for the exploration of the environment.[18,19]

Large Receptor Fields

- Large receptor fields function in gross discrimination.[18,19]

CORTICAL REPRESENTATION OF RECEPTOR FIELDS (THE HOMUNCULUS)

- Small receptor fields (eg, those of the mouth, tongue, hands, feet) are afforded a large amount of cortical representation on both the sensory and motor homunculi.
- Large receptor fields (eg, legs, abdomen, arms, back) are afforded smaller amounts of cortical representation on the homunculi.[20,21]

REFERENCES

1. Price DD, Greenspan JD, Dubner R. Neurons involved in the exteroceptive function of pain. *Pain*. 2003;106(3):215-219. doi:10.1016/j.pain.2003.10.016.

2. Craig AD. How do you feel? Interoception: the sense of the physiological condition of the body. *Nat Rev Neurosci*. 2002;3(8):655-666. doi:10.1016/S0959-4388(03)00090-4.

3. Proske U. The role of muscle proprioceptors in human limb position sense: a hypothesis. *J Anat*. 2015;227(2):178-183. doi:10.1111/joa.12289.

4. Donnelly K. Protopathic Pain. In: Kreutzer J, DeLuca J, Caplan B, eds. *Encyclopedia of Clinical Neuropsychology*. New York, NY: Springer; 2011:2061-2061. doi:10.1007/978-0-387-79948-3_777.

5. Velstra IM, Bolliger M, Baumberger M, Rietman JS, Curt A. Epicritic sensation in cervical spinal cord injury: diagnostic gains beyond testing light touch. *J Neurotrauma*. 2013;30(15):1342-1348. doi:10.1089/neu.2012.2828.

6. May-Benson TA, Koomar JA. Identifying gravitational insecurity in children: a pilot study. *Am J Occup Ther*. 2007;61(2):142-147. doi:10.5014/ajot.2015.694001.

7. Collins DF, Refshauge KM, Todd G, Gandevia SC. Cutaneous receptors contribute to kinesthesia at the index finger, elbow, and knee. *J Neurophysiol*. 2005;94(3):1699-1706. doi:10.1152/jn.00191.2005.

8. Smith JL, Crawford M, Proske U, Taylor JL, Gandevia SC. Signals of motor command bias joint position sense in the presence of feedback from proprioceptors. *J Appl Physiol*. 2009;106(3):950-958. doi:10.1152/japplphysiol.91365.2008.

9. Gebhart GF. Visceral pain—peripheral sensitisation. *Gut*. 2000;47(Suppl 4):iv54-iv55. doi:10.1136/gut.47.suppl_4.iv54.

10. Merzendorfer H. A new view of photoreceptors. *J Exper Biol*. 2013;216(3):iv-iv. doi:10.1242/ jeb.077727.

11. Jones B. Evolution: evolution of olfactory receptors in mammals. *Nat Rev Genet*. 2014;15(9):575-575. doi:10.1038/nrg3809.

12. Fettiplace R, Hackney CM. The sensory and motor roles of auditory hair cells. *Nat Rev Neurosci*. 2006;7(1):19-29. doi:10.1038/nrn1828.

13. Chaudhari N, Roper SD. The cell biology of taste. *J Cell Biol*. 2010;190(3):285-296. doi:10.1083/jcb.201003144.

14. Curthoys I. Vestibular otoliths, response to vibration and sound. In: Jaeger D, Jung R, eds. *Encyclopedia of Computational Neuroscience*. New York, NY: Springer; 2014:1-8. doi:10.1007/978-1-4614-7320-6_155-2.

15. Macefield VG. Physiological characteristics of low-threshold mechanoreceptors in joints, muscle and skin in human subjects. *Clin Exper Pharmacol Physiol*. 2005;32(1-2):135-144. doi:10.1111/j.1440-1681.2005.04143.x.

16. Schepers RJ, Ringkamp M. Thermoreceptors and thermosensitive afferents. *Neurosci Biobehav Rev*. 2010;34(2):177-184. doi:10.1016/j.neubiorev.2009.10.003.

17. Underbakke ES, Kiessling LL. Classifying chemoreceptors: quantity versus quality. *Eur Mol Biol Org J*. 2010;29(20):3435-3436. doi:10.1038/emboj.2010.246.

18. Haggard P, Christakou A, Serino A. Viewing the body modulates tactile receptive fields. *Exper Brain Res*. 2007;180(1):187-193. doi:10.1007/s00221-007-0971-7.

19. Haggard P, Iannetti GD, Longo MR. Spatial sensory organization and body representation in pain perception. *Curr Biol*. 2013;23(4):R164-R176. doi:10.1016/j.cub.2013.01.047.

20. Eickhoff SB, Grefkes C, Fink GR, Zilles K. Functional lateralization of face, hand, and trunk representation in anatomically defined human somatosensory areas. *Cerebral Cortex*. 2008;18(12):2820-2830. doi:10.1093/cercor/bhn039.

21. Fabri M, Polonara G, Salvolini U, Manzoni T. Bilateral cortical representation of the trunk midline in human first somatic sensory area. *Hum Brain Mapp*. 2005;25(3):287-296. doi:10.1002/hbm.20099.

Neurons and Action Potentials

Neuron

- A neuron is the electrically excitable nerve cell and fiber of the nervous system.
- Neurons are composed of the following[1-3]:
  - Cell body (soma), nucleus, dendrites, main axon branch (with possible axon collaterals), and terminal boutons.

Cell Body

- The cell body contains the nucleus of the neuron, which stores the genetic codes of the organism.[1-3]

Dendrites

- Dendrites are the tree-like processes that attach to the cell body.
- They receive messages from the terminal boutons of a presynaptic neuron.
- Dendrites can bifurcate, or produce additional dendritic branches.
- Bifurcation increases the neuron's receptor sites.[1-3]

Axon Hillock

- The axon hillock is the region where the cell body and axon attach.
- Axon hillocks can function as tight junctions between 2 cells (or an impermeable barrier).[1-3]

Axon

- An axon is the fiber emerging from the axon hillock and extending to the terminal boutons.
- Axons transmit action potentials, or nerve signals, to the terminal boutons.[1-3]

Myelin

- Axons are covered by a cellular sheath called *myelin*.
- Myelin is composed of lipids and proteins and acts as an insulating substance of the axon. The myelin conducts nerve signals down the axon, away from the neural cell body.
- The more myelin the axon has, the faster its conduction rate.[1-3]
- There are 2 primary types of myelin:
  1. *Schwann cells*: Schwann cells are located in the peripheral nervous system (PNS) and are able to be regenerated if damaged.[4-6]
  2. *Oligodendrocytes*: Oligodendrocytes are located in the central nervous system (CNS) and cannot regenerate if damaged.[7]

Nodes of Ranvier

- Nodes of Ranvier are spaces between the myelin where nerve signals jump from one node to the next in the process of conduction.
- At the node of Ranvier, the axon is unmyelinated and able to generate the electrical activity needed for nerve conduction.[8]

Gutman SA. *Quick Reference Neuroscience for Rehabilitation Professionals: The Essential Neurologic Principles Underlying Rehabilitation Practice, Third Edition* (pp 106-112). © 2017 Taylor & Francis Group.

Multiple Sclerosis: Disease of the Myelin

- Multiple sclerosis (MS) involves random demyelination of the CNS.
- The disease is characterized by periods of exacerbation and remission over many years.
- In the early stages of MS, there is normal or near-normal neurologic function between exacerbations. As the disease progresses, remissions grow shorter and are marked by less improvement.
- Signs and symptoms can be variable because demyelination can occur in a wide variety of locations in the CNS.[9]
- Sensory symptoms:
  - Numbness, paresthesias, and Lhermitte sign (causalgia radiating down the back and lower extremities, elicited by neck flexion)
- Motor symptoms:
  - Abnormal gait, bladder and sexual dysfunction, vertigo, nystagmus, fatigue, and speech disturbance
  - MS of the spinal cord produces asymmetrical weakness secondary to plaques that interfere with the descending motor tracts.
  - Ataxia of the limbs occurs secondary to an interruption of nerve signal conduction in the dorsal columns.
  - MS is considered to be a disease process that affects the upper motor neurons (UMN).
- Commonly affected areas:
  - Optic nerve —————▶ visual field acuity
  - Corticospinal tracts —————▶ muscle strength
  - Corticobulbar tracts —————▶ speech and swallowing functions
  - Cerebellar tracts —————▶ gait and coordination
  - Spinocerebellar tracts —————▶ balance
  - Medial longitudinal fasciculus—▶ conjugate gaze of the extraocular eye muscles
  - Dorsal columns —————▶ discriminative touch, pressure, vibration, proprioception, kinesthesia

Amyotrophic Lateral Sclerosis: Death of Upper and Lower Motor Neurons

- Amyotrophic lateral sclerosis (ALS) is a severe degenerative neurologic disorder affecting motor function.
- ALS is a disease of both the CNS and the PNS. The UMNs of the cerebral cortex and the lower motor neurons (LMNs) of the ventral horn of the spinal cord are both affected.
- Sensory and cognitive functions remain intact.
- The death of UMNs and LMNs leads to denervation, causing muscle atrophy and spasticity.
- UMN lesions result in the following:
  - Muscle weakness
  - Spasticity
  - Loss of fine motor control
- Either UMN or LMN lesions can account for the following:
  - Dysphagia (difficulty swallowing)
  - Dysarthria (difficulty articulating words clearly)
  - Dysphonia (difficulty projecting one's voice audibly)
- LMN lesions result in the following:
  - Fasciculations
  - Muscle weakness
  - Muscle atrophy
  - Hyporeflexia
- Common early symptoms:
  - Muscle cramps involving the distal legs
  - A slow, progressive weakness and atrophy of the distal muscle groups of one upper extremity
- These early symptoms are then followed by a wider spread of muscle weakness in surrounding body areas.
- Eventually, UMNs and LMNs involving multiple limbs and the head are affected.
- In advanced stages of the disease, muscles of the palate, pharynx, tongue, neck, and shoulders are affected.
- Death commonly occurs from denervation of the respiratory musculature.[10]

Myasthenia Gravis: Disorder of the Neuromuscular Junction

- Myasthenia gravis is a chronic autoimmune disorder that affects the neuromuscular junction of voluntary muscles.
- The disease process is characterized by production of acetylcholine receptor antibodies that destroy acetylcholine receptors at the neuromuscular junction. Essentially, acetylcholine receptor antibodies block the transmission of acetylcholine across the neuromuscular junction. The production of acetylcholine receptor antibodies is thought to be an autoimmune response.
- This results in severe muscular weakness and fatigue.
- Typically, the disease first affects eye and head musculature. Progression continues to the limbs and sometimes to respiratory muscles.
- Anticholinesterase agents are commonly used to reduce the breakdown of acetylcholine in the neuromuscular synaptic space.
- Increased availability of acetylcholine in the synaptic space enhances muscular contraction.
- Corticosteroid drugs are used to suppress the immune response if anticholinesterase agents are ineffective.[11]

Axon Collaterals

- Axon collaterals project from the main axon structure.
- They serve to transmit nerve signals to several parts of the nervous system simultaneously.[1-3]

Terminal Boutons (Synaptic Boutons)

- Terminal boutons emerge from the end branches of the axon and contain neurotransmitter substances.[1-3]

Synaptic Cleft

- The synaptic cleft is the space between a presynaptic neuron's terminal boutons and a postsynaptic neuron's dendrites.
- The terminal boutons release their neurotransmitter substances into the synaptic cleft.[1-3]

Neurotransmitter

- The neurotransmitter is a chemical stored in the terminal boutons.
- It is released into the synaptic cleft to transmit messages to another neuron.[12]

Presynaptic Neuron

- The presynaptic neuron is the first order neuron that releases its neurotransmitter into the synaptic cleft.[1-3]

Postsynaptic Neuron

- The postsynaptic neuron is the second order neuron.
- It receives the presynaptic neuron's neurotransmitter substance from the synaptic cleft, but only if the neurotransmitter possesses the specific molecules that can bind to the postsynaptic neuron's receptor sites.[1-3]

Neurotransmitter Activity Termination

- Neurotransmitters must be broken down or removed after reaching the postsynaptic cell to prevent continued signal conduction and allow further cycles of neurotransmitter release and signaling.
- There are 3 primary ways through which neurotransmitter activity can be terminated.

Diffusion

- The neurotransmitter detaches from the postsynaptic receptor, drifts out of the synaptic cleft, and is absorbed by glial cells.[13]

Enzymatic Degradation
- An enzyme is a chemical substance that breaks down a neurotransmitter so that the postsynaptic neuron can repolarize in order to fire again; these are also called *antitransmitters*.
- Enzymes are located in the synaptic cleft and terminate the postsynaptic neuron's response.
- Example: Acetylcholinesterase (AChE) is the enzymatic antitransmitter for acetylcholine (ACh). ACh is a neurotransmitter important for activating neuromuscular-joint movements.[12]

Re-Uptake Process
- Re-uptake is the process by which a neurotransmitter is reabsorbed into the presynaptic neuron's terminal boutons.[14]

Down Regulation
- Down regulation is a decrease in the number of receptors on the postsynaptic neuron (for a specific neurotransmitter), often due to long-term exposure to the neurotransmitter.
- In response to too much neurotransmitter, the receptor sites on the second order neuron will decrease.[15]

Synaptic Delay
- Synaptic delay is the time required for the neurotransmitter to diffuse across a postsynaptic neuron's membrane.
- Average synaptic delay is 1 to 2 milliseconds.[16]

Post-Tetanic Potentiation
- Post-tetanic potentiation occurs in synapses that are frequently used.
- When the presynaptic bouton becomes excited, it releases greater amounts of neurotransmitter substance.
- The postsynaptic neuron then has prolonged and repetitive discharge after firing due to too much neurotransmitter release or too slow enzymatic degradation.[17]

Decreases in Synaptic Transmission

Anoxia
- Anoxia is lack of oxygen.
- When the neural cell body experiences anoxia, synaptic transmission begins to fail within 45 seconds.[18]

Paralysis Due to Poison
- Paralysis due to poison, such as snake venom or plant poison (eg, curare), occurs because the poison blocks ACh at the neuromuscular junction.
- This causes a decreased postsynaptic potential at the cell membrane of the muscle.
- Example: Botulism (food poisoning) is a condition in which the release of ACh at the presynaptic bouton is blocked, causing fatigue of the neurotransmitters at the neuromuscular junction and resulting in skeletal paralysis.[19]

Spasms Due to Cholinergic Drugs
- The term *cholinergic* refers to neurological systems that use ACh. Cholinergic drugs are chemicals that bind with and activate the same neuronal receptors as ACh.
- Cholinergic drugs increase the effects of ACh at the neuromuscular junction, thus producing spasms in the muscle.
- Tardive dyskinesia is a condition caused by cholinergic drugs in which patients may experience full body spasms, lip smacking, and tongue protrusion.[20]

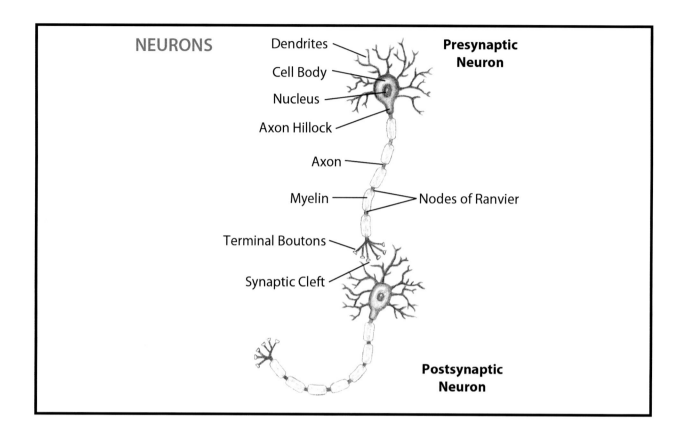

Synaptic Fatigue

- Synaptic fatigue occurs as a result of a neurotransmitter depletion due to the repetitive stimulation of a presynaptic neuron.
- Synaptic fatigue underlies the addiction process. Every time an individual uses an addictive substance, the CNS is abnormally flooded with the neurotransmitter dopamine. This causes the brain to decrease its own natural production of dopamine, leading to cravings for the addictive substance.[21]

Electrical Potentials at Synapses

- The release of neurotransmitters into the synaptic cleft results in the stimulation of receptors on the postsynaptic neuron's cell membrane.
- The chemical stimulation of these receptors can cause the membrane ion channel to open.
- The flux of ions across the postsynaptic membrane generates a postsynaptic potential.[1-3,12]

Postsynaptic Potentials

- Postsynaptic potentials are changes in ion concentration on the postsynaptic membrane.
- When a neurotransmitter binds to a receptor site on a postsynaptic membrane, the result may be either depolarization or hyperpolarization of the postsynaptic membrane.
- Depolarization of the cell membrane causes the neuron to become excited. An excitatory postsynaptic potential is generated.
- Hyperpolarization of the cell membrane causes inhibition of the neuron. An inhibitory postsynaptic potential is generated.[1-3,12]

Membrane Potentials

- The membrane potential is the electrical charge that travels across the cell membrane.
- It is the difference between the chemical composition inside and outside the cell; in other words, the sodium potassium balance inside and outside the cell.
- If the membrane potential is strong enough, it causes an action potential.[1-3,12]

Action Potentials

- An action potential is the brief electrical impulse that provides the basis for conduction of nerve signals along the axon.
- It results from the brief changes in the cell's membrane permeability to sodium and potassium ions. A strong enough action potential will cause the neuron to become excited and start the conduction process.[22]

Sequence of Events of Synaptic Transmission

- An action potential arrives at the presynaptic terminal boutons.
- The membrane of the presynaptic terminal boutons depolarizes, thus causing the opening of the voltage-gated calcium (CA^{2+}) channels.
- The influx of CA^{2+} (in the terminal boutons) triggers the release of neurotransmitters into the synaptic cleft.
- If the neurotransmitter has compatible molecules, it will bind to the receptor sites of the postsynaptic neuron.[23]

Events of Excitatory Postsynaptic Potentials

- Sodium (Na^+) channels remain closed during the state of a resting membrane.
- The Na^+ channels open when a neurotransmitter, released into the synaptic cleft, binds to the membrane receptors of the postsynaptic cell membrane.
- The resulting influx of Na^+ depolarizes the membrane and causes excitation of the postsynaptic neuron.[24]

Events of Inhibitory Postsynaptic Potentials

- Chloride (Cl^-) channels remain closed during the state of a resting membrane.
- Cl^- channels open when a neurotransmitter is released into the synaptic cleft and binds to receptor sites of the postsynaptic cell membrane.
- The resulting influx of Cl^- hyperpolarizes the cell membrane, thus causing inhibition of the postsynaptic neuron.[25]

REFERENCES

1. Levitan IB, Kaczmarek LK. *The Neuron: Cell and Molecular Biology*. 4th ed. New York, NY: Oxford University Press; 2015.

2. Nicholls JG, Martin AR, Wallace BG, Fuchs PA. *From Neuron to Brain*. 5th ed. Sunderland, MA: Sinauer; 2011.

3. Price DJ, Jarman AP, Mason JO, Kind PC. *Building Brains: An Introduction to Neural Development*. Oxford, UK: Wiley-Blackwell; 2011.

4. Tzvetanova ID, Nave KA. Axons hooked to Schwann cell metabolism. *Nat Neurosci*. 2014;17(10):1293-1295. doi:10.1038/nn.3825.

5. Sulaiman OA, Gordon T. Effects of short-and long-term Schwann cell denervation on peripheral nerve regeneration, myelination, and size. *Glia*. 2000;32(3):234-246. doi:10.1002/1098-1136(200012).

6. Jessen KR, Mirsky R, Lloyd AC. Schwann cells: development and role in nerve repair. *Cold Spring Harb Perspect Biol*. 2015;7(7):a020487. doi:10.1101/cshperspect.a020487.

7. Silver J, Schwab ME, Popovich PG. Central nervous system regenerative failure: role of oligodendrocytes, astrocytes, and microglia. *Cold Spring Harb Perspect Biol*. 2015;7(3):a020602. doi:10.1101/cshperspect.a020602.

8. Arancibia-Carcamo IL, Attwell D. The node of Ranvier in CNS pathology. *Acta Neuropathol*. 2014;128(2):161-175. doi:10.1007/s00401-014-1305-z.

9. Frischer JM, Weigand SD, Guo Y, et al. Clinical and pathological insights into the dynamic nature of the white matter multiple sclerosis plaque. *Ann Neurol*. 2015;78(5):710-721. doi:10.1002/ana.24497.

10. Kiernan MC, Vucic S, Cheah BC, et al. Amyotrophic lateral sclerosis. *Lancet*. 2011;377(9769):942-955. doi:10.1016/S0140-6736(10)61156-7.

11. Kumar V, Kaminski HJ. Treatment of myasthenia gravis. *Curr Neurol Neurosci Rep*. 2011;11(1):89-96. doi:10.1007/s11910-010-0151-1.

12. von Bohlen und Halbach O, Dermietzel H. *Neurotransmitters and Neuromodulators: Handbook of Receptors and Biological Effects*. 2nd ed. Weinheim, Germany: Wiley; 2006.

13. Petrini EM, Barberis A. Probing the lateral diffusion of individual neurotransmitter receptors. In: Benfenati F, Fabrizio ED, Torre V, eds. *Novel Approaches for Single Molecule Activation and Detection*. New York, NY: Springer; 2014:203-219. doi:10.1007/978-3-662-43367-6_11.

14. Amara SG, Kuhar MJ. Neurotransmitter transporters: recent progress. *Annu Rev Neurosci*. 1993;16(1):73-93. doi:10.1146/annurev.ne.16.030193.000445.

15. Taylor C, Fricker AD, Devi LA, Gomes I. Mechanisms of action of antidepressants: from neurotransmitter systems to signaling pathways. *Cell Signal*. 2005;17(5):549-557. doi:10.1016/j.cellsig.2004.12.007.

16. Steuber V, Willshaw D. A biophysical model of synaptic delay learning and temporal pattern recognition in a cerebellar Purkinje cell. *J Comput Neurosci*. 2004;17(2):149-164. doi:10.1023/B:JCNS.0000037678.26155.b5.

17. Xue L, Wu LG. Post-tetanic potentiation is caused by two signalling mechanisms affecting quantal size and quantal content. *J Physiol*. 2010;588(24):4987-4994. doi:10.1113/jphysiol.2010.196964.

18. Brown GC, Neher JJ. Inflammatory neurodegeneration and mechanisms of microglial killing of neurons. *Mol Neurobiol*. 2010;41(2-3):242-247. doi:10.1007/s12035-010-8105-9.

19. Cherington M. Botulism: update and review. *Sem Neurol*. 2004;24(2):155-163. doi:10.1055/s-2004-830901.

20. Kim J, MacMaster E, Schwartz TL. Tardive dyskinesia in patients treated with atypical antipsychotics: case series and brief review of etiologic and treatment considerations. *Drugs Context*. 2014;3:212259. doi:10.7573/dic.212259.

21. Koob GF, Volkow ND. Neurocircuitry of addiction. *Neuropsychopharmacology*. 2010;35(1):217-238. doi:10.1038/npp.2009.110.

22. Barnett MW, Larkman PM. The action potential. *Pract Neurol*. 2007;7(3):192-197.

23. Greengard P. The neurobiology of slow synaptic transmission. *Science*. 2001;294(5544):1024-1030. doi:10.1126/science.294.5544.1024.

24. Catterall WA. From ionic currents to molecular mechanisms: the structure and function of voltage-gated sodium channels. *Neuron*. 2000;26(1):13-25. doi:10.1016/S0896-6273(00)81133-2.

25. Nilius B, Droogmans G. Amazing chloride channels: an overview. *Acta Physiol Scand*. 2003;177(2):119-147. doi:10.1046/j.1365-201X.2003.01060.x.

Special Sense Receptors

- The special sense receptors are designed to transmit sensory information for olfaction, gustation, vision, audition, and equilibrium.

OLFACTION

Olfactory Receptors

- The olfactory receptors are the cilia, or hair cells, located in the nostrils and nasal membranes.[1]

Physiology

- Some chemical stimulus (an odor) is received by the hair cell receptors.
- The odor molecules dissolve in the mucous that bathes the receptors on the cilia.
- The dissolution of the molecules causes a membrane potential in the receptor endings.
- If the membrane potential is strong enough, an action potential will be generated.
- The action potential is then propagated down cranial nerve (CN) 1, the olfactory nerve.[1]

Olfactory Pathway

- The olfactory pathway leads from the nasal membrane to the olfactory bulb and tract, and travels to the olfactory cortex (pyriform cortex in the temporal lobe).
- The olfactory cortex is part of the limbic system, along with the amygdala and hippocampus.
- The amygdala and hippocampus play roles in the storage of long-term memories.
- The olfactory cortex takes information from the hippocampus and projects it to the hypothalamus.
- From the hypothalamus, the olfactory information is then projected to the dorsomedial thalamus and finally to the orbitofrontal cortex for conscious association of the odor with previously stored memories.
- The connection between the olfactory pathway and the hippocampus is phylogenetically old. This is the connection that triggers the remembrance of old memories in response to odors. Examples are the memories of one's grandmother elicited in response to the smell of the kind of cookies she baked, or the memories of playing softball as a child elicited in response to the smell of freshly cut grass on a summer day.
- The memories that are elicited as a result of the connection between the olfactory tract and hippocampus have a strong emotional component. This results because the limbic system has a key role in the regulation of emotion.[1]

Therapeutic Significance

- Olfactory stimulation is used with comatose patients to facilitate central nervous system (CNS) arousal and activity.
- Aromatherapy is based on the principle that odors can elicit enhanced moods as a result of the limbic-olfactory connection.

Olfactory Lesions

A Bilateral Lesion of the Olfactory Nerves

- A bilateral lesion of the olfactory nerves will result in the loss of smell (anosmia). This type of lesion occurs frequently in patients with traumatic brain injury (TBI) secondary to brainstem involvement.

Gutman SA. *Quick Reference Neuroscience for Rehabilitation Professionals:*
The Essential Neurologic Principles Underlying Rehabilitation Practice,
Third Edition (pp 114-132).
© 2017 Taylor & Francis Group.

- A unilateral lesion of an olfactory nerve will result in loss of smell on the ipsilateral side but will commonly go undetected by the patient because the sense of smell continues to be perceived by the opposite, undamaged olfactory nerve.[1,2]

A Lesion of the Olfactory Cortex (Pyriform Cortex)

- A lesion to the olfactory cortex may result in seizures because this region is often the origin of seizure activity. Commonly, the perception of odors that are not present (olfactory hallucinations) may antecede seizure activity. This clinical phenomenon is referred to as a *seizure aura*.[1,2]

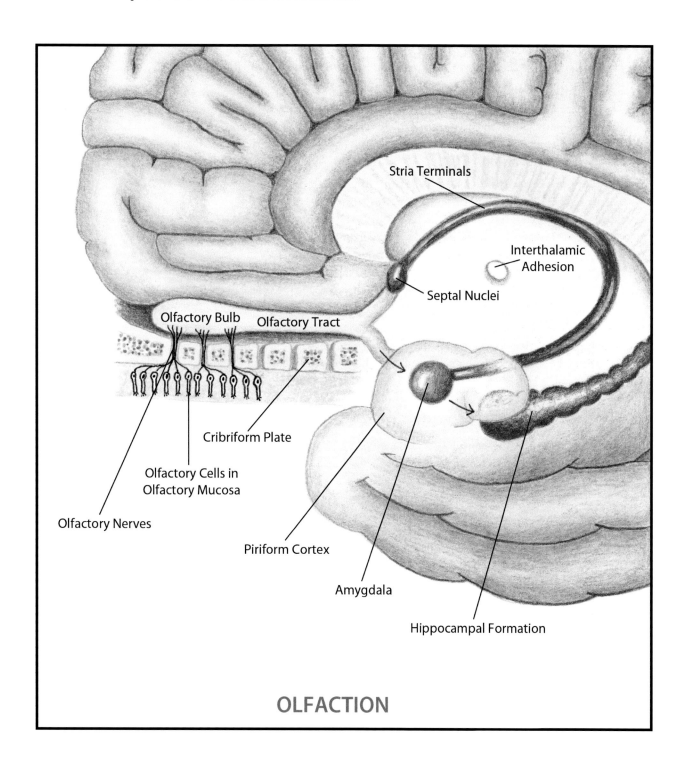

OLFACTION

GUSTATION

Gustatory Receptors
- The gustatory receptors are the taste buds found on the folds of papillae located on the surface of the tongue.
- Papillae are the small protuberances on which the taste buds lie.
- The taste buds form synapses with the sensory neurons that convey taste information to the brain.[3]

Physiology
- Saliva dissolves food in the mouth.
- Dissolved ions enter the pores of the papillae and taste buds.
- This causes a membrane potential.
- If the membrane potential is strong enough, it will cause an action potential.[3]

Gustatory Pathway
- The gustatory pathway leads from the taste bud receptors to the solitary nucleus in the medulla.
- Gustatory information is then propagated to the amygdala, hypothalamus, and thalamus.
- From the thalamus, gustatory information then travels to the primary gustatory cortex (located in the frontal insula) for conscious interpretation.[3,4]

The Connection Between Taste and Smell
- The sense of smell is critical for the function of taste.
- If the sense of smell is lost, the sense of taste will also be lost.
- The orbitofrontal cortex is a brain region that integrates gustatory and olfactory information.
- When the orbitofrontal cortex cannot integrate olfactory and gustatory information, gustation is lost.
- Example: Gustation is lost during common colds when olfaction is severely diminished due to respiratory congestion.
- Damage to the orbitofrontal region is common in TBI and may account for the lost sense of smell and taste that many individuals with TBI experience.[4,5]

Therapeutic Significance
- Gustatory stimulation is used in the sensory stimulation treatment of comatose patients.
- It is also used to facilitate oral motor function in children and adults with oral musculature dysfunction.

Gustatory Information Is Received From Cranial Nerves 7, 9, and 10

- The taste receptors on the anterior of the tongue are mediated by CN 7.
- The taste receptors on the posterior of the tongue are mediated by CN 9.
- The taste receptors on the palate and epiglottis are mediated by CN 10.

Super Tasters vs Nontasters

- Humans fall into at least 3 primary categories of tasters: super tasters, medium tasters, and nontasters.
- Super tasters can detect phenylthiocarbamide, a pungent substance that can be synthesized in a lab, while nontasters cannot detect the substance, and medium tasters can only partially detect the substance.
- Heightened taste sensitivity may be related to the presence of the TAS2R38 gene.
- Super tasters are more sensitive to the 4 basic tastes: sweet, sour, salty, and bitter. They are also able to detect a proposed fifth taste called *umami*. Umami is a Japanese word meaning meaty or hearty.
- While the tongue normally contains 100 to 200 papillae per square centimeter, super tasters may have twice as many. Nontasters have half the normal number of papillae, but each papillae seems to be much larger.
- Other studies have found that super tasters tend to be thinner than medium and nontasters. Because super tasters can detect taste more acutely, they may be able to feel satiated more quickly and eat less than medium and nontasters.
- It is estimated that 25% of the population are super tasters, another 25% are nontasters, and 50% are medium tasters.[6,7]

Specific Taste Regions of the Tongue

- The tip of the tongue can detect all tastes but predominantly detects sweet tastes.
- Salty tastes are detected on the sides of the tongue.
- Bitter and sour tastes are detected on the posterior of the tongue.
- Although the majority of taste buds are located on the tongue, taste buds are also found on the palate, pharynx, and epiglottis.

GUSTATION

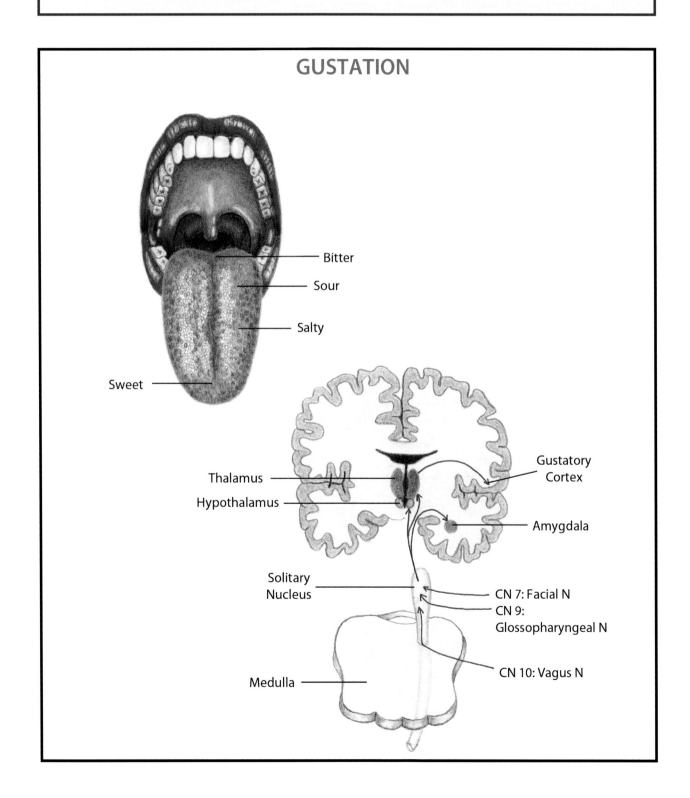

VISION (ACUITY)

Anatomy of the Eyeball

Sclera

- The sclera is the outer layer of the eyeball.[8,9]

Cornea

- The transparent anterior portion of the sclera is called the *cornea*.
- The cornea lies in front of the iris and pupil.[8,9]

Choroid

- The choroid is the middle layer of the eyeball.
- It contains the iris and lens and extends behind the retina.[8,9]
  - *Iris*
    - The iris is the circular structure that forms the colored portion of the eye.
    - It controls the size of the pupil opening.
  - *Lens*
    - The lens is the structure that focuses light rays on the retina.

Anterior Chamber

- The anterior chamber contains the gelatinous fluid between the cornea and lens called *aqueous humor*.[8,9]

Posterior Chamber

- The posterior chamber is located directly behind the lens and extends to the retina.
- It contains both aqueous humor and vitreous humor.[8,9]

Pupil

- The pupil is the circular black opening in the center of the iris.
- Light enters through the pupil.
- The amount of light permitted is controlled by the constriction of the iris.[8,9]

Fovea Centralis

- The fovea is the central region of the retina.
- It primarily contains cone receptors.
- The fovea is the location upon which incoming visual images are focused.[8,9]

Retina

- The retina is the photosensitive layer at the posterior of the eyeball.
- It contains the rods and cones: the photoreceptors.[8,9]
- *Rods*
  - Rods are specialized receptors for peripheral vision and function in dim light.
- *Cones*
  - Cones are specialized receptors for color vision and acuity.
  - These visual receptors function optimally in bright light.
  - In dim light, humans are color blind and lack acuity.

Visual Receptor Pathway

- Light waves enter the eye and are refracted by the cornea and lens.
- The light waves are then focused upon either the fovea (where the cones are located) or the peripheral retina (where the rods are located).
- A chemical reaction occurs in the rods and cones, and a membrane potential is generated.
- If the membrane potential is strong enough, an action potential is then propagated along CN 2, the optic nerve.
- Visual signals are then propagated down the optic nerve to the optic chiasm.

VISION

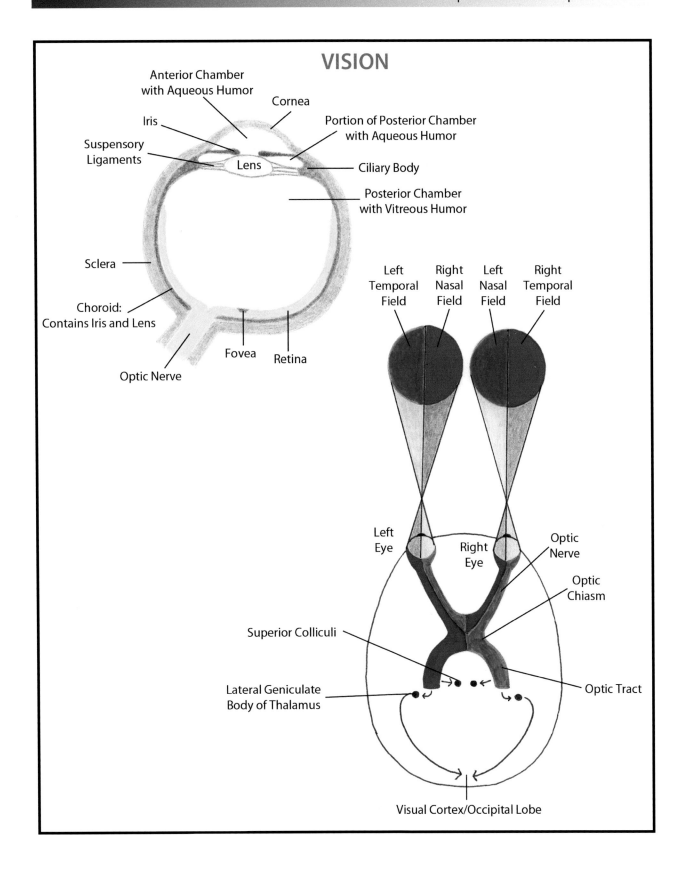

Light-Sensitive Receptors in the Eye: Role in Setting the Internal Clock

- A third type of receptor cell has been found in the retina and is composed of photoreceptive ganglion cells.
- These cells contain a light-sensitive protein called *melanopsin*, a protein that helps convert light into an electrochemical signal that is sent to the pineal gland and hypothalamus.
- The hypothalamus and pineal gland regulate the body's circadian rhythms, or internal clock.
- Melatonin is produced by the pineal gland and plays a role in the ability to fall asleep and maintain sleep. Melatonin production ceases when the photoreceptive ganglion cells in the eye detect light.
- Researchers suggest that the photoreceptors may help regulate the body's circadian rhythms. Without the ability to detect light, the internal clock quickly begins to dysfunction. This may underlie such conditions as seasonal affective disorder and sleep disturbances.[10,11]
- Researchers have begun to experiment with functional applications that use certain types of light to enhance health and cognitive stimulation. For example, some hospitals now use warm, reddish light in patient rooms for its calming effect. Similarly, bluer, alertness-enhancing light is used in work settings where employees need to maintain a high level of vigilance for lengthy periods of time.[10,11]

- The optic chiasm is the area where the optic nerves join together at the base of the brain. The optic chiasm is a midline structure that joins the optic tracts.
- Visual signals then project from the optic tracts to 2 locations: the superior colliculi of the midbrain and the lateral geniculate nucleus of the thalamus.
- The fibers that project to the superior colliculi then travel along the medial longitudinal fasciculus back to the thalamus.
- All visual fibers that travel through the thalamus then continue on to the occipital lobe.
- In the occipital lobe, visual signals first travel to the primary visual cortex (V1). V1 is responsible for the detection of a visual stimulus.
- Visual signals then travel from V1 to the visual association cortices for interpretation of the visual stimulus.[8,9,12]

Visual Field Pathways

- Visual information from the nasal fields is refracted by the lens. As a result, visual information from the nasal fields travels along the lateral aspect of the optic nerves and tracts.
- Visual information from the temporal fields is also refracted by the lens. As a result, visual information from the temporal fields travels along the medial aspect of the optic nerves and tracts.
- Visual information from the temporal fields crosses at the optic chiasm.
- The lens also inverses the visual image on the retina. As a result, visual information from the right visual field is focused on the left region of the retina.
- Visual information from the left visual field is focused on the right region of the retina.
- Each cerebral hemisphere receives visual information from the contralateral visual field.
  - The right cerebral hemisphere receives visual information from the left visual field.
  - The left cerebral hemisphere receives visual information from the right visual field.
  - Thus, if the left visual field is lost, it is due to a lesion in the right optic tract or right cerebral hemisphere. If the right visual field is lost, it is due to a lesion in the left optic tract or left cerebral hemisphere.[8,9]

Primitive Visual System

The visual pathways that travel from the optic tracts to the superior colliculi (of the midbrain) and lateral geniculate nucleus (of the thalamus) allow the brain to process and interpret visual data on an unconscious (noncortical) level. These pathways form a primitive visual system that enables organisms to respond quickly to visual stimuli without conscious interpretation. For example, it has been documented that patients with cortical blindness, in which the occipital lobe cannot interpret visual data but the external visual anatomy remains intact and can process visual stimuli, are able to identify images with greater accuracy than chance. The evolutionary significance of these pathways may have been to allow organisms the ability to respond to danger more quickly than the time required for the occipital lobes to consciously detect and interpret visual data and send that information to the frontal lobe for conscious decision making.[13]

VISUAL PATHWAYS

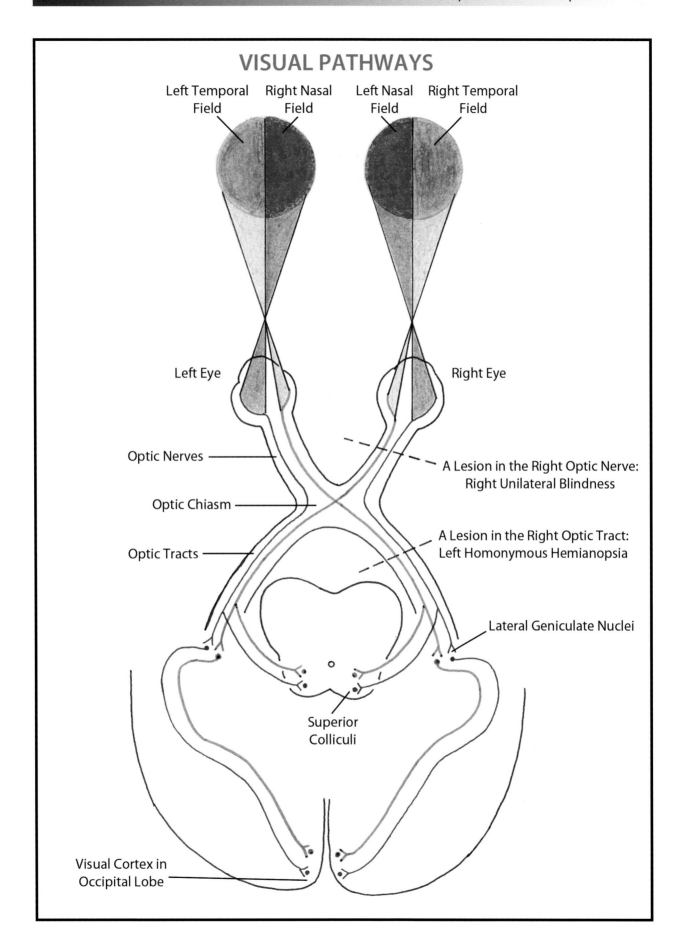

Left Temporal Field

Right Nasal Field

Left Nasal Field

Right Temporal Field

Left Eye

Right Eye

Optic Nerves

A Lesion in the Right Optic Nerve:
Right Unilateral Blindness

Optic Chiasm

Optic Tracts

A Lesion in the Right Optic Tract:
Left Homonymous Hemianopsia

Lateral Geniculate Nuclei

Superior Colliculi

Visual Cortex in Occipital Lobe

PATHOLOGY OF THE VISUAL PATHWAYS

Contralateral Homonymous Hemianopia

- A contralateral homonymous hemianopia is a loss of the visual field on the opposite side of the lesion.
- A left visual field cut, or left contralateral homonymous hemianopia, results from a lesion in the right optic tract.
- A right visual field cut, or right contralateral homonymous hemianopia, results from a lesion in the left optic tract.[14]

Bitemporal Hemianopia

- A bitemporal hemianopia occurs when the temporal fields in both eyes have been lost.
- It results from a lesion to the central optic chiasm.
- Bitemporal hemianopia results in tunnel vision.[15]

Blindness as a Result of Optic Pathway Damage

- Unilateral blindness can result from a lesion to the ipsilateral optic nerve.
- Bilateral blindness can result from a large lesion that knocks out the entire optic chiasm.[16]

A Blind Spot in the Visual Field

- A blind spot inside a visual field suggests retinal damage (not optic nerve or tract damage).[17]

AUDITION

Auditory Receptor Anatomy

Cochlea

- The cochlea is a fluid-filled structure located in the inner ear.
- It contains a structure called the *organ of Corti*.[18,19]

Organ of Corti

- The organ of Corti contains the auditory receptors, or hair cells, that are attached to the basilar membrane at the base of the organ of Corti.[18,19]

Auditory Pathway

- Sound, or *vibration*, is the stimulus for the organ of Corti.
- Sound waves travel through the external auditory meatus (the ear canal) to the tympanic membrane (the eardrum).
- When sound waves reach the tympanic membrane, the membrane vibrates and causes the ossicles to vibrate.
- The ossicles are the bones of the middle ear: the malleus (hammer), incus (anvil), and stapes (stirrup).
- The stapes presses against the oval window, causing it to vibrate.
- Cochlear vibration then causes the basilar membrane to flex back and forth.
- Pressure changes of the cochlear fluid are then transmitted to the round window.
- In response, the round window flexes back and forth in a manner opposite to the movement of the oval window.
- The hair cells of the basilar membrane begin to bend, causing a membrane potential to be generated.
- If the membrane potential is strong enough, an action potential will be propagated down CN 8, the vestibulocochlear nerve.
- The auditory message is then sent to the cochlear nucleus in the medulla. From here, fibers project to the superior olivary nucleus (medulla level), the inferior colliculus (midbrain level), and to the medial geniculate nucleus of the thalamus.
- From the thalamus, auditory fibers project to the primary auditory cortex (A1) in the temporal lobe. A1 is responsible for the detection of auditory stimuli.
- The auditory messages are then sent to the auditory association areas (A2+) for interpretation.[18,19]

AUDITORY RECEPTOR ANATOMY AND PATHWAY

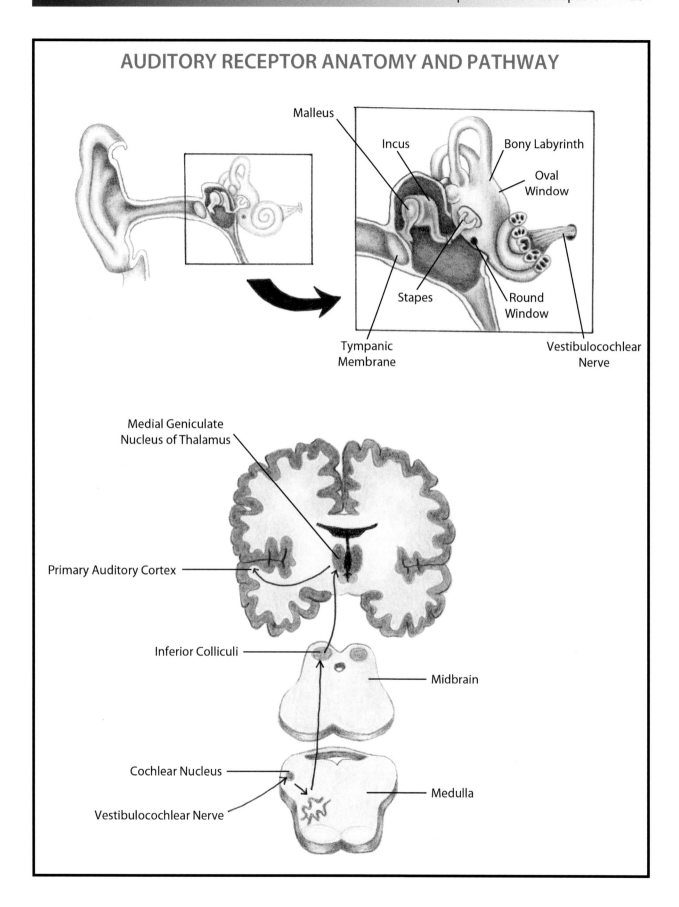

Hearing Impairment

Sensorineural

- Sensorineural hearing impairment involves damage to the inner ear, vestibulocochlear nerve, and/or the brain.[20]

Conductive

- Conductive hearing impairment involves damage to the outer and/or middle ear structures.[21]

Lesion to the Auditory Portion of the Vestibulocochlear Nerve

- This causes deafness or tinnitus.[22]

Lesion to the Primary Auditory Cortex

- This causes cortical deafness; the structures of the auditory pathway are intact, but A1 cannot detect incoming auditory stimuli.[23]

Lesion to the Auditory Association Cortices

- This may cause *auditory agnosia*, the inability to interpret sounds.[24]

EQUILIBRIUM

Equilibrium Receptor Anatomy

- The receptors of equilibrium are the hair cells of the semicircular canals, utricle, and saccule located in the inner ear.[25]

Three Semicircular Canals

- The 3 semicircular canals are as follows:
  1. Superior semicircular canal
  2. Posterior semicircular canal
  3. Horizontal semicircular canal
- The semicircular canals are a system of canals called the *bony labyrinth and* respond to movement of the head.
- Within the bony labyrinth is a membranous labyrinth.
- Both labyrinths contain fluid.
- Perilymph is the fluid located within the bony labyrinth.
- Endolymph is the fluid located within the membranous labyrinth.[25,26]

Ampulla

- Located at the end of each semicircular canal is a small enlargement called the *ampulla*.
- Each ampulla contains hair cells.[25,26]

Utricle

- The utricle is located just medially to the semicircular canals.[25,27]

Saccule

- The saccule is located just medial and inferior to the utricle.[25,27]

Together, the Utricle and Saccule Respond to the Following:
- Gravity
- Changes in head position

The Semicircular Canals Respond to the Following:
- Angular acceleration and deceleration (rotation)
- Linear acceleration and deceleration (moving forward on a bike or on skis)

POSTROTARY NYSTAGMUS

- Nystagmus is an involuntary, rapid, repetitive, jerky oscillating movement of the eyeballs in either a horizontal, vertical, or rotary direction.[28]
- Nystagmus can occur in the absence of pathology in response to the following:
  ○ Rotation
  ○ Optokinetic nystagmus (elicited by tracking a moving target across the visual field; once the object moves out of the visual field, the eyes will reflexively jerk back to fixate on a new moving target. An example is being on a train and watching sequential telephone poles pass by.)
  ○ Caloric testing (involves inserting cold or warm water into the external auditory canal, which results in a convective current in the semicircular canal endolymph)
- Nystagmus can also occur as a result of pathology:
  ○ Damage to the labyrinths of the inner ear
  ○ Vestibular nuclei damage at the pons-medulla junction
  ○ Vestibulocochlear nerve damage
  ○ Extraocular nuclei damage in the midbrain and pons
  ○ Extraocular cranial nerve damage
  ○ Cerebellar damage
- Postrotary nystagmus occurs normally after rotation. Patients with neurologic deficits will experience postrotary nystagmus for longer periods than normal after the rotation has stopped.
- The individual is rotated to the right (on a rotation board/swing).
- Fluid inside the labyrinths displaces toward the left due to the sudden rotation of the head to the right.
- This causes the hair cells to bend and become excited.
- An action potential is generated along the vestibular portion of the vestibulocochlear nerve.
- While the individual is rotating to the right, the fluid in the labyrinths eventually catches up to the labyrinths and begins to move at the same rate as the labyrinths.
- This causes the hair cells to stop firing; they are no longer being bent.
- The rotation board/swing is stopped.
- The fluid in the labyrinths now displaces to the right because the head has stopped, but the fluid has not yet stopped.
- This again bends the hair cells and causes them to become excited.
- An action potential is generated and travels along the vestibular portion of the vestibulocochlear nerve.
- The individual experiences nystagmus to the right and has a sensation of the room rotating to the right.
- If asked to point at a fixed object, the individual will overshoot it by pointing further right (past pointing to the right).
- The individual also experiences a tendency to fall to the right.[29]

Nystagmus Testing

- There are several standardized tests to assess whether nystagmus is pathological or normal.
- All tests must be done with caution, as they can induce nausea due to the connection between the vestibular system and the vagus nerve.

Postrotary Nystagmus Test (Section of the Sensory Integration and Praxis Test)

- This is a standardized test for children and adults.
- The individual sits on a rotating swing. The rotation is stopped, and the therapist examines the time length of nystagmus.
- A normal range for nystagmus to continue after rotation has stopped is 8 to 14 seconds.
- One disadvantage of this method is that the vestibular apparatus on both sides must be tested simultaneously.[30]

Caloric Testing

- Caloric testing is usually performed by physicians.
- The patient's head is elevated to 30 degrees.
- To induce nystagmus, 30 to 50 mL of warm or cold water is squirted into the external auditory canal.
- This procedure produces convection currents in the optic fluid that mimic the effects of angular acceleration.
- The advantage of caloric testing is that the vestibular apparatus on each side can be tested separately.[31]

Optokinetic Testing

- Optokinetic testing can be induced from prolonged, recurrent stimulation of the extraocular cranial nerves.
- When the head is held stationary, the human eye will track a moving target to a certain distance (usually to the point at which the target object moves out of the visual field).
- The eyes will then reflexively jerk back to fixate on a new moving target.
- Examples: The person observes a black and white rotating drum or watches telephone poles pass by while seated on a train.[32]

Electronystagmography

- Electronystagmography (ENG) is a precise and objective method of assessing nystagmus.
- The test is usually performed by physicians.
- Electrodes are placed on the canthus (angle) of each eye and above and below each eye. A ground electrode is placed on the forehead. This electrode placement accesses the extraocular eye muscles.
- The individual is rotated; the rotation is stopped.
- The ENG records the nystagmus on paper (as with electromyography).
- The velocity, frequency, and amplitude of nystagmus can be evaluated.
- Advantages of ENG are that it is easily administered, is noninvasive, and does not interfere with vision.[33]

Videonystagmography

- Videonystagmography (VNG) is similar to ENG but uses video to evaluate and measure nystagmus with small cameras located within a head mask.
- Advantages of VNG are its easy administration, noninvasiveness, and noninterference with vision.[34]

EQUILIBRIUM RECEPTOR ANATOMY

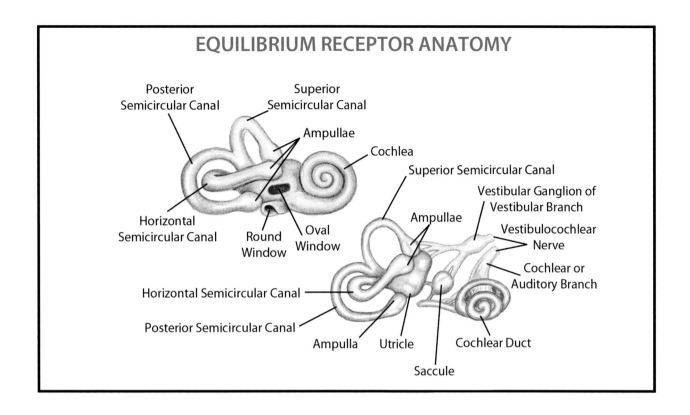

REFERENCES

1. Fleischer J, Breer H, Strotman J. Mammalian olfactory receptors. *Front Cell Neurosci.* 2009;3:45-54. doi:10.3389/neuro.03.009.2009.

2. Stevenson RJ. An initial evaluation of the functions of human olfaction. *Chem Senses.* 2010;35(1):3-20. doi:10.1093/chemse/bjp083.

3. Behrens M, Meyerhof W. Gustatory and extragustatory functions of mammalian taste receptors. *Physiol Behav.* 2011;105(1):4-13. doi:10.1016/j.physbeh.2011.02.010.

4. Small DM. Taste representation in the human insula. *Brain Struct Funct.* 2010;214(5-6):551-561. doi:10.1007/s00429-010-0266-9.

5. Toepel U, Murray MM. Human gustation: when the brain has taste. *Curr Biol.* 2015;25(9):R381-R383. doi:10.1016/j.cub.2015.03.002.

6. Reed DR. Birth of a new breed of supertaster. *Chem Senses.* 2008;33(6):489-491. doi:10.1093/chemse/bjn031.

7. Hayes JE, Keast RS. Two decades of supertasting: where do we stand? *Physiol Behav.* 2011;104(5):1072-1074. doi:10.1016/j.physbeh.2011.08.003.

8. Remington LA. *Clinical Anatomy and Physiology of the Visual System.* 3rd ed. St. Louis, MO: Butterworth-Heinemann; 2012.

9. Schiller PH, Tehovnik EJ. *Vision and the Visual System.* New York, NY: Oxford University Press; 2015.

10. Gooley JJ, Chamberlain K, Smith KA, et al. Exposure to room light before bedtime suppresses melatonin onset and shortens melatonin duration in humans. *J Clin Endocrinol Metab.* 2010;96(3):E463-E472. doi:10.1210/jc.2010-2098.

11. Lucas RJ, Peirson SN, Berson DM, et al. Measuring and using light in the melanopsin age. *Trends Neurosci.* 2014;37(1):1-9. doi:10.1016/j.tins.2013.10.004.

12. Kravitz DJ, Saleem KS, Baker CI, Ungerleider LG, Mishkin M. The ventral visual pathway: an expanded neural framework for the processing of object quality. *Trends Cogn Sci.* 2013;17(1):26-49. doi:10.1016/j.tics.2012.10.011.

13. Hall N, Colby C. S-cone visual stimuli activate superior colliculus neurons in old world monkeys: implications for understanding blindsight. *J Cogn Neurosci.* 2014;26(6):1234-1256. doi:doi:10.1162/jocn_a_00555.

14. Perez C, Chokron S. Rehabilitation of homonymous hemianopia: insight into blindsight. *Front Integr Neurosci.* 2014;8:82. doi:10.3389/fnint.2014.00082.

15. Peli E, Satgunam P. Bitemporal hemianopia; its unique binocular complexities and a novel remedy. *Ophthalmic Physiol Opt.* 2014;34(2):233-242. doi:10.1111/opo.12118.

16. Shofty B, Constantini S, Bokstein F, et al. Optic pathway gliomas in adults. *Neurosurgery.* 2014;74(3):273-280. doi:10.1227/NEU.0000000000000257.

17. Spaide RF, Koizumi H, Freund KB. Photoreceptor outer segment abnormalities as a cause of blind spot enlargement in acute zonal occult outer retinopathy–complex diseases. *Am J Ophthalmol.* 2008;146(1):111-120. doi:10.1016/j.ajo.2008.02.027.

18. Moller AR. *Hearing: Anatomy, Physiology, and Disorders of the Auditory System.* 3rd ed. San Diego, CA: Plural; 2012.

19. Fritzsch B, Knipper M, Friauf E. Auditory system: development, genetics, function, aging, and diseases. *Cell Tissue Res.* 2015;361(1):1-6. doi:10.1007/s00441-015-2218-4.

20. Schreiber BE, Agrup C, Haskard DO, Luxon LM. Sudden sensorineural hearing loss. *Lancet.* 2010;375(9721):1203-1211. doi:10.1016/S0140-6736(09)62071-7.

21. Grant JR, Arganbright J, Friedland DR. Outcomes for conservative management of traumatic conductive hearing loss. *Otol Neurotol.* 2008;29(3):344-349. doi:10.1097/MAO.0b013e3181690792.

22. Eggermont JJ, Roberts LE. The neuroscience of tinnitus: understanding abnormal and normal auditory perception. *Front Syst Neurosci.* 2012;6:53. doi:10.3389/fnsys.2012.00053.

23. Brody RM, Nicholas BD, Wolf MJ, Marcinkevich PB, Artz GJ. Cortical deafness: a case report and review of the literature. *Otol Neurotol.* 2013;34(7):1226-1229. doi:10.1097/MAO.0b013e31829763c4.

24. Suh H, Shin YI, Kim SY, et al. A case of generalized auditory agnosia with unilateral subcortical brain lesion. *Ann Rehabil Med.* 2012;36(6):866-870. doi:10.5535/arm.2012.36.6.866.

25. Goldberg JM, Wilson VJ, Cullen KE, et al. *The Vestibular System: A Sixth Sense.* New York, NY: Oxford University Press; 2012.

26. Agrawal Y, Zuniga MG, Davalos-Bichara M, et al. Decline in semicircular canal and otolith function with age. *Otol Neurotol.* 2012;33(5):832-839. doi:10.1097/MAO.0b013e3182545061.

27. Tribukait A, Rosenhall U, Österdahl B. Morphological characteristics of the human macula sacculi. *Audiol Neurotol.* 2005;10(2):90-96. doi:10.1159/000083364.

28. Strupp M, Kremmyda O, Brandt T. Pharmacotherapy of vestibular disorders and nystagmus. *Sem Neurol.* 2013;33(3): 286-296. doi:10.1055/s-0033-1354594.

29. Mulligan S. Validity of the postrotary nystagmus test for measuring vestibular function. *OTJR.* 2011;31(2):97-104. doi:10.3928/15394492-20100823-02.

30. Ayres AJ. *Sensory Integration and Praxis Test (SIPT).* Los Angeles, CA: Western Psychological Services; 1989.

31. Rohrmeier C, Richter O, Schneider M, et al. Triple test as predictive screen for unilateral weakness on caloric testing in routine practice. *Otol Neurotol.* 2013;34(2):297-303. doi:10.1097/MAO.0b013e31827d0901.

32. Papanagnu E, Brodsky MC. Is there a role for optokinetic nystagmus testing in contemporary orthoptic practice? Old tricks and new perspectives. *Am Orthopt J.* 2014;64(1):1-10. doi:10.3368/aoj.64.1.1.

33. Szirmai A, Keller B. Electronystagmographic analysis of caloric test parameters in vestibular disorders. *Eur Arch Otorhinolaryngol.* 2013;270(1):87-91. doi:10.1007/s00405-012-1939-1.

34. Miłoński J, Pietkiewicz P, Bielińska M, Kuśmierczyk K, Olszewski J. The use of videonystagmography head impulse test (VHIT) in the diagnostics of semicircular canal injuries in patients with vertigo. *Int J Occup Med Environ Health.* 2014;27(4):583-590. doi:10.2478/s13382-014-0278-4.

CLINICAL TEST QUESTIONS

Sections 9 to 11

1. Mr. Weinholtz has seen his physician for an upper respiratory infection. He becomes dizzy upon standing and lists to his right side when attempting to walk. Which special sense receptors may have been affected?
    1. visual receptors (rods and cones of the retina)
    2. auditory receptors (hair cells of the cochlea)
    3. equilibrium receptors (semicircular canals, utricles, and saccules of the inner ear)
    4. cutaneous receptors
    5. proprioceptors
    6. visceral receptors
    a. 1, 4
    b. 2, 5
    c. 3, 5
    d. 3, 6

2. Ms. Chaudhari has a neurological disorder caused by demyelination of neurons in the CNS. The disease process is characterized by periods of exacerbation and remission over many years. Sensory symptoms include numbness, paresthesias, and causalgia. Motor symptoms include abnormal gait, bladder and sexual dysfunction, vertigo, and fatigue. This disease is known as:
    a. amyotrophic lateral sclerosis
    b. multiple sclerosis
    c. myasthenia gravis
    d. muscular dystrophy

3. Mr. Greenspan was diagnosed with a severe degenerative neurological disorder affecting both the central and peripheral nervous systems. Upper and lower motor neurons denervate, resulting in muscle atrophy, spasticity (of upper motor neurons), and flaccidity (of lower motor neurons). In advanced stages of the disease, a wider spread of muscle weakness in the throat, neck, head, and shoulders occurs. Death commonly follows denervation of the respiratory muscles. This disease is known as:
    a. amyotrophic lateral sclerosis
    b. multiple sclerosis
    c. myasthenia gravis
    d. muscular dystrophy

4. Ms. Lee was diagnosed with a chronic autoimmune disorder affecting the neuromuscular junction of voluntary muscles. In this disease, acetylcholine receptor antibodies destroy acetylcholine receptors at the neuromuscular junction, resulting in severe muscular weakness and fatigue. The disease first affects the eye and head musculature and then progresses to the limbs and respiratory muscles. This disease is known as:
    a. amyotrophic lateral sclerosis
    b. multiple sclerosis
    c. myasthenia gravis
    d. muscular dystrophy

5. After 5 years of taking a cholinergic drug to reduce the symptoms of schizophrenia, Frank has developed tardive dyskinesia, a condition causing muscular spasms and involuntary motor movements such as lip smacking, tongue protrusion, head snapping, and jerking of the arms and legs. This disorder results from:
    a. an increased effect of acetylcholine (ACh) at the neuromuscular junction due to long-term cholinergic drug use
    b. blockage of acetylcholine at the neuromuscular junction causing neurotransmitter fatigue and resulting in skeletal paralysis
    c. anoxia, or lack of oxygen, at the neuromuscular junction resulting in failed synaptic transmission and muscle weakness
    d. denervation of the ACh receptors causing muscle atrophy and weakness

6. Ms. Mendoza was diagnosed with a tumor in her right optic tract. Her occupational therapist has detected a contralateral homonymous hemianopia causing:
   a. a right visual field cut
   b. a left visual field cut
   c. complete blindness
   d. tunnel vision

7. Mr. Takahashi was diagnosed with tunnel vision, in which the temporal fields in both eyes have been lost. This condition results from:
   a. a lesion to the right optic tract
   b. a lesion to the left optic tract
   c. a lesion to the lateral regions of the optic chiasm
   d. a lesion to the central region of the optic chiasm

8. Ms. Vaccarino has intact auditory anatomy of the outer, middle, and inner ear. However, she cannot accurately interpret sounds. For example, when she heard a door close in the clinic setting, she asked if someone fell. This condition likely results from _____ and is called _____.
   1. a lesion to the primary auditory area (A1)
   2. a lesion to the auditory association areas
   3. auditory agnosia
   4. auditory hemianopia
   a. 1, 3
   b. 1, 4
   c. 2, 3
   d. 2, 4

9. If Ms. Vaccarino, in the above question, could not hear despite intact outer, middle, and inner ear structures, her therapist might suspect pathology in the _____. This is referred to as a _____ hearing impairment.
   1. primary auditory area
   2. auditory association areas
   3. sensorineural
   4. conductive
   a. 1, 3
   b. 1, 4
   c. 2, 3
   d. 2, 4

10. Ms. Maniadakis is being tested for the presence of abnormal nystagmus. Which of the following is not used to assess nystagmus?
    a. caloric testing
    b. electroencephalography
    c. optokinetic testing
    d. videonystagmography

Answers

1. c
2. b
3. a
4. c
5. a
6. b
7. d
8. c
9. a
10. b

Vestibular System

FUNCTION OF THE VESTIBULAR SYSTEM

- The vestibular system functions to maintain our equilibrium and balance and our head in an upright vertical position.
- The system has a role in the coordination of head and eye movements through the vestibulo-ocular reflex.
- The system also influences tone through the alpha and gamma motor neurons and the medial and lateral vestibulospinal tracts.
- The vestibular, visual, and proprioceptive systems work collaboratively to maintain an understanding of the body's position in space. When one of these systems becomes compromised, the others are used to compensate.
- When the vestibular system is impaired, patients rely more heavily on their proprioceptive and visual systems to maintain an awareness of their body's position in space.
- Disorders causing a progressive loss of vestibular function (from a degenerative disorder) may go unnoticed by the patient as the person grows increasingly reliant upon the visual and proprioceptive systems.
- Patients will experience difficulty, however, on uneven ground surfaces (such as sand) or in dim light, when visual and proprioceptive cues cannot be accurately used.[1]

VESTIBULAR SYSTEM INPUT

- The vestibular system receives sensory input from the following neural areas[2]:
  - Vestibulocochlear nerve (CN 8)
  - Vestibular nuclei in the pons-medulla junction
  - Vestibular apparatus in the inner ear (semicircular canals, utricle, and saccule)
  - Cerebellum
  - Extraocular cranial nerves and nuclei

VESTIBULAR PATHWAY

- The vestibular nuclei in the pons-medulla junction receive vestibular information about balance and equilibrium from the following:
  - Vestibular apparatus in the inner ear
  - Extraocular nuclei in the midbrain and pons
  - Cerebellum

Gutman SA. *Quick Reference Neuroscience for Rehabilitation Professionals:*
The Essential Neurologic Principles Underlying Rehabilitation Practice,
Third Edition (pp 134-139).
© 2017 Taylor & Francis Group.

- The vestibular nuclei send the information they receive to the alpha and gamma motor neurons in the ventral horn of the spinal cord.
- This information is sent via the vestibulospinal tracts.
- The motor neurons in the ventral horn synapse with spinal nerves in the periphery.
- The spinal nerves in the periphery project to antigravity muscles, the muscles that maintain the body's upright position against gravity. These are the extensors in the legs, trunk, and back.
- The muscle spindles, Golgi tendon organs, and joint receptors then send information about the body's position in space back to the cerebellum in a feedback loop.
- The cerebellum uses this information to make ongoing decisions about the modification of muscular activity in order to enhance balance.
- There are also motor neurons in the ventral horn that project to the head and neck musculature via the medial longitudinal fasciculus.
- These structures mediate the head righting and tonic neck reflexes, which remain present throughout the lifespan to maintain the head in an upright position.
- Eye and head movements are also integrated by the medial longitudinal fasciculus.
- This tract allows feedback about the head's position to be continuously sent back to the extraocular nuclei in the midbrain and pons.[1,3]

RELATIONSHIP BETWEEN THE RETICULAR FORMATION AND THE VESTIBULAR SYSTEM

- The reticular formation is diffusely located in the brainstem and is composed of the reticular activating and inhibiting systems.
- The reticular activating system screens sensory information to alert the brain to attend to important incoming sensory data. It also responds to excitatory vestibular stimulation by arousing the brain and body.
- The reticular inhibiting system acts as a mechanism to calm the brain/body in response to inhibitory sensory information.
- The reticular formation in the brainstem integrates information from the vestibular system via the medial longitudinal fasciculus tract and the vestibulospinal tracts.
- Vestibular sensory data, such as slow rocking, are integrated by the reticular formation and calm the individual.
- Excitatory vestibular sensory data, such as fast dancing, spinning (rotary acceleration), and roller coasters (linear acceleration), are integrated by the reticular formation and arouse the brain/body.
- Children seek this kind of inhibitory and excitatory vestibular sensation to facilitate the development and organization of their nervous systems.
- The need for intense vestibular stimulation decreases as humans age. Often, adults cannot tolerate the same kind of intense vestibular stimulation they craved as children and adolescents.[4]

RELATIONSHIP BETWEEN THE AUTONOMIC NERVOUS SYSTEM AND THE VESTIBULAR SYSTEM

- The autonomic nervous system (ANS) mediates cranial nerve (CN) 10, the vagus nerve.
- The visceral branches of the vagus nerve conduct signals to and from the gastrointestinal tract.
- Because the vagus nerve has connections to the vestibular pathways, these connections may explain why overexcitation of the vestibular system can induce nausea and vomiting.[5]

Two Categories of Vestibular Dysfunction

Peripheral Nervous System

- Peripheral nervous system dysfunction of the vestibular system involves the vestibular apparatus in the inner ear[6]:
  - Semicircular canals
  - Utricle
  - Saccule

Central Nervous System

- Central nervous system (CNS) dysfunction of the vestibular system involves the vestibular pathways and structures of the CNS[7]:
  - Vestibulocochlear nerve
  - Vestibular nuclei in the pons-medulla junction
  - Cerebellum
  - Extraocular cranial nerve nuclei

Signs and Symptoms of Vestibular Impairment

- Nystagmus
- Tinnitus
- Vertigo
- Hearing loss
- Loss of balance and possible falls
- Broad-based stance (to accommodate for imbalance)
- Sweating, nausea, and vomiting (due to ANS involvement)

Motion Sickness: Disorder of the Vestibular System

- Motion sickness is a disorder of the vestibular system that is caused by repeated rhythmic stimulation (eg, car, plane, or boat travel).
- Symptoms include vertigo, nausea, vomiting, lowered blood pressure, tachycardia, and sweating.
- Pooling of blood in the lower extremities commonly leads to postural hypotension and fainting.
- Motion sickness can sometimes be alleviated by obtaining a match between visual and motion signals reaching the vestibular system.
- For example, observing the upcoming traffic conditions in a car, rather than reading a book, can suppress feelings of motion sickness.
- Motion sickness usually decreases in severity with repeated exposure.
- Anti-motion sickness drugs suppress the activity of the vestibular system.[8]

Romberg Test

- The Romberg test is used to assess disequilibrium.
- The patient is asked to stand with his or her feet together and shoulders flexed to 90 degrees (and positioned in front of the patient).
- The patient is then asked to close his or her eyes. When visual cues are removed, the patient's postural stability is based on vestibular and proprioceptive information.
- The therapist observes the patient's degree of postural sway, balance, and arm stability.
- Impaired vestibular function is indicated by postural sway and a tendency for the arms to drift toward the affected side.
- If the vestibular system is severely impaired, the patient will fall toward the affected side.[9]

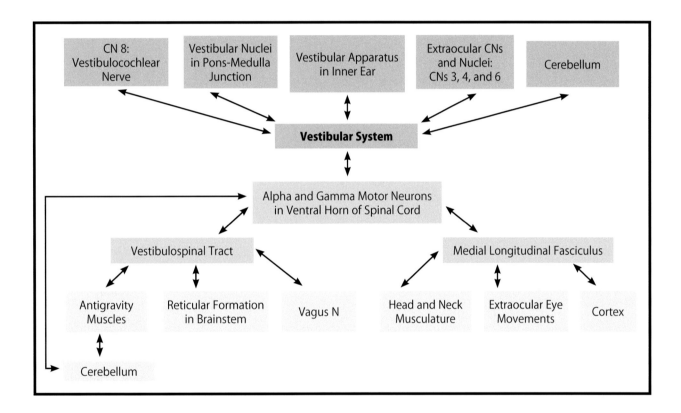

Vestibulo-Ocular Reflex

The vestibulo-ocular reflex is an eye movement reflex that maintains stable images on the retina despite head movement. When the head moves, the reflex becomes activated and produces an eye movement in the opposite direction from that of the head. When the head moves in one direction, the eyes will reflexively move in the opposite direction. Impairment of the vestibulo-ocular reflex can result in difficulty reading during movement (eg, reading street signs or smartphone information while walking) because such patients cannot stabilize eye movement while the head moves. The vestibulo-ocular reflex can be tested by rapidly moving a patient's head to one side. This is called the *rapid head impulse test* (also *Halmagyi-Curthoys test*). Normally, the patient's eyes will move in the opposite direction of the head's movement. Impairment of the reflex is indicated by the patient's inability to reposition the eyes in the opposite direction during passively forced head movement. The reflex functions in light or total darkness and when the eyes are open or closed.[10]

REFERENCES

1. Dieterich M, Brandt T. The bilateral central vestibular system: its pathways, functions, and disorders. *Ann NY Acad Sci.* 2015;1343(1):10-26. doi:10.1111/nyas.12585.

2. Cullen KE. The vestibular system: multimodal integration and encoding of self-motion for motor control. *Trends Neurosci.* 2012;35(3):185-196. doi:10.1016/j.tins.2011.12.001.

3. Sadeghi SG, Minor LB, Cullen KE. Neural correlates of sensory substitution in vestibular pathways following complete vestibular loss. *J Neurosci.* 2012;32(42):14685-14695. doi:10.1523/JNEUROSCI.2493-12.2012.

4. Steinbacher BC, Yates BJ. Processing of vestibular and other inputs by the caudal ventrolateral medullary reticular formation. *Am J Physiol Regul Integr Comp Physiol.* 1996;271(4):R1070-R1077.

5. Yates BJ, Bronstein AM. The effects of vestibular system lesions on autonomic regulation: observations, mechanisms, and clinical implications. *J Vestib Res.* 2005;15(3):119-130.

6. Agrawal Y, Bremova T, Kremmyda O, Strupp M. Semicircular canal, saccular and utricular function in patients with bilateral vestibulopathy: analysis based on etiology. *J Neurol.* 2013;260(3):876-883. doi:10.1007/s00415-012-6724-y.

7. De Foer B, Kenis C, Van Melkebeke D, et al. Pathology of the vestibulocochlear nerve. *Eur J Radiol.* 2010;74(2):349-358. doi:10.1016/j.ejrad.2009.06.033.

8. Oman CM, Cullen KE. Brainstem processing of vestibular sensory exafference: implications for motion sickness etiology. *Exper Brain Res.* 2014;232(8):2483-2492. doi:10.1007/s00221-014-3973-2.

9. Agrawal Y, Carey JP, Hoffman, HJ, Sklare DA, Schubert MC. The modified Romberg balance test: normative data in US adults. *Otol Neurotol.* 2011;32(8):1309-1311. doi:10.1097/MAO.0b013e31822e5bee.

10. Welgampola MS, Migliaccio AA, Myrie OA, Minor LB, Carey JP. The human sound-evoked vestibulo-ocular reflex and its electromyographic correlate. *Clin Neurophysiol.* 2009;120(1):158-166. doi:10.1016/j.clinph.2008.06.020.

SECTION 13

Autonomic Nervous System

FUNCTION OF THE AUTONOMIC NERVOUS SYSTEM

- The autonomic nervous system (ANS) is a subdivision of the peripheral nervous system that independently regulates critical life body functions without the need for cortical input.[1]
- The ANS does the following:
  - Innervates the internal organs, blood vessels, and glands
  - Regulates cardiac and smooth muscle (muscle of glands and organs)
  - Regulates secretion from glands
  - Controls vegetative functions (functions that allow the body to continue functioning despite severe brain damage):
    - Temperature
    - Digestion
    - Heart rate
    - Respiration
    - Metabolism
    - Maintenance of internal organ homeostasis
    - Blood pressure
- Influences muscle tone through the vestibulospinal, rubrospinal, and reticulospinal tracts

CENTRAL COMPONENTS OF AUTONOMIC NERVOUS SYSTEM

- The central portion of the ANS consists of parts of the cerebral cortex, hypothalamus, thalamus, limbic system, cerebellum, and spinal cord.
- Efferent fibers that originate in the cortex project descending fibers through the thalamus and hypothalamus.
- These fibers end on a cranial nerve nuclei to influence involuntary muscles, vessels, and glands.[2]

Anterior and Posterior Hypothalamus

- The hypothalamus is a major control center of the ANS and regulates temperature, thirst, feeding behaviors, and endocrine functions (eg, the secretion of glands).
- The anterior hypothalamus projects pathways to the parasympathetic nervous system.
- The posterior hypothalamus projects pathways to the sympathetic nervous system.
- The hypothalamus exerts autonomic regulation over various brainstem centers that control vegetative functions (ie, life-sustaining functions such as cardiovascular and respiratory functions).[3]

Brainstem Centers: The Reticular Formation

- The reticular formation consists of interconnected neurons that are diffusely located throughout the midbrain, pons, and medulla.
- The reticular formation sends and receives projections to and from the diencephalon, cortex, and spinal cord.
- This brain center is an evolutionarily old part of the nervous system and is involved in the control of posture, visceral motor function, sleep, and arousal/wakefulness.

Gutman SA. *Quick Reference Neuroscience for Rehabilitation Professionals: The Essential Neurologic Principles Underlying Rehabilitation Practice, Third Edition* (pp 140-146).
© 2017 Taylor & Francis Group.

- The brains of primitive vertebrates are made up primarily of a reticular-type formation designed for survival functions.
- There are respiratory and cardiovascular centers in the reticular formation that control vital functions and reflexes such as the gag, cough, sneeze, swallow, and vomit reflexes.
- Severe injury to the brainstem often results in death or poor prognosis.
- If the brainstem remains intact but the cortex is no longer active, patients can still survive but are considered to be in a persistent vegetative state (because the brainstem controls vegetative functions).[4]
- The reticular formation also receives sensory fibers from the somatic and visceral systems (including vision and olfaction). This sensory information is then relayed to the thalamus and cortex for CNS regulation.
- The reticular formation's motor fibers synapse with (a) motor neurons of the pyramidal and extrapyramidal systems and (b) motor neurons that synapse with preganglionic autonomic motor neurons.
- The reticulospinal tracts (descending extrapyramidal tracts of the spinal cord that inhibit and facilitate antigravity muscles and thereby influence muscle tone) originate in the reticular formation.[5]

Reticular Activating System

- The reticular activating system (RAS) is the portion of the reticular formation that is responsible for arousal, alertness, and wakefulness.
- It filters all incoming sensory information and alerts the cortex to attend to important sensory input.
- This results in a sharpening of attention to important sensory information from the environment.
- The RAS is diffusely located throughout the brainstem but is believed to be primarily located in the midbrain, with connections to the thalamus and hypothalamus.[6]

Lesions to the Reticular Activating System

- Disorders of the RAS can result in disrupted sleep-wake cycles and attentional problems (eg, severe inability to focus and concentrate, impulsivity).
- Significant lesions to the RAS can result in stuporous states of consciousness. When the RAS is lost, the reticular inhibitory system may become dominant and produce heightened somnolence.[7]

Reticular Inhibitory System

- The reticular inhibitory system (RIS) is involved in producing calming states and sleep. Certain types of sensory input, such as slow rocking or deep pressure, can activate the RIS to calm the body.
- The counterpart system to the RAS, the RIS is considered to be diffusely located in the midbrain and medulla, with connections to the thalamus and hypothalamus.[8]

Lesions to the Reticular Inhibitory System

- Lesions to the RIS can result in constant wakefulness and vigilance. When the RIS is damaged, the RAS may become dominant and cause heightened arousal.[9]

Limbic Lobe

- The limbic lobe has a role in the relationship between our emotions and the ANS.
- Heightened emotional states can cause the sympathetic nervous system to become activated and dampen parasympathetic nervous system activity.
- When humans are agitated or nervous, they may experience loss of appetite because the sympathetic nervous system is geared up and has shut down the digestive system (regulated by the parasympathetic nervous system).
- When humans or animals are frightened, loss of bladder control can occur; fear can interfere with ANS regulation.
- When individuals are in great pain, nausea may occur as a result of the connections between the ANS, the vagus nerve, and the limbic lobe.
- Similarly, blushing, heart palpitations, clammy hands, and dry mouth are emotional responses that are mediated by limbic system structures and the ANS.[10]

Spinal Cord

- The spinal cord contains important ANS reflexes that are modulated by higher CNS centers.
- When there is lost communication between spinal cord reflexes and higher CNS centers, as in spinal cord injury, such reflexes function in an unmodified manner.
- For example, uncontrolled sweating, vasomotor instability, and reflex bowel and bladder functions occur when regulation of ANS spinal cord level reflexes are lost.[11]

PERIPHERAL COMPONENTS OF THE AUTONOMIC NERVOUS SYSTEM

- The peripheral components of the ANS consist of pre- and postganglionic fibers that innervate the viscera.

Preganglionic Fibers

- Preganglionic fibers are a collection of neurons in the peripheral nervous system.
- They are also called *presynaptic neurons* (or *first order neurons*).
- Preganglionic fibers have their cell bodies in the brainstem (cranial nerves [CN] 3, 7, 9, 10, 11) and spinal cord (in the intermediolateral horn of the thoracic sections and first 2 lumbar sections).[12]

Postganglionic Fibers

- Postganglionic fibers are also called *postsynaptic* (or *second order neurons*).
- These ganglionic fibers are located in the periphery.
- Their cell bodies are located in the autonomic ganglia (groups of ANS organs and tissues).[12]

Sympathetic Nervous System

- The sympathetic nervous system's preganglionic neurons have their cell bodies located in the intermediolateral horn of the thoracic and first 2 lumbar sections of the spinal cord.[13]

Parasympathetic Nervous System

- The parasympathetic nervous system's preganglionic fibers emerge from the brainstem and sacral spinal cord.[13]

SYMPATHETIC NERVOUS SYSTEM

Function

- The sympathetic nervous system activates the fight/flight response. This response occurs during situations of stress and involves the following[14-16]:
  - Accelerated heart rate
  - Increased blood pressure
  - Shift of blood flow from the skin and gastrointestinal (GI) tract to the skeletal muscles and brain
  - Increased blood sugar level
  - Dilation of the bronchioles and pupils
  - Constriction of the stomach, intestine, and internal sphincter of the urethra

Location of Cell Bodies

- The sympathetic nervous system is also called the *thoracolumbar division* because its preganglionic neurons have their cell bodies located in the intermediolateral horn of the thoracic and first 2 lumbar sections of the spinal cord.[14-16]

Sympathetic Chain Ganglia

- The sympathetic chain ganglia are a series of interconnected sympathetic ganglia that lie adjacent to the vertebral column (on both sides).
- The chain ganglia receive input from the preganglionic sympathetic fibers.
- The chain ganglia project postganglionic sympathetic fibers to specific target organs and tissues.[14-16]

Preganglionic Sympathetic Fibers

- Preganglionic sympathetic fibers extend from their cell bodies (in the intermediolateral horn of T1-L2) to the chain ganglia.[14-16]

Postganglionic Sympathetic Fibers

- Postganglionic sympathetic fibers extend from the chain ganglia to (1 of 3) collateral ganglia (located outside the chain).
- A collateral ganglion is a collection of cell bodies located outside the sympathetic chain ganglia.
- There are 3 main collateral ganglia in the body (3 on each side of the vertebral column):
  1. Celiac ganglion
  2. Superior mesenteric ganglion
  3. Inferior mesenteric ganglion

- The postganglionic sympathetic fibers ascend or descend through the chain ganglia before synapsing on 1 of the collateral ganglia.
- After synapsing on one of the collateral ganglia, the postganglionic sympathetic fibers project to a target or end organ.[14-16]

Neurotransmitters of the Sympathetic Division

- The preganglionic fibers use acetylcholine (ACh).
- The postganglionic fibers use norepinephrine (noradrenalin).[14-16]

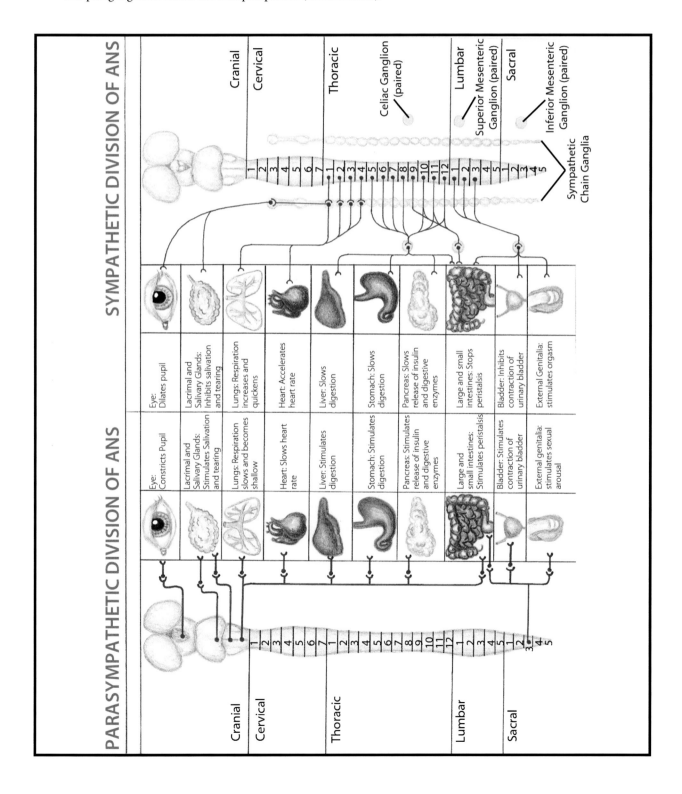

PARASYMPATHETIC NERVOUS SYSTEM

Function

- The parasympathetic nervous system is responsible for energy conservation, storage, and replenishment.
- This subdivision of the ANS maintains heart rate, respiration, metabolism, and digestion in a state of homeostasis.[14-16]

Location of Cell Bodies

- The parasympathetic nervous system is also called the *craniosacral division* because its cell bodies are located in the brainstem and sacral spinal cord.[14-16]

Preganglionic Parasympathetic Fibers

- The preganglionic parasympathetic fibers extend directly from their cell bodies to the terminal ganglia located within or very near the organs that they supply.[14-16]

Postganglionic Parasympathetic Fibers

- The postganglionic parasympathetic fibers are short in length. They extend from the terminal ganglia to the target end organ.[14-16]

Neurotransmitters of the Parasympathetic Division

- Both the pre- and postganglionic fibers use ACh.[14-16]

COMPARISON OF THE PARASYMPATHETIC AND SYMPATHETIC NERVOUS SYSTEMS

Function

- The sympathetic nervous system activates the fight/flight response and prepares the body for action.
- The parasympathetic nervous system regulates homeostasis and slows the body down.[14-16]

Cell Bodies

- Sympathetic nervous system cell bodies are located in the intermediolateral horn of the thoracic and first 2 lumbar segments of the spinal cord.
- Parasympathetic nervous system cell bodies are located in the brainstem and sacral sections of the spinal cord.[14-16]

Pathways

- Preganglionic sympathetic fibers extend from their cell bodies to the sympathetic chain ganglia. Postganglionic sympathetic fibers then travel from the chain ganglia to a collateral ganglion and finally synapse on a target organ.
- Preganglionic parasympathetic fibers extend from their cell bodies to a terminal ganglion. Postganglionic parasympathetic fibers then travel from the terminal ganglia to the target organ.[14-16]

Neurotransmitters

- Preganglionic sympathetic fibers use ACh. Pre- and postganglionic parasympathetic fibers use ACh.
- Postganglionic sympathetic fibers use norepinephrine (noradrenalin).[14-16]

AUTONOMIC NERVOUS SYSTEM AND DISEASE/ILLNESS

Stress, Illness, and Disease

- Studies have shown that individuals with chronic stress are more prone to disease, illness, and physical and mental health disorders.
- Stress activates the sympathetic nervous system, causing increased release of norepinephrine, epinephrine (adrenaline), and corticosteroids (stress hormones).
- Chronic activation of the sympathetic nervous system can cause blood vessel constriction, increased heart rate, heightened cholesterol production, and hypertension.
- Continued overactivation of the sympathetic nervous system has been linked to cardiovascular disease, immune suppression, depression, anxiety, inflammatory responses, sleep disturbances, and pain.[17,18]

Stress and Healing

- Stress promotes sympathetic nervous system activity and decreased cellular repair.
- Parasympathetic nervous system activity promotes homeostasis and facilitates cellular repair and tissue restoration.

Autonomic Neuropathy
- Autonomic neuropathy is an ANS disorder that affects involuntary body functions such as heart rate, blood pressure, and sweating.
- Autonomic nerve damage disrupts messages sent between the brain and ANS.
- Signs and symptoms vary depending on which structures of the ANS are involved but may include the following:
  - Orthostatic hypotension
  - Urinary and bowel incontinence
  - Gastrointestinal disorders
  - Inability to regulate temperature
  - Decreased pupillary response
- Causes can be related to a large number of diseases affecting the ANS including autoimmune diseases, nerve injury, diabetes, and some infectious diseases.[19]

Horner Syndrome
- Horner syndrome is an ANS disorder that results from a transection of the oculomotor sympathetic pathway (CN 3).
- Symptoms of Horner syndrome are ipsilateral and include the following[20]:
  - Ipsilateral miosis (constriction of the pupil)
  - Partial ptosis (drooping of the ipsilateral eyelid)
  - Flushed dry skin on the ipsilateral face
  - Ipsilateral sunken eyeball

- Parasympathetic nervous system activity is heightened during restorative sleep, or stage 4 sleep.
- Some research has linked illnesses such as chronic fatigue syndrome and fibromyalgia to deficiencies of stage 4 restorative sleep.[21]

Denervation
- Denervation is an interruption of neuronal innervation in which the injured neuron experiences hypersensitivity to its own neurotransmitter.
- Denervation can result in dysregulation of the ANS.[22]

AUTONOMIC NERVOUS SYSTEM CHARACTERISTICS

Sympathetic
- Activated in short bursts when an individual is stressed, angry, frightened, or excited. May be activated continuously if an individual has chronic stress.
- Fight/flight response
- Pupils dilate
- Increased vigilance of event/environment
- Heart rate increases
- Blood pressure increases
- Respiration increases and quickens
- Vasoconstriction of arteries to bring blood to heart faster
- Saliva thickens
- Blood is diverted away from the GI tract and shifts to skeletal muscles and brain
- Digestive juices stop production
- Peristalsis stops
- Activation of all muscle groups
- Cell destruction
- Body temperature changes

Parasympathetic
- Activated continuously to maintain homeostasis of body systems. Will shut down when sympathetic nervous system takes over.
- Homeostasis
- Pupils contract
- Decreased vigilance of environment
- Heart rate slows
- Blood pressure decreases
- Respiration slows and becomes shallow
- Vasodilation of arteries
- Saliva thins
- Blood returns to viscera in GI tract
- Digestive juices begin to be secreted again
- Peristalsis is continuous unless sympathetic nervous system shuts parasympathetic nervous system down
- Relaxation of most muscle groups
- Cell repair
- Body temperature is maintained at a constant level (98.6°F)

REFERENCES

1. Mathias CJ, Bannister R, eds. *Autonomic Failure: A Textbook of Clinical Disorders of the Autonomic Nervous System.* 5th ed. Oxford, UK: Oxford University Press; 2013.

2. Cechetto DF. Cortical control of the autonomic nervous system. *Exper Physiol.* 2014;99(2):326-331. doi:10.1113/expphysiol.2013.075192.

3. Kalsbeek A, Bruinstroop E, Yi CX, Klieverik LP, La Fleur SE, Fliers E. Hypothalamic control of energy metabolism via the autonomic nervous system. *Ann N Y Acad Sci.* 2010;1212(1):114-129.

4. Brisson CD, Hsieh YT, Kim D, Jin AY, Andrew RD. Brainstem neurons survive the identical ischemic stress that kills higher neurons: insight to the persistent vegetative state. *PLoS One.* 2014;9(5):e96585. doi:10.1371/journal.pone.0096585.

5. Yeo SS, Chang PH, Jang SH. The ascending reticular activating system from pontine reticular formation to the thalamus in the human brain. *Front Hum Neurosci.* 2013;7:416. doi:10.3389/fnhum.2013.00416.

6. Jang SH, Kwon HG. The ascending reticular activating system from pontine reticular formation to the hypothalamus in the human brain: a diffusion tensor imaging study. *Neurosci Lett.* 2015;590:58-61. doi:10.1016/j.neulet.2015.01.071.

7. Jang SH, Kim SH, Lim HW, Yeo SS. Injury of the lower ascending reticular activating system in patients with hypoxic–ischemic brain injury: diffusion tensor imaging study. *Neuroradiology.* 2014;56(11):965-970. doi:10.1007/s00234-014-1419-y.

8. Clément O, Garcia SV, Libourel PA, Arthaud S, Fort P, Luppi PH. The Inhibition of the dorsal paragigantocellular reticular nucleus induces waking and the activation of all adrenergic and noradrenergic neurons: a combined pharmacological and functional neuroanatomical study. *PLoS One.* 2014;9(5):e96851. doi:10.1371/journal.pone.0096851.

9. Brevig HN, Watson CJ, Lydic R, Baghdoyan HA. Hypocretin and GABA interact in the pontine reticular formation to increase wakefulness. *Sleep.* 2010;33(10):1285-1293.

10. Levenson RW. The autonomic nervous system and emotion. *Emot Rev.* 2014;6(2):100-112. doi:10.1177/1754073913512003.

11. Krassioukov A. Autonomic function following cervical spinal cord injury. *Respir Physiol Neurobiol.* 2009;169(2):157-164. doi:10.1016/j.resp.2009.08.003.

12. McCorry LK. Physiology of the autonomic nervous system. *Am J Pharm Educ.* 2007;71(4):78.

13. Sohn JW, Harris LE, Berglund ED, et al. Melanocortin 4 receptors reciprocally regulate sympathetic and parasympathetic preganglionic neurons. *Cell.* 2013;152(3):612-619. doi:10.1016/j.cell.2012.12.022.

14. Benarroch EE. Central autonomic network. In: Low PA, Benarroch EE, eds. *Clinical Autonomic Disorders.* 3rd ed. Philadelphia, PA: Lippincott, Williams, and Wilkins; 2008:17-28.

15. Hamill RW, Shapiro RE, Vizzard MA. Peripheral autonomic nervous system. In: Robertson D, Biaggioni I, Burnstock G, Low PA, Pain JFR, eds. *Primer on the Autonomic Nervous System.* 3rd ed. London, UK: Academic Press; 2012:17-37.

16. Janig W, McLachlan EM. Neurobiology of the autonomic nervous system. In: Mathias CJ, Bannister R, eds. *Autonomic Failure: A Textbook of Clinical Disorders of the Autonomic Nervous System.* 5th ed. Oxford, UK: Oxford University Press; 2013:21-34.

17. Malpas SC. Sympathetic nervous system overactivity and its role in the development of cardiovascular disease. *Physiol Rev.* 2010;90(2):513-557. doi:10.1152/physrev.00007.2009.

18. Dragomir AI, Gentile C, Nolan RP, D'Antono B. Three-year stability of cardiovascular and autonomic nervous system responses to psychological stress. *Psychophysiology.* 2014;51(9):921-931. doi:10.1111/psyp.12231.

19. Koike H, Hashimoto R, Tomita M, et al. The spectrum of clinicopathological features in pure autonomic neuropathy. *J Neurol.* 2012;259(10):2067-2075. doi:10.1007/s00415-012-6458-x.

20. Trobe JD. The evaluation of Horner syndrome. *J Neuroophthalmol.* 2010;30(1):1-2. doi:10.1097/WNO.0b013e3181ce8145.

21. Pejovic S, Natelson BH, Basta M, Fernandez-Mendoza J, Mahr F, Vgontzas AN. Chronic fatigue syndrome and fibromyalgia in diagnosed sleep disorders: a further test of the "unitary" hypothesis. *BMC Neurol.* 2015;15(1):53. doi:10.1186/s12883-015-0308-2.

22. Richa FC. Autonomic hyperreflexia after spinal cord injury. *J Spine.* 2014;4(196):2.

Enteric Nervous System

- The enteric nervous system (ENS) is an independent circuit of ganglionic cells that regulate gastrointestinal (GI) system function, including GI motility, GI fluid exchange and blood flow, and gastric and pancreatic secretion.
- The ENS is loosely connected to the central nervous system (CNS) but can function independently without CNS instruction.[1]

LOCATION

- The ENS is located in sheaths of tissue that line the esophagus, stomach, small intestine, and colon.[2]

COMPOSITION

- The structure of the ENS consists of a network of neurons, neurotransmitters, and proteins. It contains approximately 400 million neurons, one-thousandth the number of neurons in the brain, and one-tenth the number of neurons in the spinal cord (SC).[3]

CHEMICAL SUBSTANCES IN THE BRAIN AND ENTERIC NERVOUS SYSTEM

- Every chemical substance that helps to control the brain has been found in the intestines, including the following[4]:
  - Major neurotransmitters such as serotonin, dopamine, glutamate, norepinephrine, acetylcholine, and nitric oxide
  - Two dozen small brain proteins called *neuropeptides*
  - *Mast cells*: cells of the immune system
  - *Enkephalins*: one class of the body's natural opiates
  - *Benzodiazepines*: the family of psychoactive chemicals that include Valium (diazepam) and Xanax (alprazolam)

DEVELOPMENT OF THE ENTERIC NERVOUS SYSTEM

- A formation of tissue called the *neural crest* develops early in embryogenesis.
- One section of the neural crest turns into the CNS (brain and SC).
- Another piece migrates to become the *ENS*.
- Only later in fetal development are the 2 systems connected via the vagus nerve (CN 10).[5]

COMMUNICATION BETWEEN THE CENTRAL AND ENTERIC NERVOUS SYSTEMS

- The CNS sends signals to the ENS through a small number of command neurons (which are decision-making neurons).
- Command neurons control the pattern of activity in the GI tract and form an independent system.
- Both the CNS and vagus nerve modify the firing rate of command neurons.

Gutman SA. *Quick Reference Neuroscience for Rehabilitation Professionals: The Essential Neurologic Principles Underlying Rehabilitation Practice, Third Edition* (pp 148-154).
© 2017 Taylor & Francis Group.

- Command neurons send signals to the ENS's interneurons (interneurons are small neurons that connect 2 major neurons).
- Both command neurons and interneurons are located in 2 layers of intestinal tissue:
  1. Myenteric plexus (regulates the velocity and intensity of muscle contractions in the GI tract)
  2. Submucosal plexus (regulates the secretion and absorption of GI tract molecules)
- The myenteric and submucosal plexuses have sensors for sugar, protein, and acidity levels. These sensors monitor the progress of digestion and determine how the intestines should mix and propel their contents.[6]

DRUG INTERACTIONS AND THE CONNECTION BETWEEN THE ENTERIC AND CENTRAL NERVOUS SYSTEMS

- When pharmacologists design a drug to have effects on the brain, the drug commonly has concomitant effects on the GI tract that are undesired (ie, negative side effects).
- The intestine contains a substantial amount of serotonin. When pressure receptors in the GI tract's lining are stimulated, serotonin is released and begins the reflexive motion of peristalsis.
- It is estimated that 25% or more of individuals taking a selective serotonin re-uptake inhibitor (SSRI, a class of antidepressants including Prozac [fluoxetine], Paxil [paroxetine], Zoloft [sertraline], and Celexa [citalopram]) experience accompanying GI problems including nausea, diarrhea, and constipation.[7]
- SSRIs act on serotonin, preventing its re-uptake by receptor cells. Although robust levels of serotonin are considered beneficial in the CNS, high serotonin levels in the GI tract can cause bowel problems.
- SSRIs double the speed at which food is passed through the colon, explaining why some people taking SSRIs experience diarrhea.
- Sometimes, too much antidepressant medication can have the effect of producing constipation.
- Similarly, some antibiotics, like erythromycin, act on the GI receptors to produce oscillations, causing cramping and nausea.[8]
- Drugs like morphine and heroin attach to the intestine's opiate receptors and can produce constipation.[7,8]
- People with Alzheimer disease and Parkinson disease often experience constipation because the pathology of their CNS disorder also causes dysregulation of the intestine's functioning.[9]
- The ENS can become addicted to drugs just like the CNS does.[10]

CENTRAL AND ENTERIC NERVOUS SYSTEM SIMILARITIES DURING SLEEP

- Both the CNS and ENS act similarly when deprived of input from the external world.
- During sleep, the CNS produces 90-minute cycles of slow wave sleep punctuated by periods of rapid eye movement (REM) sleep, in which dreams occur.
- During the night when the ENS has no food, it produces 90-minute cycles of slow wave muscle contractions punctuated by short bursts of rapid muscle movements.
- The CNS and ENS influence each other during sleep. Patients with bowel problems have been shown to have abnormal REM sleep, a finding consistent with folk wisdom suggesting that indigestion causes nightmares.[11,12]

ENTERIC AND CENTRAL NERVOUS SYSTEMS' RESPONSE TO FIGHT/FLIGHT SITUATIONS

- When individuals encounter frightening situations, the CNS releases stress hormones that prepare the body to fight or flee (via the sympathetic nervous system).
- The GI tract also contains many sensory nerves that are stimulated by this chemical surge and produce the common sensation of butterflies in the stomach.
- The CNS instructs the GI tract to shut down during fight/flight situations.
- Fear and chronic stress similarly cause the vagus nerve to increase the firing rate of serotonin circuits in the GI tract.
- When the GI tract becomes overstimulated with high levels of serotonin, bowel problems can occur (eg, colitis, irritable bowel syndrome [IBS]).
- Similarly, when nerves in the esophagus are highly stimulated by an increase in the release or production of serotonin or norepinephrine, the esophagus constricts, making swallowing difficult. The feeling of being "choked up with emotion" may have derived from the esophageal constriction that occurs in emotionally laden situations.[13,14]

DISORDERS OF THE ENTERIC NERVOUS SYSTEM

- A number of disorders can effect the ENS, including Crohn disease, colitis, diverticulitis, and IBS.

- Although these disorders may have different etiologies, they all effect intestinal motility and cause malabsorption of needed nutrients. Disorders of the ENS have common signs and symptoms including chronic abdominal pain, cramping, bloating, diarrhea, and constipation. Because signs and symptoms are so similar, differential diagnosis must be confirmed using laboratory tests and radiologic imaging. Currently, treatment aims to manage symptoms rather than cure the condition. Treatment can include dietary changes, medication, and sometimes surgery.

- IBS is an ENS disorder that effects the large intestine, causing chronic cramping, bloating, abdominal pain, diarrhea, constipation, and mucous in the stool. Unlike inflammatory bowel diseases, such as Crohn disease and colitis, IBS does not cause permanent tissue changes. The condition has no known cause but is more likely to occur after an infection or stressful life event. In some cases, small intestinal bacterial overgrowth is found to be present. Patients diagnosed with IBS are more likely to concomitantly experience disorders of chronic fatigue syndrome, fibromyalgia, headache, back pain, depression, and anxiety. Common factors of these disorders are inflammation and over-activation of microglia in the CNS.[15]

- Colitis is a form of inflammatory bowel disease (IBD) involving inflammation of the colon and/or large intestines and characterized by the formation of ulcers or open sores. Inflammation may have a clear cause, such as an infection, or a cause that may be indeterminable. Signs and symptoms include abdominal pain and tenderness, loss of appetite and weight, fatigue, bloody diarrhea, bloody stools, mucous in the stool, cramping, bloating, and urgency. Although the etiology of colitis is not well understood, some consider it to be an autoimmune disorder.[16]

- Crohn disease is also a form of IBD in which the immune system may attack the GI tract. Genetic and environmental factors have been implicated in Crohn disease, but the condition is not well understood. Signs and symptoms are similar to colitis but also include rectal bleeding. Fistulae (abnormal passageways between tissues and organs) can form in the rectal area, causing pain, leakage, and discharge from the rectum. Severe obstruction of parts of the GI tract can cause bowel perforation, which can be life threatening if not surgically addressed immediately. Due to the chronic inflammation of Crohn disease, other body areas and organs can become inflamed, including the joints, eyes, mouth, and skin. Gallstones and kidney stones may also result.[17]

- Diverticulitis is an ENS disorder involving the development of pouches or diverticula in the left bowel wall, particularly the large intestine and colon. The process of pouch formation is referred to as *diverticulosis*. When diverticula become inflamed, diverticulitis results. Signs and symptoms include abdominal pain, fever, cramping, bloating, diarrhea, constipation, nausea, and increased white blood cell count. Although the cause of diverticulitis is unknown, genetic and environmental factors have been implicated. Diagnosis is confirmed using computed tomography scan.[18]

REFERENCES

1. Furness JB. The enteric nervous system and neurogastroenterology. *Nat Rev Gastroenterol Hepatol*. 2012;9(5):286-294. doi:10.1038/nrgastro.2012.32.

2. Sasselli V, Pachnis V, Burns AJ. The enteric nervous system. *Dev Biol*. 2012;366(1):64-73. doi:10.1016/j.ydbio.2012.01.012.

3. Obermayr F, Hotta R, Enomoto H, Young HM. Development and developmental disorders of the enteric nervous system. *Nat Rev Gastroenterol Hepatol*. 2013;10(1):43-57. doi:10.1038/nrgastro.2012.234.

4. Kabouridis PS, Pachnis V. Emerging roles of gut microbiota and the immune system in the development of the enteric nervous system. *J Clin Invest*. 2015;125(3):956. doi:10.1172/JC176308.

5. Lake JI, Heuckeroth RO. Enteric nervous system development: migration, differentiation, and disease. *Am J Physiol Gastrointest Liver Physiol*. 2013;305(1):G1-G24. doi:10.1152/ajpgi.00452.2012.

6. Furness JB. The enteric nervous system: normal functions and enteric neuropathies. *Neurogastroenterol Motil*. 2008;20(s1):32-38.

7. Matthys A, Haegeman G, Van Craenenbroeck K, Vanhoenacker P. Role of the 5-HT7 receptor in the central nervous system: from current status to future perspectives. *Mol Neurobiol*. 2011;43(3):228-253. doi:10.1007/s12035-011-8175-3.

8. Rhee SH, Pothoulakis C, Mayer EA. Principles and clinical implications of the brain–gut–enteric microbiota axis. *Nat Rev Gastroenterol Hepatol*. 2009;6(5):306-314. doi:10.1038/nrgastro.2009.35.

9. Shprecher DR, Derkinderen P. Parkinson disease: the enteric nervous system spills its guts. *Neurol*. 2012;78(9):683-683. doi:10. 1212/ WNL. 0b013e31824bd195.

10. Brock C, Olesen SS, Olesen AE, Frøkjaer JB, Andresen T, Drewes AM. Opioid-induced bowel dysfunction. *Drugs*. 2012;72(14):1847-1865. doi:10.2165/11634970-000000000-00000.

11. Kumar D, Idzikowski C, Wingate DL, Soffer EE, Thompson P, Siderfin C. Relationship between enteric migrating motor complex and the sleep cycle. *Am J Physiol Gastrointest Liver Physiol*. 1990;259(6):G983-G990.

12. Jarrett ME, Burr RL, Cain KC, Rothermel JD, Landis CA, Heitkemper MM. Autonomic nervous system function during sleep among women with irritable bowel syndrome. *Digest Dis Sci*. 2008;53(3):694-703. doi:10.1007/s10620-007-9943-9.

13. Qin HY, Cheng CW, Tang XD, Bian ZX. Impact of psychological stress on irritable bowel syndrome. *World J Gastroenterol*. 2014;20(39):14126-14131. doi:10.3748/wjg.v20.i39.14126.

14. Chang L. The role of stress on physiologic responses and clinical symptoms in irritable bowel syndrome. *Gastroenterology*. 2011;140(3):761-765. doi:10.1053/j.gastro.2011.01.032.

15. Camilleri M. Peripheral mechanisms in irritable bowel syndrome. *N Engl J Med*. 2012;367(17):1626-1635. doi:10.1056/NEJMra1207068.

16. Kornbluth A, Sachar DB. Ulcerative colitis practice guidelines in adults: American college of gastroenterology, practice parameters committee. *Am J Gastroenterol*. 2010;105(3):501-523. doi:10.1038/ajg.2009.727.

17. Baumgart DC, Sandborn WJ. Crohn's disease. *Lancet*. 2012;380(9853):1590-1605. doi:10.1016/S0140-6736(12)60026-9.

18. Eglinton T, Nguyen T, Raniga S, Dixon L, Dobbs B, Frizelle FA. Patterns of recurrence in patients with acute diverticulitis. *Br J Surg*. 2010;97(6):952-957. doi:10.1002/bjs.7035.

CLINICAL TEST QUESTIONS

Sections 12 to 14

1. Mr. Stanilopolis recently fell. He told his therapist that he fell because he was not wearing his glasses. However, his daughter reports to the therapist that her father commonly walks with a broad-based gait, uses furniture in the home to help him stabilize his balance while walking, and frequently loses his balance in dim light and unlevel surfaces. The daughter also states that her father commonly complains of dizziness (vertigo), ear ringing (tinnitus), and decreased hearing. Upon examination, the therapist finds an abnormal presence of nystagmus. She suspects impairment of which neurological system?
   a. visual system
   b. proprioceptive system
   c. vestibular system
   d. autonomic nervous system

2. In the above question, Mr. Stanilopolis's therapist administers the Romberg test to assess his balance. She asks Mr. Stanilopolis to stand with eyes closed, feet together, and shoulders flexed to 90 degrees (held in front of the body). Mr. Stanilopolis begins to sway and loses his balance. When using the Romberg test and removing visual cues, a patient's postural stability is based on:
   a. vestibular and proprioceptive information
   b. reticular formation and cerebellar information
   c. parasympathetic and sympathetic nervous system information
   d. basal ganglia information

3. Ann and Amanda are in a car traveling to school. Amanda is a passenger in the front seat while Ann drives. Amanda is using this commuting time to catch up on reading for her classes. Fifteen minutes into the drive, Amanda begins to sweat and feel nauseated. She first attributes her discomfort to a lack of breakfast. Amanda continues to read but feels increasingly dizzy, faint, and nauseous. She tells Ann, who recognizes Amanda's condition as motion sickness and advises her to stop reading and instead watch the oncoming traffic. Ann recognizes that motion sickness is often caused by:
   a. an incongruence between proprioceptive and vestibular system signals reaching the cortex
   b. incongruent signals traveling to the cortex from the reticular activating and inhibiting systems
   c. parasympathetic nervous system dominance (over sympathetic nervous system activity)
   d. an incongruence between visual and motion signals reaching the vestibular system

4. James has been in a persistent vegetative state for 5 days after an auto vehicle accident. Although an electroencephalogram indicates no cortical activity, James' vegetative functions (eg, temperature, heart rate, respiration, blood pressure, and gag and cough reflexes) continue to be maintained. The neurological system responsible for the control of vegetative functions is the:
   a. vestibular system
   b. autonomic nervous system
   c. parasympathetic nervous system
   d. sympathetic nervous system

5. Ricardo is in first grade and has difficulty with attention and concentration. He becomes easily distracted by noise in the hallway or by movement and sound from his classmates. When distracted, Ricardo cannot refocus on his schoolwork and instead rises from his chair and walks around the classroom. Which neurological system plays a role in screening sensory information so that the cortex can attend to the most salient information while filtering extraneous information from the environment?
   a. vestibular system
   b. enteric nervous system
   c. limbic system
   d. reticular formation

6. Emile is walking home from work late at night. The street he is walking on is dimly lit and silent. Emile believes that he can hear someone walking behind him in the distance. He is carrying a large sum of money that he must deposit in the bank tomorrow. As he hears the footsteps growing closer, Emile's heart rate accelerates. The hunger that he felt has dissipated, as blood flow has shifted from his gastrointestinal tract to his skeletal muscles and brain. Emile's blood pressure has increased, and he feels alert and anxious. Which neurological system has become dominant and is responsible for these physiological changes?

   a. vestibular system

   b. parasympathetic nervous system

   c. sympathetic nervous system

   d. enteric nervous system

7. Adam has been taking codeine, a narcotic prescription medication for pain, after injuring himself at work. Although the narcotic controls his pain level, Adam has noticed that he has developed constipation despite having no dietary changes. Explanations accounting for Adam's constipation include all but which one of the following?

   a. Narcotics stimulate parasympathetic activity, thus shutting down peristalsis.

   b. Narcotics can change the level of serotonin in the enteric nervous system, thereby creating bowel problems.

   c. Narcotics block messages sent from the enteric nervous system to the autonomic nervous system signaling the start and stop of peristalsis.

   d. Drugs with morphine and narcotic properties attach to the intestine's opiate receptors and can produce constipation.

8. Disorders of the ENS result in chronic bowel problems, including abdominal pain, cramping, bloating, diarrhea, and constipation. Which one of the below is not an ENS disorder?

   a. Crohn disease

   b. colitis

   c. food poisoning

   d. diverticulitis

9. Since Mrs. Bonnetti was a child, she has experienced chronic pain in her abdomen, cramping and bloating, and periods of diarrhea and constipation. Mrs. Bonnetti was recently diagnosed with a form of inflammatory bowel disease in which ulcers form in the colon and large intestines. Some consider this disease to be an autoimmune disorder. This disease is known as:

   a. abdominal hernia

   b. viral gastroenteritis

   c. intestinal cancer

   d. colitis

10. Maria has been diagnosed with a form of inflammatory bowel disease involving the development of pouches or diverticula in the bowel wall of the large intestine and colon. This disease is known as:

   a. colitis

   b. diverticulitis

   c. Crohn disease

   d. irritable bowel syndrome

Answers

1. c
2. a
3. d
4. b
5. d
6. c
7. a
8. c
9. d
10. b

Pain

- Pain is the sensory experience that is unpleasant and is associated with possible tissue damage.
- The detection of pain indicates that a pathological condition may be occurring in the organism.
- Pain detection is called *nociception*; nociceptors are specialized receptors that detect harmful stimuli.

THE PROCESS OF PAIN: FOUR STAGES

Nociception Can Be Divided Into Four Stages

Transduction

- Transduction occurs when free nerve endings in the periphery (ie, nociceptors) become stimulated.
- Nociceptors are located in the skin, muscles, connective tissue, circulatory system, and viscera.
- Nociception stimulation results from damage to nerve endings or from the release of chemicals at the injury site.[1,2]

Transmission

- Transmission involves the conduction of pain signals along afferent pathways in the periphery to the spinal cord (SC) and brain.
- Two primary fibers are involved in the transmission process: A delta and C fibers.[2-4]
- A delta fibers are large, thinly myelinated fibers that transmit signals quickly in response to tissue damage. Pain signals propagated along A delta fibers are sharp, stinging, highly localized, and short-lasting.
- C fibers are small, unmyelinated, and conduct pain signals more slowly. Pain signals carried along C fibers are poorly localized, dull, aching, and longer-lasting.

Perception

- Perception is the process whereby the cortex attaches meaning to, or interprets, pain signals.
- The perception of pain involves (a) pain threshold and (b) pain tolerance.
  - Pain threshold refers to the amount of pain stimulation required before pain is perceived. Pain thresholds are generally similar among all people.[5]
  - Pain tolerance refers to the amount of pain a person is able to tolerate before seeking health care intervention.[6] Pain tolerance varies widely from person to person.
- The primary somatosensory area (SS1), secondary somatosensory area (SS2), posterior multimodal association area, and limbic system structures all have a role in the perception of pain.

Modulation

- Modulation involves the modification of pain signals by different central nervous system (CNS) and peripheral nervous system (PNS) centers along the pain pathway.
- Generally, pain can be modified at the level of the peripheral nociceptor, the SC, the brainstem, and the cortex.[7]

Gutman SA. *Quick Reference Neuroscience for Rehabilitation Professionals: The Essential Neurologic Principles Underlying Rehabilitation Practice, Third Edition* (pp 156-169).
© 2017 Taylor & Francis Group.

TYPES OF PAIN

Somatic Pain

- Somatic pain occurs from the body (eg, skin, skeletal muscles, bones) and can be divided into superficial and deep pain.
- Superficial somatic pain results from nociceptor stimulation in the skin or superficial tissues and is usually well-localized (eg, pin prick).
- Deep somatic pain results from nociceptor stimulation of the ligaments, tendons, bones, blood vessels, fasciae, and muscles, and is commonly poorly localized (eg, muscular ache).[8]

Visceral Pain

- Visceral pain occurs from the viscera (eg, internal organs, glands, smooth muscle) and is dull or diffuse and not well-localized.
- This type of pain is usually accompanied by an autonomic nervous system response (eg, changes in heart rate, respiration, and blood pressure; nausea; dilated pupils; perspiration; pallor).[9]

Qualities of Pain

- Acute pain is commonly considered to last less than 30 days and resolves quickly.
- Chronic pain lasts overtime. Some sources define chronic pain as pain that lasts longer than 3 to 6 months. Chronic pain is also defined as pain that extends beyond the expected length of recovery.[10]
- Pain can be defined as sharp or dull.
- Dull aches tend to be diffuse and long-lasting because they are carried by slow-conducting, small, unmyelinated C fibers.
- Sharp pain tends to be well-localized and short-lasting because it is carried by fast-conducting, large A delta fibers.

Pain Receptors

- Pain receptors are believed to be specialized free nerve endings, called *nociceptors*, that respond to tissue damage resulting from thermal, mechanical, and chemical stimulation.
- If stimulated intensely enough, other types of receptors may act as pain receptors as well.[11]

MAJOR PAIN PATHWAYS

Spinothalamic Spinal Cord Tracts

- The spinothalamic tracts are ascending somatic sensory pathways that receive pain information from the skin and skeletal muscles.
- Sensory nerves carry pain information from the skin and skeletal muscles in the periphery to the dorsal horn of the SC.
- When these spinal nerves synapse in the dorsal horn, they release a neurotransmitter called *substance P*. Substance P is a neuropeptide that acts as a neurotransmitter in the detection of and response to inflammatory processes and pain.
- The spinothalamic tracts travel from the SC to the thalamus and send projections to the cortex for conscious pain detection and interpretation.
- Substance P is transmitted via the spinothalamic tracts to the thalamus and cortex.[12]

Reticulospinal Tracts

- The reticulospinal tracts are descending sensory tracts that receive pain information from the periphery through afferent spinal nerves that synapse in the reticular formation of the brainstem.
- The reticulospinal tracts have their origin in the medullary reticular formation.
- There, they travel to the raphe nuclei of the brainstem. The raphe nuclei are a group of nuclei located in the medulla and situated along the midline.
- When the raphe nuclei become excited, they release endorphins through a descending pathway to the place of pain origin to decrease the pain sensation.[13]

Trigeminothalamic Tracts

- The trigeminothalamic tracts have their origin in the trigeminal lemniscus in the brainstem.
- The trigeminal lemniscus projects afferent fibers from the trigeminal nerve (CN 5) to the thalamus and then to the cortex.
- This tract specifically carries pain sensation from the face.[14]

Pathways to the Cortex for the Conscious Detection of Pain

- Pain messages from the SC tracts are projected to the thalamus and then to the cortex for conscious detection and interpretation.
- SS1, located in the postcentral gyrus, detects incoming somatosensory data from the periphery.
- Pain messages are then projected to the secondary somatosensory area (SS2) for interpretation. SS2 is located just posterior to SS1.
- Pain messages are then projected to the posterior multimodal association area for the integration of pain information with other sensory data. For example, the multimodal association area can integrate pain with smell. An individual can learn to associate the smell of spoiled food with the experience of abdominal pain to avoid ingesting spoiled food in the future.
- The multimodal association area sends projections to the limbic system for the integration of sensation, emotion, and memory. For example, an individual can remember the smell of spoiled food at later dates and recall the abdominal pain associated with eating spoiled food.[15]

HOW THE BODY CONTROLS PAIN

Gate Control Theory

- One of the first theories of pain control was the Gate Theory proposed by Melzack and Wall in 1965.
- In simple terms, the Gate Theory suggested that the transmission of pain information could be blocked in the dorsal horn, closing the gate to pain.
- Lamina II, or the substantia gelatinosa in the dorsal horn, was suggested as the site of interference with pain message transmission.
- The Gate Theory suggested that afferent sensory fibers carry pain sensation from the periphery into the dorsal horn of the SC.
- This information synapses in the substantia gelatinosa.
- T-cells, which are specialized cells in the SC, then begin to fire and cause the release of substance P.
- If the substantia gelatinosa can be facilitated by another pathway (a collateral pathway), the T-cell firing will diminish, causing a decrease in pain transmission.
- While components of the Gate Theory have been disproved, the theory continues to provide a foundation for many subsequent theories describing pain mechanisms.[16]

Counterirritant Theory of Pain Cessation

- The Counterirritant Theory of Pain Cessation has incorporated evidence-based findings first proposed by the Gate Theory.
- The Counterirritant Theory suggests that non-nociceptors in the dorsal horn inhibit the excited nociceptors (also in the dorsal horn).
- For example, pressure (such as rubbing the painful area) stimulates mechanoreceptor afferent fibers.
- The proximal branches of the mechanoreceptors in the dorsal horn activate interneurons that synapse on the excited nociceptors (in the dorsal horn).
- These interneurons release the neurotransmitter enkephalin, a chemical in the family of endorphins.
- Enkephalin binds with the excited nociceptor and diminishes the release of substance P.
- Enkephalin binding on the nociceptor inhibits the transmission of nociceptive signals, thus decreasing the sensation of pain.[17]

ANALGESIC INHIBITION OF PAIN

- Analgesia is an absence of pain in response to stimulation that would otherwise cause pain.
- Analgesic mechanisms can be activated by the following:
  - Endorphins: naturally occurring substances (ie, opioid inhibitory neuropeptides) that diminish the sensation of pain
  - Pharmaceuticals that diminish the sensation of pain
- Endorphins include enkephalin, dynorphin, and beta-endorphin.
- Opiates are the family of analgesic drugs that block nociceptor signals without affecting other sensations.
- Both endorphins and analgesic drugs bind to the same receptor site.
- The inhibition of nociceptive information can also be inhibited by the supraspinal levels of the nervous system. These are brainstem centers that provide natural analgesia and are referred to as *pain inhibiting centers*:
  - The raphe nuclei in the medulla
  - The periaqueductal gray in the midbrain
  - The locus ceruleus in the pons
- When the raphe nuclei are stimulated, axons projecting to the SC release the neurotransmitter serotonin in the dorsal horn. This release of serotonin inhibits the transmission of nociceptive signals.
- When the periaqueductal gray is stimulated, it also produces an analgesic effect by activating the raphe nuclei.
- The ceruleospinal tract originates at the locus ceruleus in the pons. When stimulated, it causes norepinephrine to bind to the spinothalamic tract in the dorsal horn. Binding of norepinephrine to the spinothalamic tract suppresses the release of substance P, thus diminishing pain messages to the cortex.
- Narcotic drugs (derived from opium or opium-like compounds) bind to receptor sites in the periaqueductal gray, the raphe nuclei, and the dorsal horn. By binding to these receptor sites, narcotic drugs induce analgesia and stupor (a state of reduced consciousness).[18]

STRESS-INDUCED ANALGESIA

- The brainstem pain inhibiting centers can be activated naturally by injury and athletic overexertion.
- Often, people injured during accidents, disasters, or athletic competition may not feel pain until the event has passed. Stress occurring during the event may trigger the pain inhibition centers.
- Stress-induced analgesia involves activation of the following:
  - The raphe nuclei descending tracts
  - The release of the hormonal endorphins from the pituitary gland (particularly beta-endorphins)
  - The release of hormonal endorphins from the adrenal medulla (particularly enkephalins)
- Hormonal endorphins bind to the opiate receptors in the brain and SC.
- Beta-endorphins are the most potent endorphins and can trigger analgesic affects that last for hours.[19]

PAIN TRANSMISSION CAN BE DIMINISHED AT SEVERAL NERVOUS SYSTEM LEVELS

The Periphery

- Non-narcotic analgesics (eg, aspirin) decrease the synthesis of prostaglandins, thus preventing prostaglandins from sensitizing peripheral pain receptors. Prostaglandins are a large group of biologically activated, carbon-20, unsaturated fatty acids.[20]
- NSAIDs (nonsteroidal anti-inflammatory drugs, such as ibuprofen and naproxen) and local anesthetic agents also produce analgesic effects by interrupting peripheral transmission at an early stage of the pain process. NSAIDs inhibit prostaglandin production, thus reducing the number of pain chemicals available to stimulate peripheral nociceptors.[21]
- Local anesthetics can be administered to nerve endings at the site of injury or to the nerve plexus supplying the area. Peripheral transmission of pain signals is interrupted by localized or regional blockade.
- The application of heat and cold to a painful area similarly reduces peripheral pain signals by altering blood flow to the area and reducing swelling.

Dorsal Horn

- Inhibitory neurons in the dorsal horn release enkephalin or dynorphin. These can diminish pain sensation through interneurons that bind to the excited nociceptor. This is the principle of the Counterirritant Theory.[17]

Supraspinal Descending Systems

- The raphe nuclei, periaqueductal gray, and locus ceruleus can inhibit nociceptive information.[22]

Hormonal System

- The hormonal system involves the release of hormonal endorphins from the pituitary gland (particularly beta-endorphins).
- It also involves the release of hormonal endorphins from the adrenal medulla (particularly enkephalins).[23]

Cortical Level

- The cortical detection and interpretation of pain can be altered by an individual's expectations, distraction level, anxiety, and belief (particularly regarding placebo effects).[15]

PAIN TRANSMISSION CAN ALSO BE INTENSIFIED AT SEVERAL NERVOUS SYSTEM LEVELS

- Edema and endogenous chemicals can sensitize free nerve endings in the periphery.
- For example, following a minor burn injury, sensory stimuli that would normally be innocuous can cause heightened pain. This is referred to as *central sensitization*.[24]
- Fear and anxiety can also heighten the experience of pain.[2]

CHRONIC PAIN AND PAIN TOLERANCE

- Prostaglandins form as a result of damaged cells. An enzyme called *phospholipase A* breaks down phospholipids in the cell membrane and converts them to arachidonic acid. A second enzyme then breaks down arachidonic acid, and, as a result, prostaglandins are formed.
- Sensitization by prostaglandins lowers the threshold of pain fibers. This results in allodynia, a condition in which nonpainful stimuli now produce pain (ie, people who once had a higher pain tolerance now experience pain more easily).
- Some theorists suggest that a synaptic memory of pain in the nociceptive pathway can be formed when glutamate binds to certain pain receptors on the postsynaptic neuron. Then, when excessive or repeated stimulation of the small, unmyelinated C fibers occurs, SC neurons become sensitized, further creating the synaptic memory of pain.
- The synaptic memory becomes easier to trigger each time it is stimulated, so that a once non-noxious stimulus can now trigger the synaptic memory of pain.
- This phenomenon is referred to as *wind-up* and may underlie the development of chronic pain.[24,25]

REFERRED PAIN

- Referred pain is pain that is perceived to originate from one body region when it actually originates from a different body region.
- Usually, referred pain occurs when visceral pain (from an internal organ or gland) is perceived as originating from a somatic area (such as the skin or skeletal muscles).
- For example, during a heart attack, the brain may misinterpret the nociceptive information as arising from the skin on the medial left arm.
- Similarly, gallbladder pain is often referred to the right subscapular region.
- The phenomenon of referred pain can be explained by the dermatomal distribution[26]:
  - In a heart attack, nociceptive information from the heart projects to and from the SC segment T1. The dermatomal sensation of the medial left arm also projects to and from T1.
  - Because the cortex is unfamiliar with pain messages received from the heart, it initially interprets the pain as originating from the left arm, until the pain becomes excruciating.
  - Some dorsal root neurons have 2 peripheral axons: 1 that innervates the skin and skeletal muscle and 1 that innervates the viscera. Stimulation of the visceral branch of a dual receptive neuron may be the source of cortical misinterpretation.

Noninvasive Pain Management Procedures

Stimulation of the Mechanoreceptors (Massage)

- Stimulation of the mechanoreceptors to reduce pain sensation is based on the Counterirritant Theory and involves rubbing or massaging the painful area.
- The proximal branches of the mechanoreceptors in the dorsal horn activate interneurons that synapse on the excited nociceptors (also in the dorsal horn).
- These interneurons release the neurotransmitter enkephalin, which binds with the excited nociceptor and diminishes the release of substance P (released from the excited nociceptors).
- Enkephalin binding on the nociceptor inhibits the transmission of nociceptive signals, thus decreasing the sensation of pain.[27]

Electrical Stimulation

- Electrical stimulation is a form of pain management that may work by (a) blocking the transmission of pain signals along the nerve, (b) promoting the release of endorphins, (c) causing vasodilation (widening of the blood vessels) allowing increased oxygenated blood to the painful area, or (d) some combination of these.
- Electrical stimulation can be applied in various forms, including (a) transcutaneous electrical nerve stimulation (TENS), (b) interferential current therapy (ICT), and microcurrent electrical neuromuscular stimulation (MENS).
- The administration of electrical stimulation commonly involves the placement of electrodes over the painful body part.
- Electrical stimulation is used to treat both acute and chronic pain conditions, including back pain, headaches, and arthritis.[28]

Transcutaneous Electrical Nerve Stimulation

- TENS involves the transmission of electrical signals to the PNS through conductive gel pads placed on the identified painful region.
- The therapist finds the dermatomal region of the pain area and applies TENS to activate the mechanoreceptors.[29]

Interferential Current Therapy

- ICT is a form of TENS in which electrical stimulation is administered directly to the muscle fibers rather than nerves, possibly improving blood flow and promoting tissue healing.
- ICT is used to treat chronic pain conditions and improve recovery time of soft-tissue and muscle damage.[30]

Microcurrent Electrical Neuromuscular Stimulation

- MENS is a device that sends weak electrical pulses to identified pain regions through electrodes placed on the skin.
- MENS is used to treat chronic pain conditions and speed recovery of damaged tissues and muscles.[31]

Thermotherapy

- Thermotherapy involves the use of heat to treat chronic and acute pain syndromes, including back pain, arthritis, tendinitis, and muscular aches.
- Thermotherapy works through vasodilation, allowing the blood vessels in the painful area to widen, thus increasing blood flow to the area. It can also relax superficial muscles, making them more elastic and decreasing joint stiffness.
- The most common forms of thermotherapy include hot packs, paraffin, ultrasound, and diathermy.[32]

Hot Packs

- Hot packs contain a silicone gel that, when immersed in hot water, has the capacity to absorb and hold a great amount of heat.
- Hot packs are not able to provide deeply penetrating heat, as is ultrasound.
- They are recommended for large body areas, such as the back, and can provide only temporary pain relief.[33]

Paraffin

- Paraffin wax baths are a method of superficial heat conduction involving heated wax into which patients immerse their hands to reduce pain, joint stiffness, and increase blood flow.
- Paraffin baths are recommended for joint tightness and pain, particularly in the hands.[34]

Ultrasound

- Ultrasound involves conversion heating, or high-frequency sound waves.
- As ultrasound is propagated through tissue, it is absorbed and converted into heat.
- Ultrasound may improve circulation, soften scar tissue and adhesions, reduce chronic inflammation, and reduce irritation of nerve roots.
- Ultrasound is one of the most effective heat modalities for deep structures; reported depths of penetration travel 5 to 6 cm below the superficial layers of the skin.[35]

Diathermy

- Diathermy is the use of high-frequency electromagnetic currents to increase blood flow, release soft tissue adhesions and scarring, reduce joint stiffness, and promote soft tissue and muscular healing.
- Ultrasound is a form of diathermy, along with short wave and microwave diathermy.
- Microwaves and shortwaves are selectively absorbed by tissues with high water content.
- Shortwave diathermy is commonly used for deep muscle and joint pain, while microwave diathermy is less deeply penetrating.
- Microwave diathermy uses higher frequencies than shortwave diathermy, and penetration depth is not as deep as that achieved through shortwave diathermy.[36]

Cryotherapy (Cold Packs)

- Cold packs are useful for anesthetizing sensory receptors to relieve pain. The analgesic effects of ice result from decreased nerve conduction along pain fibers.
- Cold therapy also produces vasoconstriction, which slows circulation, thus reducing inflammation and relieving pain.
- Because cold reduces muscle spindle activity and decreases the velocity of nerve conduction, cold application can be used to reduce muscle spasms and tightness.[37]

Hydrotherapy

- Hydrotherapy is a method of convection heat using water and can be considered a type of thermotherapy.
- It can be performed in swimming pools, whirlpools, showers, or immersion tanks that allow patients to (a) exercise with reduced stress to joints and (b) relax tight or spastic muscle groups.
- This is particularly useful for large body areas, such as the back and legs.[38]

Fluidotherapy

- Fluidotherapy (DJO Global Inc) is a dry superficial thermal modality that transfers heat to soft tissue through heated air and particles (corn husks ground to the size of sand grains).
- Fluidotherapy is much like a dry whirlpool, with particles instead of water as the heating medium.
- The particles are circulated by hot air blown within the fluidotherapy machine. The particles agitate around the body part at a temperature of approximately 108°F to 124°F.
- Fluidotherapy may work via vasodilation and mechanical stimulation. Vasodilation causes increased oxygenated blood flow to the painful area. Mechanical stimulation may help to desensitize skin and scar pain after injury.
- This technique is useful for pain relief in the extremities, particularly in the hand, wrist, forearm, and ankle.[39]

Kinesio Tape

- Kinesio taping involves using a special elastic tape over the muscles to (a) assist function and provide support, (b) prevent over-use, and (c) reduce pain and inflammation.
- Kinesio tape is used for muscular disorders and lymphedema reduction.
- This technique involves a nonrestrictive type of taping that allows for full range of motion in functional activities, in contrast to traditional sports taping in which tape is wrapped fully around a joint for stabilization and limits both range of motion and vascular circulation.[40]

Acupuncture

- Acupuncture is part of traditional Chinese medicine (TCM) and is one of the oldest documented medical treatments in the world.

REFERRED PAIN

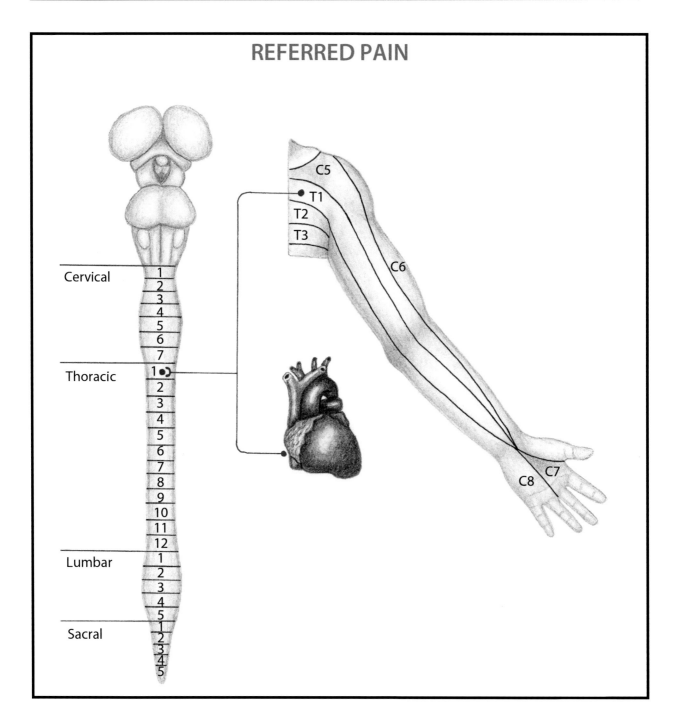

- In TCM, the body is believed to be in a state of health when its 2 forces, yin and yang, are balanced. When one force dominates the other, an imbalance occurs, causing disease states. An imbalance between yin and yang is said to cause a blockage in the flow of qi, the vital life force. Such blockage is believed to result in pain and disease.
- In order to restore health and relieve pain, specific acupuncture points (called *meridians*) need to be stimulated. The most common form of acupuncture involves inserting hair-thin needles into the skin along the meridian points.
- While the mechanism through which acupuncture works is unknown, it is suggested that it stimulates the release of naturally occurring opioids in the body.
- Acupuncture has been shown to provide lasting pain relief if the procedure is applied over time.[41]

Stress Management and Meditation

- Stress management and meditation techniques involve learning how to release the body's naturally occurring endorphins and raise pain thresholds by using visual imagery.
- Such techniques can involve deep and slow breathing to reduce pain-related anxiety, and guided imagery to promote pain management and analgesia.[42]

Biofeedback

- Biofeedback is the process in which patients learn to consciously control body functions that are typically involuntary, such as muscle tension and heart rate, through the use of instruments that provide feedback about the body's activity.
- For example, biofeedback may involve learning to release tension in muscles that may be contracted because the individual is using those muscles to guard or protect a painful region.
- Biofeedback can help patients to better manage pain sensations.[43]

INVASIVE PAIN MANAGEMENT PROCEDURES

Nerve Blocks

- Nerve blocks involve injections of local anesthetics and steroids in the area of a spinal nerve in an attempt to decrease pain; effects are often short-lasting.
- There are several different types of nerve blocks.

Facet and Medial Branch Blocks

- A facet block involves an injection of local anesthetic and/or steroid, using x-ray guidance, into a joint space in the spine to relieve pain.
- A medial branch block is similar, but the anesthetic is injected outside of the joint space near the nerve that supplies the joint (called the *medial branch*).
- A series of injections over time is commonly required to provide effective and lasting relief of pain.[44]

Root Blocks

- A root block involves the injection of anesthetic and/or steroid, using x-ray guidance, into the area where the nerve exits the SC.
- A root block is performed to alleviate pain in the extremities that follows the distribution of a single nerve.
- Root blocks can be repeated if good results are initially obtained.[45]

Epidural Steroid Injections

- Epidural steroid injections involve the administration of a local anesthetic and steroid into the subdural space to provide pain relief by reducing the inflammation of the nerve roots as they exit the SC.
- The injections are commonly administered in a series of 3 injections. The length of time between each injection depends on the type of steroid administered. If pain is substantially reduced after the first injection, further injections are not needed unless the pain returns at a later date.[46]

Spinal Surgery

- Surgery of the spine may be considered as an option when back pain cannot be relieved through noninvasive methods.

Discogram

- A discogram is a diagnostic procedure used to determine the anatomical source of low back pain. The procedure is most frequently used to determine whether degenerative disc disease is the cause of a patient's pain.
- A needle is inserted into the center of the suspected discs, one at a time. Radiographic dye is then injected into each disc. The patient is awakened at this time and asked to indicate present pain level. If the injection of dye recreates the patient's pain in a specific disc(s), that disc is determined to be the source of pain.
- Frequently, after the discogram is completed, a CT scan is performed to further examine the identified disc(s).[47]

Discectomy

- Back pain is most commonly caused by herniation of the disc; in other words, the disc ruptures, moves out of place, and may impinge upon nearby structures (such as nerve roots).
- A discectomy involves the removal of a herniated disc and the replacement of the disc with synthetic material.[48]

Laminectomy

- A laminectomy involves the partial or total removal of the lamina, the small bony plate that sits at the back of each vertebrae.
- This procedure is commonly performed for conditions of spinal stenosis, narrowing of the spinal canal causing impingement of the cord and nerves.[49]

Foraminotomy

- A foraminotomy is a surgical procedure used to enlarge foraminal openings, the openings through which the nerves exit the SC.
- It is commonly performed to alleviate a compressed or impinged nerve.[50]

Spinal Fusion

- A spinal fusion is a surgical technique used to join 2 or more vertebrae to eliminate pain caused by degenerative spinal conditions and deformities.
- Spinal fusion involves the use of synthetic and natural bone material; metal devices (such as cages, plates, screws, and rods) are used to stabilize the vertebrae.
- The bone grafts will grow around the metal instrumentation and strengthen the vertebral architecture.[51]

Intrathecal Pumps (Indwelling Pain Pump)

- Intrathecal pumps are surgically implanted mechanical devices used to deliver medications to the SC region. The instrumentation consists of a computerized pump, a reservoir, and a catheter.
- Intrathecal pumps must be implanted surgically, usually under the skin of the lower abdomen. The catheter is placed into the spinal fluid space and connected to the reservoir.
- The pump is programmed to deliver pain medication in a controlled fashion.
- Intrathecal pumps are considered for patients who have not responded to oral opioid treatment.[52]

PHARMACEUTICAL MANAGEMENT OF PAIN

Nonsteroidal Anti-Inflammatory Drugs

- NSAIDs can reduce swelling and the secondary damage that can occur as a result of swelling.
- These drugs do not alter cognitive functions, cause respiratory depression, or cause nausea; NSAIDs are non-narcotic and nonaddictive. Long-term side effects include gastrointestinal problems.
- NSAIDs include aspirin, ibuprofen, and naproxen.[21]

Acetaminophen

- Acetaminophen is a group of analgesic medications that are most commonly used as alternatives to NSAIDs. They can be used alone or in combination with NSAIDs.
- Potential long-term side effects include liver and kidney damage.
- Name brand acetaminophen includes Tylenol, Anacin, and Valadol.[53]

Opioids

- Opioid drugs bind to opioid receptors in the CNS, PNS, and enteric nervous system (gastrointestinal tract).
- Because of their highly addictive qualities, opioids are only indicated after other pharmacological options have been exhausted.
- Side effects include sedation, respiratory depression, constipation, and addiction.
- Opioids include morphine, codeine, Demerol (meperidine), and Oxycontin (oxycodone).[54]

Muscle Relaxants

- Muscle relaxants are indicated to alleviate severe musculoskeletal pain and muscle spasticity.
- They function by blocking transmission in the neuromuscular junction.
- Side effects include dizziness, sedation, nausea, and dependence with long-term use.
- Common muscle relaxants include Flexeril (cyclobenzaprine), Valium (diazepam), and Robaxin (methocarbamol).[55]

Anticonvulsants

- Anticonvulsants, a type of antiseizure medication, have been increasingly used in the treatment of neuropathic pain (ie, pain derived from damage to the CNS or PNS, such as diabetic neuropathy, post-herpetic neuralgia, and fibromyalgia).
- Anticonvulsant effectiveness in neuropathic pain management may relate to these drugs' interaction with voltage-gated calcium channels and ability to bind with neurotransmitters associated with pain perception.
- Side effects include dizziness, sedation, weight gain, and heightened risk of seizure.[56]

Fibromyalgia

- Fibromyalgia is a chronic pain syndrome that does not have a clear etiology.
- Some studies suggest that changes occur in the CNS, leading to heightened sensitivity of pain fibers. The primary symptom of fibromyalgia, widespread chronic pain, may result from a neurochemical imbalance causing an inflammatory process and allodynia (heightened pain in response to non-noxious tactile stimuli). This is commonly known as a *wind-up phenomenon*, in which the body's pain mechanisms become oversensitized to tactile stimuli with repeated exposure.[57]
- Other studies suggest that deficient restorative sleep periods may contribute to the disorder. Restorative sleep occurs in deep stage 4 sleep, the period of rapid eye movement (REM). Humans generally experience two 90-minute cycles of stage 4 sleep each night. Cellular repair is believed to occur most efficiently in this stage. People who are chronically deficient of stage 4 sleep appear more likely to develop the symptoms of fibromyalgia.[58]
- Studies have also implicated genetic factors and dysfunction of the hypothalamic-pituitary-adrenal axis as causes of fibromyalgia.[59]
- Primary symptoms include tenderness of muscles and adjacent soft tissues, stiffness of muscles, and aching pain. Other symptoms can include fatigue, sleep dysfunction, numbness and tingling, headache, and short-term memory and concentration difficulties.
- Patients may have no accompanying disease; it is also likely for patients to concomitantly have rheumatoid arthritis, osteoarthritis, irritable bowel syndrome, Lyme disease, or sleep apnea.[60]
- Multiple tender points can be found on palpation. Such painful areas follow a regional rather than a dermatomal or peripheral nerve distribution.
- Increased restorative sleep and appropriate exercise have been found to benefit patients with fibromyalgia. Anticonvulsant drug therapy to treat neuropathic pain, serotonin norepinephrine reuptake inhibitor administration, and growth hormone supplemental therapy have also provided benefit. The effectiveness of these agents suggests that fibromyalgia has a neurochemical and hormonal basis.[61]

REFERENCES

1. Dussor G, Koerber HR, Oaklander AL, Rice FL, Molliver DC. Nucleotide signaling and cutaneous mechanisms of pain transduction. *Brain Res Rev.* 2009;60(1):24-35. doi:10.1016/j.brainresrev.2008.12.013.

2. Stucky CL, Gold MS, Zhang X. Mechanisms of pain. *Proc Natl Acad Sci U S A.* 2001;98(21):11845-11846. doi:10.1073/pnas.211373398.

3. DeLeo JA. Basic science of pain. *J Bone Joint Surg.* 2006;88(Suppl 2):58-62. doi.org/10.2106/JBJS.E.01286.

4. Argoff C. Mechanisms of pain transmission and pharmacologic management. *Curr Med Res Opin.* 2011;27(10):2019-2031. doi:10.1185/03007995.2011.614934.

5. Chesterton LS, Barlas P, Foster NE, Baxter GD, Wright CC. Gender differences in pressure pain threshold in healthy humans. *Pain.* 2003;101(3):259-266. doi:10.1016/S0304-3959(02)00330-5.

6. Hayes SC, Bissett RT, Korn Z, et al. The impact of acceptance versus control rationales on pain tolerance. *Psychol Rec.* 2012;49(1):3.

7. Yarnitsky D. Conditioned pain modulation (the diffuse noxious inhibitory control-like effect): Its relevance for acute and chronic pain states. *Curr Opin Anesthesiol.* 2010;23(5):611-615. doi: 10.1097/ACO.0b013e32833c348b.

8. Paine P, Kishor J, Worthen SF, Gregory LJ, Aziz Q. Exploring relationships for visceral and somatic pain with autonomic control and personality. *Pain.* 2009;144(3):236-244.

9. Strigo IA, Duncan GH, Boivin M, Bushnell MC. Differentiation of visceral and cutaneous pain in the human brain. *J Neurophysiol.* 2003;89(6):3294-3303. doi:10.1152/jn.01048.2002.

10. Ferrari LF, Bogen O, Reichling DB, Levine JD. Accounting for the delay in the transition from acute to chronic pain: Axonal and nuclear mechanisms. *J Neurosci.* 2015;35(2):495-507. doi:10.1523/JNEUROSCI.5147-13.2015.

11. Burnstock G. Purinergic receptors and pain. *Curr Pharm Des.* 2009;15(15):1717-1735.

12. Hong JH, Son SM, Jang SH. Identification of spinothalamic tract and its related thalamocortical fibers in human brain. *Neurosci Lett.* 2010;468(2):102-105. doi:10.1016/j.neulet.2009.10.075.

13. Eippert F, Bingel U, Schoell ED, et al. Activation of the opioidergic descending pain control system underlies placebo analgesia. *Neuron.* 2009;63(4):533-543. doi:10.1016/j.neuron.2009.07.014.

14. Zakrzewska JM, McMillan R. Trigeminal neuralgia: the diagnosis and management of this excruciating and poorly understood facial pain. *Postgrad Med J.* 2011;87(1028):410-416. doi:10.1136/pgmj.2009.080473.

15. Gustin SM, Peck CC, Cheney LB, Macey PM, Murray GM, Henderson LA. Pain and plasticity: is chronic pain always associated with somatosensory cortex activity and reorganization? *J Neurosci.* 2012;32(43):14874-14884. doi:10.1523/JNEUROSCI.1733-12.2012.

16. Moayedi M, Davis KD. Theories of pain: from specificity to gate control. *J Neurophysiol.* 2013;109(1):5-12. doi:10.1152/jn.00457.2012.

17. Piché M, Arsenault M, Rainville P. Cerebral and cerebrospinal processes underlying counterirritation analgesia. *J Neurosci.* 2009;29(45):14236-14246. doi:10.1523/JNEUROSCI.2341-09.2009.

18. Ossipov MH, Dussor GO, Porreca, F. Central modulation of pain. *J Clin Invest.* 2010;120(11):3779. doi:10.1172/JCI43766.

19. Parikh D, Hamid A, Friedman TC, et al. Stress-induced analgesia and endogenous opioid peptides: the importance of stress duration. *Eur J Pharmacol.* 2011;650(2):563-567. doi:10.1016/j.ejphar.2010.10.050.

20. Perchyonok VT, Reher V, Zhang S, Grobler SR, Oberholzer TG, Massey W. Insights and relative effect of aspirin, naproxen and ibuprofen containing hydrogels: from design to performance as a functional dual capacity restorative material and build in free radical defense: in-vitro studies. *Open J Stomatol.* 2014;4(3):43159. doi:10.4236/ojst.2014.42013.

21. Conaghan PG. A turbulent decade for NSAIDs: update on current concepts of classification, epidemiology, comparative efficacy, and toxicity. *Rheumatol Int.* 2012;32(6):1491-1502. doi:10.1007/s00296-011-2263-6.

22. Condés-Lara M, Martínez-Lorenzana G, Rubio-Beltrán E, Rodríguez-Jiménez J, Rojas-Piloni G, González-Hernández A. Hypothalamic paraventricular nucleus stimulation enhances c-Fos expression in spinal and supraspinal structures related to pain modulation. *Neurosci Res.* 2015;98:59-63. doi:10.1016/j.neures.2015.04.004.

23. Sprouse-Blum AS, Smith G, Sugai D, Parsa FD. Understanding endorphins and their importance in pain management. *Hawaii Med J.* 2010;69(3):70-71.

24. Latremoliere A, Woolf CJ. Central sensitization: a generator of pain hypersensitivity by central neural plasticity. *J Pain.* 2009;10(9):895-926. doi:10.1016/j.jpain.2009.06.012.

25. Harding LM, Kristensen JD, Baranowski AP. Differential effects of neuropathic analgesics on wind-up-like pain and somatosensory function in healthy volunteers. *Clin J Pain.* 2005;21(2):127-132.

26. Alonso-Blanco C, Fernández-de-Las-Peñas C, de-la-Llave-Rincón AI, Zarco-Moreno P, Galán-del-Río F, Svensson P. Characteristics of referred muscle pain to the head from active trigger points in women with myofascial temporomandibular pain and fibromyalgia syndrome. *J Headache Pain.* 2012;13(8):625-637. doi:10.1007/s10194-012-0477-y.

27. Roques BP, Fournié-Zaluski MC, Wurm M. Inhibiting the breakdown of endogenous opioids and cannabinoids to alleviate pain. *Nat Rev Drug Discov.* 2012;11(4):292-310. doi:10.1038/nrd3673.

28. Koyuncu E, Nakipoğlu-Yüzer GF, Doğan A, Özgirgin N. The effectiveness of functional electrical stimulation for the treatment of shoulder subluxation and shoulder pain in hemiplegic patients: a randomized controlled trial. *Disabil Rehabil.* 2010;32(7):560-566. doi:10.3109/09638280903183811.

29. Moran F, Leonard T, Hawthorne S, et al. Hypoalgesia in response to transcutaneous electrical nerve stimulation (TENS) depends on stimulation intensity. *J Pain.* 2011;12(8):929-935. doi:10.1016/j.jpain.2011.02.352.

30. Suh HR, Han HC, Cho HY. Immediate therapeutic effect of interferential current therapy on spasticity, balance, and gait function in chronic stroke patients: a randomized control trial. *Clin Rehabil.* 2014;28(9):885-91. doi:10.1177/0269215514523798.

31. Park RJ, Son H, Kim K, Kim S, Oh T. The effect of microcurrent electrical stimulation on the foot blood circulation and pain of diabetic neuropathy. *J Phys Ther Sci.* 2011;23(3):515-518. doi.org/10.1589/jpts.23.515.

32. Cramer H, Baumgarten C, Choi KE, et al. Thermotherapy self-treatment for neck pain relief—a randomized controlled trial. *Eur J Integr Med.* 2012;4(4):e371-e378. doi:10.1016/j.eujim.2012.04.001.

33. Rabini A, Piazzini DB, Tancredi G, et al. Deep heating therapy via microwave diathermy relieves pain and improves physical function in patients with knee osteoarthritis: a double-blind randomized clinical trial. *Eur J Phys Rehabil Med.* 2012;48(4):549-59.

34. Dilek B, Gözüm M, Şahin E, et al. Efficacy of paraffin bath therapy in hand osteoarthritis: a single-blinded randomized controlled trial. *Arch Phys Med Rehabil.* 2013;94(4):642-649. doi:10.1016/j.apmr.2012.11.024.

35. Ilter L, Dilek B, Batmaz I, et al. Efficacy of pulsed and continuous therapeutic ultrasound in myofascial pain syndrome: a randomized controlled study. *Am J Phys Med Rehabil.* 2015;94(7):547-54. doi:10.1097/PHM.0000000000000210.

36. Ortega JAA, Fernández EC, Llorent RG, González MR, Martínez ADD. Microwave diathermy for treating nonspecific chronic neck pain: a randomized controlled trial. *Spine J.* 2014;14(8):1712-1721. doi:10.1016/j.spinee.2013.10.025.

37. Wittig-Wells D, Johnson I, Samms-McPherson J, et al. Does the use of a brief cryotherapy intervention with analgesic administration improve pain management after total knee arthroplasty? *Orthop Nurs.* 2015;34(3):148-153. doi:10.1097/NOR.0000000000000143.

38. Cuesta-Vargas AI, Travé-Mesa A, Vera-Cabrera A, et al. Hydrotherapy as a recovery strategy after exercise: a pragmatic controlled trial. *BMC Complement Altern Med.* 2013;13(1):180. doi:10.1186/1472-6882-13-180.

39. Kelly R, Beehn C, Hansford A, Westphal KA, Halle JS, Greathouse DG. Effect of fluidotherapy on superficial radial nerve conduction and skin temperature. *J Orthop Sports Phys Ther.* 2005;35(1):16-23. doi:10.2519/jospt.2005.35.1.16.

40. Lim ECW, Tay MGX. Kinesio taping in musculoskeletal pain and disability that lasts for more than 4 weeks: is it time to peel off the tape and throw it out with the sweat? A systematic review with meta-analysis focused on pain and also methods of tape application. *Br J Sports Med.* 2015;49(24):1558-66. doi:10.1136/bjsports-2014-094151.

41. Vickers AJ, Linde K. Acupuncture for chronic pain. *JAMA.* 2014;311(9):955-956. doi:10.1001/jama.2013.285478.

42. Wright CJ, Schutte NS. The relationship between greater mindfulness and less subjective experience of chronic pain: mediating functions of pain management self-efficacy and emotional intelligence. *Aust J Psychol.* 2014;66(3):181-186. doi:10.1111/ajpy.12041.

43. Willmarth E, Davis F, Fitzgerald K. Biofeedback and integrative medicine in the pain clinic setting. *Biofeedback.* 2014;42(3):111-114. doi:10.5298/1081-5937-42.03.10.

44. Cohen SP, Moon JY, Brummett CM, White RL, Larkin TM. Medial branch blocks or intra-articular injections as a prognostic tool before lumbar facet radiofrequency denervation: a multicenter, case-control study. *Reg Anesth Pain Med.* 2015;40(4):376-383. doi:10.1097/AAP.0000000000000229.

45. Bensler S, Sutter R, Pfirrmann CW, Peterson CK. Long term outcomes from CT-guided indirect cervical nerve root blocks and their relationship to the MRI findings—a prospective study. *Eur Radiol.* 2015;25(11):3405-13. doi:10.1007/s00330-015-3758-4.

46. Wilkinson IM, Cohen SP. Epidural steroid injections. *Curr Pain Headache Rep.* 2012;16(1):50-59. doi:10.1007/s11916-011-0236-9.

47. Kim SM, Lee SH, Lee BR, Hwang JW. Analysis of the correlation among age, disc morphology, positive discography and prognosis in patients with chronic low back pain. *Ann Rehabil Med.* 2015;39(3):340-346. doi:10.5535/arm.2015.39.3.340.

48. Manchikanti L, Singh V, Falco FJ, et al. An updated review of automated percutaneous mechanical lumbar discectomy for the contained herniated lumbar disc. *Pain Physician.* 2013;16(2 Suppl):SE151-84.

49. Li G, Patil CG, Lad SP, Ho C, Tian W, Boakye M. Effects of age and comorbidities on complication rates and adverse outcomes after lumbar laminectomy in elderly patients. *Spine.* 2008;33(11):1250-1255. doi:10.1097/BRS.0b013e3181714a44.

50. Prasher A, Tay B. Treatment of spinal conditions in the young adult: endoscopic cervical foraminotomy. *Oper Tech Orthop.* 2015;25(3):217-224. doi:10.1053/j.oto.2015.05.004.

51. Mannion AF, Leivseth G, Brox JI, Fritzell P, Hägg O, Fairbank JC. Long-term follow-up suggests spinal fusion is associated with increased adjacent segment disc degeneration but without influence on clinical outcome: results of a combined follow-up from 4 randomized controlled trials. *Spine.* 2014;39(17):1373-1383. doi:10.1097/BRS.0000000000000437.

52. Wilkes D. Programmable intrathecal pumps for the management of chronic pain: recommendations for improved efficiency. *J Pain Res.* 2014;7:571-577. doi:10.2147/JPR.S46929.

53. Anderson BJ. Paracetamol (acetaminophen): mechanisms of action. *Pediatr Anesth.* 2008;18(10):915-921. doi:10.1111/j.1460-9592.2008.02764.x.

54. Chaparro LE, Furlan AD, Deshpande A, Mailis-Gagnon A, Atlas S, Turk DC. Opioids compared with placebo or other treatments for chronic low back pain: an update of the Cochrane review. *Spine.* 2014;39(7):556-563. doi:10.1097/BRS.0000000000000249.

55. Malanga G, Wolff E. Evidence-informed management of chronic low back pain with nonsteroidal anti-inflammatory drugs, muscle relaxants, and simple analgesics. *Spine J.* 2008;8(1):173-184. doi.10.1016/j.spinee.2007.10.013.

56. Moore A, Wiffen P, Kalso E. Antiepileptic drugs for neuropathic pain and fibromyalgia. *JAMA.* 2014;312(2):182-183. doi:10.1001/jama.2014.6336.

57. Clauw DJ. Fibromyalgia: An overview. *Am J Med.* 2009;122(12):S3-S13. doi:10.1016/j.amjmed.2009.09.006.

58. Pejovic S, Natelson BH, Basta M, Fernandez-Mendoza J, Mahr F, Vgontzas AN. Chronic fatigue syndrome and fibromyalgia in diagnosed sleep disorders: a further test of the 'unitary' hypothesis. *BMC Neurol.* 2015;15(1):53. doi:10.1186/s12883-015-0308-2.

59. Ablin JN, Buskila D. Update on the genetics of the fibromyalgia syndrome. *Best Pract Res Clin Rheumatol.* 2015;29(1):20-28. doi:10.1016/j.berh.2015.04.018.

60. Podell RN. Fibromyalgia syndrome's new paradigm: neural sensitization and its implications for treatment. *J Musculoskelet Pain.* 2007;15(2):45-54. doi:10.1300/J094v15n02_08.

61. Malemud CJ. Regulation of pain in fibromyalgia by selective serotonin and serotonin norepinephrine reuptake inhibition. *Int J Phys Med Rehabil.* 2013;1(5):1000144. doi:10.4172/2329-9096.1000144.

Peripheral Nerve Injury and Regeneration

Neuropathy

- *Neuropathy* is a general term for pathology involving one or more peripheral nerves.

Dermatomal Distribution

- The dermatomes are skin segments that are innervated by specific peripheral nerves.
- The dermatomal skin distribution corresponds closely to the skeletal muscles that are innervated by a specific peripheral nerve.
- When a therapist evaluates sensation, the therapist will test each dermatomal skin segment to identify possible loss of sensation.
- Identification of a specific dermatomal skin segment that has lost sensation will indicate the lesion level.
- For example, a loss of sensation on the *lateral* forearm and the lateral hand may result from C6 peripheral nerve loss.[1,2]

Complete Severance of a Peripheral Nerve

- A completely severed peripheral nerve results in a loss of sensation, motor control, and reflexes in the structures innervated by that specific peripheral nerve.[1,2]

Nerve Compression

- Nerve compression results in a loss of proprioception and discriminative touch.
- Pain and temperature initially remain intact. This occurs because compression of a nerve affects the large myelinated fibers first: the fibers that carry proprioceptive and discriminative touch information. There is initial relative sparing of the smaller fibers that carry pain and temperature.[3]
- When compression of a nerve occurs, sensory loss proceeds in the following order:
  - Conscious proprioception and discriminative touch
  - Cold
  - Fast pain or sharp pain
  - Heat
  - Slow pain or dull, diffuse, aching pain

When Compression Resolves

- When the compression is relieved, abnormal sensations called *paresthesias* occur as the blood supply increases.
- Paresthesias include burning, pricking, and tingling sensations.[4]
- After compression is resolved, sensation returns in the reverse order in which it was lost:
  - Slow pain or dull, diffuse, aching pain
  - Heat
  - Fast pain or sharp stinging sensations

Gutman SA. *Quick Reference Neuroscience for Rehabilitation Professionals: The Essential Neurologic Principles Underlying Rehabilitation Practice, Third Edition* (pp 170-179).
© 2017 Taylor & Francis Group.

- ○ Cold
- ○ Conscious proprioception and discriminative touch
- This process can be observed when one of the body's limbs "falls asleep" as a result of nerve compression.

Flaccidity

- When a peripheral nerve is injured, the muscles that are innervated by that nerve become flaccid and gradually atrophy. Flaccidity is reduced tone of a muscle, causing weakness or paralysis.
- Paralysis and loss of sensation occur just distal to the lesion.[5]

Schwann Cells

- Schwann cells are a type of glial cell that form myelin and produce nerve growth factor (NGF) in the peripheral nervous system (PNS).
- The production of NGF allows peripheral nerve damage in the PNS to resolve (unlike damage in the central nervous system [CNS]).
- Nerve regrowth occurs approximately 1 mm per day or 1 inch per month.
- A C6 peripheral nerve injury in the upper arm could take a year or more to fully regenerate.
- Compression injuries recover more quickly than complete severance of a nerve because damage is not as severe.[6]

Terminology of Sensory Pathology

Hypoesthesia
- A decrease in sensory *perception*. Also referred to as *hypesthesia*.[7]

Hyperesthesia
- An increase in sensory perception (eg, heightened perception of pain and temperature).[8]

Paresthesia
- The occurrence of unusual feelings such as pins and needles, tingling, and burning.[9]

Dysesthesia
- Unpleasant sensation, such as burning. *Causalgia* is an intense burning pain accompanied by trophic skin changes. Causalgia usually runs along the distribution of a nerve.[10]

Thermesthesia
- The ability to perceive temperature (hot and cold). Thermesthesia can also refer to a heightened sensitivity to heat.[11]

Thermohyperesthesia
- An increase in temperature perception (ie, hot and cold sensations become heightened).[11]

Thermohypoesthesia
- A decrease in temperature perception.[11]

Analgesia
- Loss of pain sensation.[12]

Hypalgesia
- A decrease in the ability to perceive pain.[12]

Hyperalgesia
- An increase in the ability to perceive pain (ie, pain sensation becomes heightened).[12]

Allodynia
- A condition in which an otherwise innocuous stimulus causes pain.[13]

Autonomic Dysfunction

- Autonomic dysfunction may result in vasomotor nerve disturbances.
- Vasomotor nerves are nerves that have muscular control over the blood vessel walls and control vasodilation and constriction of blood vessels.
- Autonomic trophic changes (also called *nutritional changes*) affect the skin, hair, and nails. The skin may become smooth and glossy, the nails can become thickened, and the hair on the denervated skin area thins or falls out.[14]

Complex Regional Pain Syndrome

- An example of autonomic dysfunction is complex regional pain syndrome (CRPS), also referred to as *reflex sympathetic dystrophy*. CRPS is a chronic neurovascular disease characterized by skin changes (eg, sweating, heightened sensitivity, changes in skin temperature, and redness), debilitating pain, edema, restricted movement, and muscle atrophy over time. Burning, stabbing, and throbbing sensations can make touch to the affected limb intolerable. There is currently no known etiology; however, the onset of CRPS can occur after injury or surgical procedure. Rehabilitation therapy to treat CRPS may include tactile sensitization (to help reduce pain through progressive exposure to intolerable sensations), progressive weightbearing activities, and remobilization of the limb in daily living activities. Mirror box therapy (in which the patient's brain interprets movement of the nonaffected limb as derived from the impaired side) has been shown to be beneficial. Drug therapies include antidepressants, anti-inflammatories, anticonvulsants, and local anesthetic injections.[15]

Brachial Plexus

- The brachial plexus is a network of peripheral spinal nerves including C5, C6, C7, C8, and T1.
- The nerves that supply the upper extremities emerge from the brachial plexus.
- The brachial plexus is a site of common compression syndromes:
  - Radial nerve compression can cause the following[16]:
    - Wrist and finger drop (compression of the radial nerve, causing an inability to extend the wrist and fingers)
    - Tennis elbow (chronic inflammation of the extensor muscles and tendons of the forearm at the lateral epicondyle of the elbow; also referred to as *lateral epicondylitis*)
    - Saturday night palsy (damage to the radial nerve from falling asleep with the axillary area of an arm draped over the edge of a bench compressing the radial nerve)
  - Median nerve compression can cause the following[17]:
    - Carpal tunnel syndrome (compression of the medial nerve as it travels through the carpal tunnel; symptoms include pain, numbness, and paresthesias of the thumb, index finger, third digit, and radial half of the fourth digit
  - Ulnar nerve compression can cause the following[18]:
    - Clawhand deformity (compression of the ulnar nerve resulting in hyperextension of the metacarpophalangeal joints of the fourth and fifth digits and flexion of the DIP and PIP joints of the fourth and fifth digits causing a claw-like appearance)
    - Cubital tunnel syndrome (impingement of the ulnar nerve as it travels through the cubital tunnel at the elbow medial edge; causes pain and paresthesias in the fourth and fifth digits)
    - Guyon canal syndrome (compression of the ulnar nerve as it travels through the Guyon canal in the wrist; causes pain, weakness, and paresthesias in the fourth and fifth digits)

Lumbar Plexus

- The lumbar plexus is a network of peripheral spinal nerves formed by L1 through L4.
- It is also a common site of compression syndromes:
  - Sciatic nerve compression can cause sciatica (compression of the sciatic nerve, usually on one side, causing radiating pain in the lumbosacral, buttock, leg, and foot regions, depending on severity).[19]
  - Peroneal nerve compression can cause foot drop (compression of the peroneal nerve, resulting in toe dragging or a steppage gait, in which the patient lifts his or her bent knees high enough to avoid dragging the foot).[20]

TYPES OF PERIPHERAL NEUROPATHY

Mononeuropathy

- Mononeuropathy involves damage to a single nerve.[21]
- It is usually due to compression or entrapment. Examples include the following:
  - *Wrist drop*: caused by radial nerve entrapment
  - *Foot drop*: caused by peroneal nerve entrapment

Radiculopathy

- Radiculopathy is a nerve root impingement that results from a lesion affecting the dorsal or ventral roots.
- Radiculopathy commonly results from herniated vertebral discs, degenerative disc disease, osteoarthritis, facet joint dysfunction, and spondylolisthesis.[22]

Plexopathy

- Plexopathy is caused by damage to one of the plexuses, brachial or lumbar, and involves multiple peripheral nerve damage.[23]

Polyneuropathy

- Polyneuropathy usually involves bilateral damage to more than one peripheral nerve.[24]
- Example: Stocking and glove polyneuropathy. Usually caused by a disease process such as diabetes
- With mild disease, only the distal lower extremities are involved.
- With more severe disease, the distal upper extremities are also involved.

DEEP TENDON REFLEXES

- When a peripheral neuropathy occurs, the individual often presents with an absence of distal deep tendon reflexes.
- An asymmetric decrease in deep tendon reflexes occurs in the following[25]:
  - Radiculopathy (nerve root impingement on one side)
  - Plexopathy (brachial or lumbar plexus involvement)
  - Mononeuropathy (unilateral spinal nerve injury)

POLYNEUROPATHY OF STOCKING AND GLOVE SYNDROME

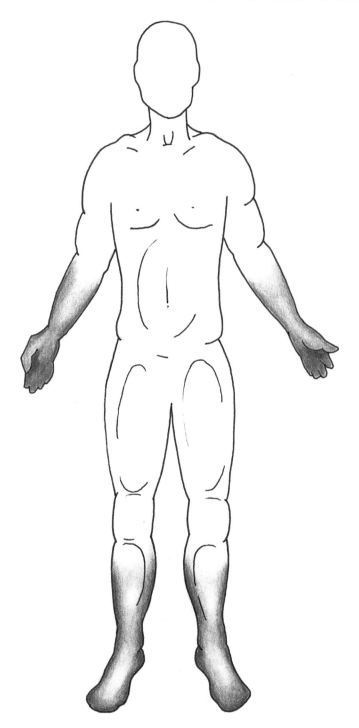

The blue indicates polyneuropathy involvement of the upper and lower extremities.

Neuropathies Caused by a Disease Process

Guillain-Barré Syndrome

- Guillain-Barré is an acute inflammatory polyradiculopathy.
- It is preceded by an infectious illness that usually resolves before the neurologic dysfunction becomes evident.
- The disease is characterized by edema and demyelination of peripheral spinal roots.
- Guillain-Barré involves progressive ascending muscular weakness of the limbs (as in stocking and glove neuropathy). This produces flaccid paralysis that has a symmetric pattern.
- Paresthesia and numbness often accompany motor function loss.
- Guillain-Barré also involves complete tendon areflexia.
- Autonomic nervous system (ANS) involvement can result in postural hypotension (when one rises from a horizontal position, blood pressure may drop to precariously low levels), arrhythmias, facial flushing, diarrhea, erectile dysfunction, urinary retention, and increased sweating.
- Although progress is commonly slow, most patients experience complete recovery.[26]

Diabetes Mellitus

- Diabetes mellitus is an endocrine disorder involving insulin deficiency or intolerance.
- Diabetic neuropathy is one of the most common complications of the disease process and affects at least 50% of patients with both type I and type II diabetes.
- While the exact mechanisms underlying diabetic neuropathy are unknown, damage to the peripheral nerves is thought to be a primary cause. This damage is mediated by inflammation and demyelination of large peripheral nerves, leaving smaller nerves intact. This results in lost inhibitory pain control from the spinal cord centers.
- Common symptoms include pain, numbness and tingling, and mild weakness, and diminished proprioception, vibration, and discriminative touch. Patients commonly report burning pain in the distal lower extremities (bilaterally).
- Polyneuropathies, mononeuropathies, plexopathies, and autonomic neuropathies can all occur in diabetes.
- Diabetes can be associated with abnormalities at any level of the PNS.
- Autonomic neuropathies involve the gastrointestinal, cardiovascular, and genitourinary systems.
- ANS involvement can result in postural hypotension, arrhythmias, facial flushing, diarrhea, erectile dysfunction, urinary retention, and increased sweating.
- In addition to pain and the loss of sensory and motor function, diabetic neuropathies can severely impair everyday function[27]:
  - Patients are at an increased risk for falls, due to the loss of sensation and position sense.
  - Burns and injuries to the feet are problematic, due to the loss of temperature and pain sensation.
  - Impaired vasomotor reflexes may result in dizziness and syncope (fainting) when the patient moves from a supine to standing position.
  - Urinary retention can increase the risk for bladder infection and renal complications.

PERIPHERAL NERVE INJURY AND REGENERATION PROCESS

Severed Axon

- When an axon is severed, the portion connected to the cell body is referred to as the *proximal segment*.
- The portion that is now disconnected from the cell body is called the *distal segment*.[28]

Leakage of Protoplasm

- Immediately after injury, protoplasm leaks out of each severed end, and the 2 segments retract away from each other.[28]

Wallerian Degeneration

- The distal segment undergoes a process called *Wallerian degeneration.*
- The myelin sheath pulls away from the distal segment.
- The distal segment swells and breaks into smaller segments.
- The axon terminals degenerate rapidly.
- The entire distal segment dies.
- Glial cells and microphages scavenge the area and clean up the debris from the degenerated distal segment.[29]

Central Chromatolysis

- Sometimes the cell body of the proximal segment undergoes degenerative changes called *central chromatolysis.* This may lead to cell death.
- Simultaneously, the postsynaptic *neuron,* no longer innervated by the presynaptic neuron, may also degenerate and die.[30]

Sprouting

- The regrowth of damaged axons is called *sprouting.*
- Sprouting takes 2 forms[31]:
    1. Collateral
    2. Regenerative

Collateral Sprouting

- Collateral sprouting occurs when a denervated postsynaptic neuron is re-innervated by branches of an intact axon located near the damaged axon.
- In other words, another neuron projects a collateral axon branch to the cell body of the postsynaptic neuron.[32]

Regenerative Sprouting

- Regenerative sprouting occurs when an axon and its postsynaptic neuron have both been damaged.
- The proximal segment of the damaged neuron projects side sprouts to form new synapses with other undamaged postsynaptic neurons.[33]

Functional Regeneration Occurs in the Peripheral Nervous System

- Regeneration of axons occurs primarily in the PNS.
- This is partly due to the production of NGF by Schwann cells.
- Schwann cells are the myelin around the PNS axons; Schwann cells do not exist in the CNS.
- Oligodendrites are the myelin cells that wrap around the CNS axons; oligodendrites do not produce NGF.
- There is little or no recovery in most areas of the CNS.[28]

Recovery Speed in the Periphery

- Regeneration of damaged axons in the PNS is slow: 1 mm of growth per day or 1 inch of recovery per month.
- A severed nerve in the upper arm, such as C6, will take at least a year to recover.[28]

Problems That Can Occur in the Nerve Regeneration Process

- Sometimes an axon will innervate a new postsynaptic neuron that is inappropriate.
- For example, after injury of a peripheral nerve, motor axons may innervate different muscles than before the injury.
- When the neuron fires, this results in unintended movements called *synkineses.*
- Synkineses are usually short-lived, as the person relearns muscle control.
- Similarly, in the sensory systems, innervation of a sensory receptor by axons that previously innervated a different type of sensory receptor can cause confusion of sensory modalities.[34]

SYNAPTIC CHANGES AFTER INJURY

Synaptic Effectiveness

- Local edema in the injured area causes compression of the presynaptic neuron's cell body or axon.
- When the edema is resolved, synaptic effectiveness returns.[28]

Denervation Hypersensitivity

- Denervation hypersensitivity occurs when the postsynaptic neuron of an injured presynaptic neuron becomes hypersensitized to its own neurotransmitter.
- This occurs because the postsynaptic neuron develops new receptor sites that can respond to neurotransmitters released by other nearby neurons.
- This occurs only for a short time and produces temporary muscle twitches and pain.[35]

Synaptic Hypereffectiveness

- Synaptic hypereffectiveness occurs when only some branches of a presynaptic axon are destroyed, leaving the majority of branches intact.
- The remaining axon branches receive all of the neurotransmitter substance that would normally be shared among only the terminal end branches.
- This results in a larger than normal amount of neurotransmitter being released onto postsynaptic receptors.[31]

Unmasking of Silent Synapses

- In the normal PNS, many synapses seem to be unused unless other pathways become injured.
- Unmasking of silent synapses occurs when previously unused synapses become active after other pathways have been damaged.[36]

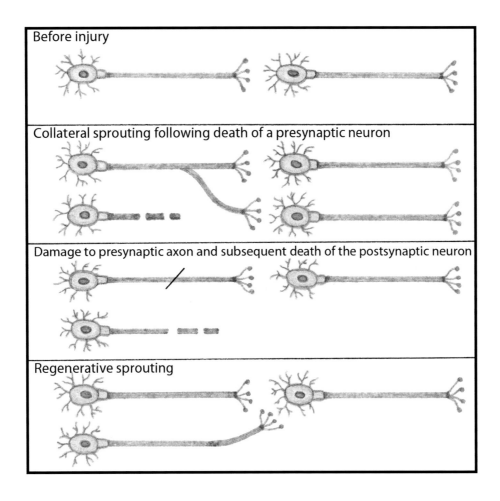

REFERENCES

1. Lee MWL, McPhee RW, Stringer MD. An evidence-based approach to human dermatomes. *Clin Anat.* 2008;21(5): 363-373. doi:10.1002/ca.20636.

2. Apok V, Gurusinghe NT, Mitchell JD, Emsley HCA. Dermatomes and dogma. *Pract Neurol.* 2011;11(2):100-105. doi:10.1136/jnnp.2011.242222.

3. Lundborg G, Dahlin LB. Anatomy, function, and pathophysiology of peripheral nerves and nerve compression. *Hand Clin.* 1996;12(2):185-193.

4. Grøvle L, Haugen AJ, Keller A, Natvig B, Brox JI, Grotle M. The bothersomeness of sciatica: patients' self-report of paresthesia, weakness and leg pain. *Eur Spine J.* 2010;19(2):263-269. doi:10.1007/s00586-009-1042-5.

5. Latronico N, Bolton CF. Critical illness polyneuropathy and myopathy: a major cause of muscle weakness and paralysis. *Lancet Neurol.* 2011;10(10):931-941. doi:10.1016/S1474-4422(11)70178-8.

6. Madduri S, Gander B. Schwann cell delivery of neurotrophic factors for peripheral nerve regeneration. *J Peripher Nerv Syst.* 2010;15(2):93-103. doi:10.1111/j.1529-8027.2010.00257.x.

7. Amanieu C, Hermier M, Peyron N, Chabrol A, Deiana G, Manera L. Hypoesthesia type sensory disorders. *Diagn Interv Imaging.* 2014;95(6):641-643. doi:10.1016/j.diii.2013.08.006.

8. Graven-Nielsen T, Wodehouse T, Langford RM, Arendt-Nielsen L, Kidd BL. Normalization of widespread hyperesthesia and facilitated spatial summation of deep-tissue pain in knee osteoarthritis patients after knee replacement. *Arthritis Rheum.* 2012;64(9):2907-2916. doi:10.1002/art.34466.

9. Ang CL, Foo LSS. Multiple locations of nerve compression: an unusual cause of persistent lower limb paresthesia. *J Foot Ankle Surg.* 2014;53(6):763-767. doi:10.1053/j.jfas.2014.06.013.

10. Landerholm ÅH, Hansson PT. Mechanisms of dynamic mechanical allodynia and dysesthesia in patients with peripheral and central neuropathic pain. *Eur J Pain.* 2011;15(5):498-503. doi:10.1016/j.ejpain.2010.10.003.

11. Coombes BK, Bisset L, Vicenzino B. Thermal hyperalgesia distinguishes those with severe pain and disability in unilateral lateral epicondylalgia. *Clin J Pain.* 2012;28(7):595-601. doi:10.1097/AJP.0b013e31823dd333.

12. Yates D. Pain: Reversing hyperalgesia. *Nat Rev Neurosci.* 2014;15(8):495-495. doi:10.1038/nrn3790.

13. Gangadharan V, Kuner R. Unravelling spinal circuits of pain and mechanical allodynia. *Neuron.* 2015;87(4):673-675. doi:10.1016/j.neuron.2015.08.013.

14. Low PA, Vernino S, Suarez, G. Autonomic dysfunction in peripheral nerve disease. *Muscle Nerve.* 2003;27(6):646-661. doi:10.1002/mus.10333.

15. Koh TT, Daly A, Howard W, Tan C, Hardidge A. Complex regional pain syndrome. *J Bone Joint Surg Rev.* 2014;2(7):e5. doi:10.2106/JBJS.RVW.M.00085.

16. Dang AC, Rodner CM. Unusual compression neuropathies of the forearm, part I: radial nerve. *J Hand Surg.* 2009;34(10):1906-1914. doi:10.1016/j.jhsa.2009.10.016.

17. Dang AC, Rodner CM. Unusual compression neuropathies of the forearm, part II: median nerve. *J Hand Surg.* 2009;34(10):1915-1920. doi:10.1016/j.jhsa.2009.10.017.

18. Elhassan B, Steinmann SP. Entrapment neuropathy of the ulnar nerve. *J Am Acad Orthop Surg.* 2007;15(11):672-681.

19. Ropper AH, Zafonte RD. Anatomy of the sciatic nerve. *N Engl J Med.* 2015;372:1240-1248. doi:10.1056/NEJMra1410151.

20. Myers RJ, Murdock EE, Farooqi M, Van Ness, G, Crawford DC. A unique case of common peroneal nerve entrapment. *Orthopedics.* 2015;38(7):e644-646. doi:10.3928/01477447-20150701-91.

21. Boon AJ, Harper CM. Ultrasound in the diagnosis of mononeuropathy: future directions. *Muscle Nerve.* 2011;44(6): 851-853. doi:10.1002/mus.22242.

22. Corey DL, Comeau D. Cervical radiculopathy. *Med Clin North Am.* 2014;98(4):791-799. doi:10.1016/j.mcna.2014.04.001.

23. Dyck PJB, Thaisetthawatkul P. Lumbosacral plexopathy. *Continuum (Minneap Minn).* 2014;20(5):1343-1358. doi:10.1212/01.CON.0000455877.60932.d3.

24. Kerasnoudis A, Pitarokoili K, Behrendt V, Gold R, Yoon MS. Nerve ultrasound score in distinguishing chronic from acute inflammatory demyelinating polyneuropathy. *Clin Neurophysiol.* 2014;125(3):635-641. doi:10.1016/j.clinph.2013.08.014.

25. Sharma KR, Saadia D, Facca AG, Resnick S, Ayyar DR. Diagnostic role of deep tendon reflex latency measurement in small-fiber neuropathy. *J Peripher Nerv Syst.* 2007;12(3):223-231. doi:10.1111/j.1529-8027.2007.00143.x.

26. van den Berg B, Walgaard C, Drenthen J, Fokke C, Jacobs BC, van Doorn PA. Guillain-Barre syndrome: pathogenesis, diagnosis, treatment and prognosis. *Nat Rev Neurol.* 2014;10(8):469-482. doi:10.1038/nrneurol.2014.121.

27. American Diabetes Association. Diagnosis and classification of diabetes mellitus. *Diabetes Care.* 2014;37(Suppl 1): S81-S90. doi:10.2337/dc14-S081.

28. Whalley K. Axon regeneration: splicing up repair mechanisms. *Nat Rev Neurosci.* 2015;16(7):374-375. doi:10.1038/nrn3981.

29. Conforti L, Gilley J, Coleman MP. Wallerian degeneration: an emerging axon death pathway linking injury and disease. *Nat Rev Neurosci.* 2014;15(6):394-409. doi:10.1038/nrn3680.

30. McIlwain DL, Hoke VB. The role of the cytoskeleton in cell body enlargement, increased nuclear eccentricity and chromatolysis in axotomized spinal motor neurons. *BMC Neurosci.* 2005;6(1):19. doi:10.1186/1471-2202-6-19.

31. Allodi I, Udina E, Navarro X. Specificity of peripheral nerve regeneration: interactions at the axon level. *Prog Neurobiol.* 2012;98(1):16-37. doi:10.1016/j.pneurobio.2012.05.005.

32. Koob JW, Moradzadeh A, Tong A, et al. Induction of regional collateral sprouting following muscle denervation. *Laryngoscope.* 2007;117(10):1735-1740. doi:10.1097/MLG.0b013e31812383af.

33. Cafferty WB, McGee AW, Strittmatter SM. Axonal growth therapeutics: regeneration or sprouting or plasticity? *Trends Neurosci.* 2008;31(5):215-220. doi:10.1016/j.tins.2008.02.004.

34. Pourmomeny AA, Zadmehre H, Mirshamsi M, Mahmodi Z. Prevention of synkinesis by biofeedback therapy: a randomized clinical trial. *Otol Neurotol.* 2014;35(4):739-742. doi:10.1097/MAO.0000000000000217.

35. Golder M, Burleigh DE, Belai A, et al. Smooth muscle cholinergic denervation hypersensitivity in diverticular disease. *Lancet.* 2003;361(9373):1945-1951. doi:10.1016/S0140-6736(03)13583-0.

36. Hanse E, Seth H, Riebe I. AMPA-silent synapses in brain development and pathology. *Nat Rev Neurosci.* 2013;14(12):839-850. doi:10.1038/nrn3642.

Phantom Limb Phenomenon

PHANTOM LIMB PHENOMENON

- Phantom limb phenomenon is the sensation that an amputated body part still remains.
- If the sensation is painful, it is called *phantom pain.*

Phantom Limb

- Any nonpainful sensation in the amputated limb[1]

Phantom Pain

- Painful sensations that seem to occur in the lost limb[2]

Stump Pain

- Painful sensations localized to the stump of an amputated body part[3]

Phantom Pain

- Phantom pain is a cortically generated phenomenon; there is no peripheral component.
- Phantom pain cannot be ended by nerve blocks because the mechanism of damage is not in the peripheral nervous system.
- Patients with phantom pain describe the pain as excruciating, sticking, cramping, burning, and squeezing.[4]

Phantom Pain and Phantom Limb Are Central Nervous System Phenomena

- Phantom pain is not mediated by peripheral nerve signals, as is stump pain.
- Phantom pain and phantom limb sensations are largely due to central nervous system phenomena.
- The cortical map of the body (the sensory and motor homunculi) still retains the anatomical image of the amputated body part.
- The brain believes that the amputated body part still remains.
- On transcranial magnetic stimulation (TMS), no change can be observed in the cortical map area after the amputation.[5]

Gutman SA. *Quick Reference Neuroscience for Rehabilitation Professionals: The Essential Neurologic Principles Underlying Rehabilitation Practice, Third Edition* (pp 180-186).
© 2017 Taylor & Francis Group.

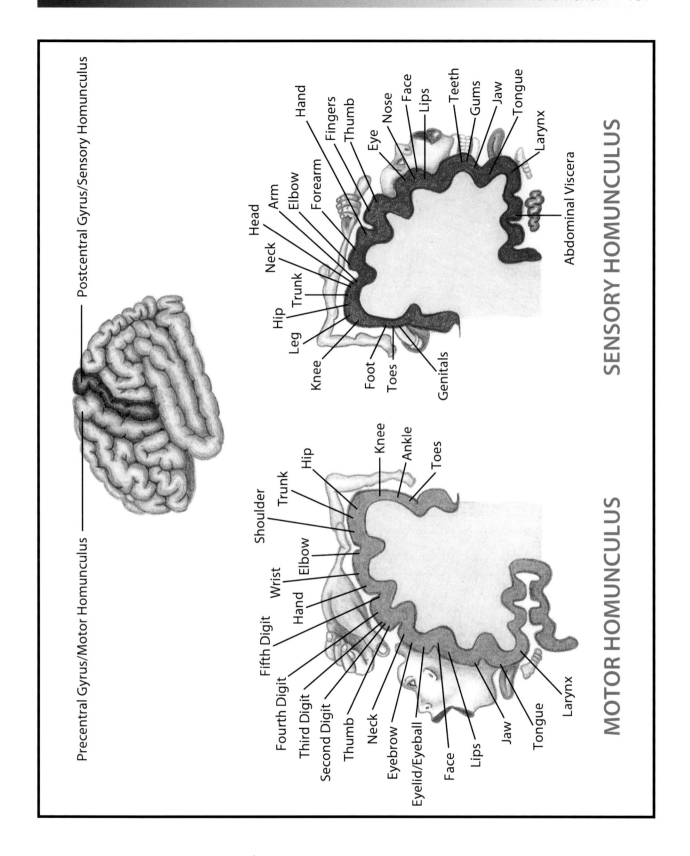

Precentral Gyrus/Motor Homunculus

Postcentral Gyrus/Sensory Homunculus

SENSORY HOMUNCULUS

Head
Neck
Arm
Elbow
Forearm
Hand
Fingers
Thumb
Eye
Nose
Face
Lips
Teeth
Gums
Jaw
Tongue
Larynx

Trunk
Hip
Leg
Knee
Foot
Toes
Genitals
Abdominal Viscera

MOTOR HOMUNCULUS

Shoulder
Trunk
Hip
Knee
Ankle
Toes

Fifth Digit
Fourth Digit
Third Digit
Second Digit
Thumb
Neck
Eyebrow
Eyelid/Eyeball
Face
Lips
Jaw
Tongue
Larynx

Wrist
Hand
Elbow

Phantom Sensations Lessen Over Time

- Other areas of the cortical map eventually appropriate the cortical region that once mediated sensation and movement of the amputated limb.
- At this time, TMS will show change in the cortical map.[6]

Phantom Limb Sensation Can Aid in Gait Training

- Patients with phantom sensations that are not painful report that they can use the phantom image to propel their prosthesis.
- Conversely, phantom pain interferes with gait training.[7]

Treatment of Phantom Pain

- Treatment for phantom pain is often ineffective.
- Transcutaneous electrical nerve stimulation works to a moderate degree.
- Vibration to the stump may work temporarily.
- Analgesics or painkillers work to a moderate degree and only temporarily.[8]

Phantom Limb Sensation Can Be Experienced in Spinal Cord Injuries

- The phantom limb sensation that people with spinal cord injury (SCI) experience tends to resolve quickly.
- Other areas of the cortical map appropriate the areas once used to mediate the paralyzed limbs.
- This may relate to the fact that in SCI, no peripheral stimulation can continue, as it might in an amputee who still retains some portion of the limb.[9]

Mirror Box

- Ramachandran and Rogers-Ramachandran have shown that, by using a mirrored box, the brain can be tricked into believing that the amputated limb is present again. The patient places his intact limb in a box with a mirror. The mirrored reflection of the intact limb appears as the amputated limb. The patient believes that he is looking down upon both his right and left hands and forearms, even though his left hand is actually amputated. When the patient is instructed to open and stretch his intact hand, it appears that the amputated hand is present and also stretching. The brain is tricked into perceiving that the amputated hand has responded to neural signals to open. Patients report that this phenomenon alleviates phantom limb pain and cramping in the amputated hand. Mirror box therapy has shown to be effective in the treatment of phantom limb pain.[10,11]

Phantom Limb Phenomena of the Hands and Feet

- Some patients with hand amputations report that if their amputated limb is touched, they experience the sensation of their face being touched.
- This phenomenon likely results from the organization of the sensory homunculus (ie, somatosensory cortex or primary somatosensory area [SS1]).
- On the somatosensory cortex, areas representing the face and hands are mapped next to each other.
- This organization may have formed in utero when the fetus's face and hands, and genitals and feet, lay next to each other in a fetal position.
- The topographical organization of the sensory homunculus then formed with these adjacent body parts mapped next to each other on SS1.
- When a hand is amputated, the contralateral area of the sensory homunculus representing the amputated hand becomes appropriated by adjacent areas of SS1 (ie, the face). This may account for the sensation of the face being touched when the amputated upper extremity limb is stimulated.
- Researchers have shown that when a prosthetic hand is grafted onto the amputated limb, the phenomenon often disappears.
- Therapists have also noted that techniques that enhance a patient's fine motor hand skills can often stimulate oral motor function. This, again, may result from the organization of the sensory homunculus.[12]

REFERENCES

1. Jerath R, Crawford MW, Jensen M. Etiology of phantom limb syndrome: insights from a 3D default space consciousness model. *Med Hypotheses.* 2015;85(2):153-159. doi:10.1016/j.mehy.2015.04.025.

2. Hommer DH, McCallin JP, Goff BJ. Advances in the treatment of phantom limb pain. *Curr Phys Med Rehabil Rep.* 2014;2(4):250-254. doi:10.1007/s40141-014-0062-1.

3. Mulvey MR, Bagnall AM, Marchant PR, Johnson MI. Transcutaneous electrical nerve stimulation (TENS) for phantom pain and stump pain following amputation in adults: an extended analysis of excluded studies from a Cochrane systematic review. *Phys Ther Rev.* 2014;19(4);234-244. doi:10.1179/1743288X13Y.0000000128.

4. Makin TR, Scholz J, Slater DH, Johansen-Berg H, Tracey I. Reassessing cortical reorganization in the primary sensorimotor cortex following arm amputation. *Brain.* 2015;138(8):2140-2146. doi:10.1093/brain/awv161.

5. Taub E, Uswatte G, Mark VW. The functional significance of cortical reorganization and the parallel development of CI therapy. *Front Hum Neurosci.* 2014;8:396. doi:10.3389/fnhum.2014.00396.

6. Lenggenhager B, Arnold CA, Giummarra MJ. Phantom limbs: pain, embodiment, and scientific advances in integrative therapies. *Wiley Interdiscip Rev Cogn Sci.* 2014;5(2):221-231. doi:10.1002/wcs.1277.

7. Sinha R, van den Heuvel WJ, Arokiasamy P. Adjustments to amputation and an artificial limb in lower limb amputees. *Prosthet Orthot Int.* 2014;38(2):115-121. doi:10.1177/0309364613489332.

8. Mulvey MR, Bagnall AM, Marchant PR, Johnson MI. Transcutaneous electrical nerve stimulation (TENS) for phantom pain and stump pain following amputation in adults: an extended analysis of excluded studies from a Cochrane systematic review. *Phys Ther Rev.* 2014;19(4):234-244. doi:10.1179/1743288X13Y.0000000128.

9. Fuentes CT, Pazzaglia M, Longo MR, Scivoletto G, Haggard P. Body image distortions following spinal cord injury. *J Neurol Neurosurg Psychiatry.* 2013;84(2):201-207. doi:10.1136/jnnp-2012-304001.

10. Miller C, Seckel E, Ramachandran VS. Using mirror box therapy to treat phantom pain in Haitian earthquake victims. *J Vision.* 2012;12(9):1323-1323. doi:10.1167/12.9.1323.

11. Ramachandran VS, Rogers-Ramachandran D. Synaesthesia in phantom limbs induced with mirrors. *Proc R Soc Lond B Biol Sci.* 1996;263(1369):377-386. doi:10.1098/rspb.1996.0058.

12. Weiss T, Miltner WH, Adler T, Brückner L, Taub E. Decrease in phantom limb pain associated with prosthesis-induced increased use of an amputation stump in humans. *Neurosci Lett.* 1999;272(2):131-134. doi:10.1016/S0304-3940(99)00595-9.

CLINICAL TEST QUESTIONS

Sections 15 to 17

1. Mr. Nunez has chronic pain in his lumbar section after a fall from a ladder. The therapist applies electrical stimulation through conductive gel pads placed on the identified painful region. This procedure is referred to as:
   a. cryotherapy
   b. hydrotherapy
   c. transcutaneous electrical nerve stimulation
   d. fluidotherapy

2. Ms. Lehmann has chronic neck and back pain with an unknown origin. She is learning to manage her pain by consciously becoming aware of and modifying the tension in and position of her muscles and joints based on feedback from an instrument that measures physiological functions such as muscular tension. This is referred to as:
   a. stress management and visualization
   b. biofeedback
   c. nerve blocks
   d. acupuncture

3. Sophia has chronic pain and tenderness throughout her neck, back, shoulders, and legs. She also reports extreme fatigue, sleep dysfunction, common headaches, and periods of cognitive fog. Sophia's physicians cannot find an anatomical cause of her pain. Patients with this condition are also likely to be diagnosed with chronic fatigue syndrome, rheumatoid arthritis, Lyme disease, and irritable bowel syndrome. This condition is known as:
   a. lupus
   b. myasthenia gravis
   c. Epstein-Barr virus
   d. fibromyalgia

4. Mr. Shibata has intense burning that extends down both legs. This condition is called _____ and is a form of _____.
   a. causalgia; dysesthesia
   b. thermohypoesthesia; thermesthesia
   c. paresthesia; hyperalgesia
   d. allodynia; hyperalgesia

5. After a soccer injury in which 16-year-old Tommy injured his left shoulder and arm, he developed a chronic neurovascular disease characterized by debilitating pain, edema, restricted movement, and muscular atrophy in his left upper extremity. Tommy also experiences burning, stabbing, and throbbing sensations that make touch to his left upper extremity intolerable. This syndrome is called:
   a. fibromyalgia syndrome
   b. causalgia
   c. stocking and glove syndrome
   d. complex regional pain syndrome

6. Mr. Zimmerman has foot drop and a steppage gait in which he lifts his right bent knee high enough to avoid dragging his foot. Compression of which nerve results in foot drop?
   a. sciatic nerve
   b. peroneal nerve
   c. ulnar nerve

7. After an acute infectious illness, Mr. Benfenati has developed a progressive ascending muscular weakness in his limbs (flaccid paralysis occurs first in his lower extremities and progresses to his upper extremities), with a symmetric pattern. He also reports paresthesias and numbness in his distal extremities. After 1 month, Mr. Benfenati experiences a complete recovery. This disease process is called:
   a. diabetes neuropathy
   b. poliomyelitis
   c. Guillain-Barré syndrome
   d. myasthenia gravis

8. Mr. Kaminski, who has diabetes, presents with weakness, numbness, paresthesia, and causalgia in his lower and upper extremities. He reports that this condition first developed bilaterally in his feet and legs, and then progressed to both hands and arms. This type of peripheral neuropathy is called _____ and results from _____.
   a. plexopathy; damage to the brachial or lumbar plexus
   b. radiculopathy; nerve root impingement
   c. polyneuropathy; bilateral damage to multiple peripheral nerves
   d. mononeuropathy; damage to one peripheral nerve

9. Mr. Kaminski, in the above question, was diagnosed with:
   a. stocking and glove neuropathy
   b. radial nerve compression
   c. sciatic nerve compression
   d. reflex sympathetic dystrophy

10. After his below-the-knee amputation, Bill reports that he can still feel his lower left leg and foot. The phenomenon of phantom limb sensation is likely caused by which of the following:
    a. peripheral damage to the nerves that were surgically severed during amputation.
    b. the formation of nerve fibromas in the residual limb of the amputated body part.
    c. the cortical map of the body (homunculus) still retains the anatomical image of the amputated body part.

Answers

1. c
2. b
3. d
4. a
5. d
6. b
7. c
8. c
9. a
10. c

Spinal Cord Tracts

REVIEW OF SPINAL CORD ANATOMY

- There are 31 pairs of spinal nerves[1-5]:
  - 8 cervical
  - 12 thoracic
  - 5 lumbar
  - 5 sacral
  - 1 coccygeal

ASCENDING SPINAL NERVES

- Ascending spinal nerves carry sensory information from the periphery (beginning with a sensory receptor) to the spinal cord (SC).
- The sensory spinal nerves enter the SC through the dorsal root and rootlets (in the peripheral nervous system [PNS]).
- Once in the dorsal horn (in the central nervous system [CNS]), the spinal nerves synapse with an interneuron.
- The interneuron synapses with an ascending sensory SC tract (in the CNS).[1-5]

ASCENDING SPINAL CORD TRACTS

- Ascending SC tracts carry the sensory information up the SC, to the brainstem, thalamus, and cortex.
- Some sensory SC tracts carry sensory information from the brainstem to the cerebellum.[1-5]

DESCENDING SPINAL CORD TRACTS

- Descending SC tracts carry motor information from the cortex, through the internal capsule, thalamus, and brainstem, to the SC (in the CNS).
- Some motor SC tracts originate in the cerebellum and brainstem.
- When descending motor SC tracts are ready to exit the cord, they synapse on an interneuron in the ventral horn of the SC.
- The interneuron then synapses on a motor neuron in the ventral horn (in the PNS).
- The motor neuron in the ventral horn synapses on a descending motor spinal nerve and exits the cord through the ventral rootlets and root (in the PNS).
- The motor spinal nerve then travels to a target muscle in the PNS.[1-5]

SPINAL CORD TRACT NAMES

- SC tract names indicate the tract's place of origin and destination.

Gutman SA. *Quick Reference Neuroscience for Rehabilitation Professionals: The Essential Neurologic Principles Underlying Rehabilitation Practice, Third Edition* (pp 188-219).
© 2017 Taylor & Francis Group.

ASCENDING SENSORY SPINAL CORD TRACTS

- Dorsal columns
- Lateral spinothalamic
- Anterior spinothalamic
- Posterior spinocerebellar
- Anterior spinocerebellar
- Cuneocerebellar
- Rostral spinocerebellar

CORTICALLY ORIGINATED DESCENDING MOTOR TRACTS

- Lateral corticospinal
- Anterior corticospinal
- Corticobulbar

MIXED PATHWAYS ORIGINATING IN THE BRAINSTEM

- Medial longitudinal fasciculus (MLF)

DESCENDING MOTOR TRACTS ORIGINATING IN THE BRAINSTEM

- Vestibulospinal
- Rubrospinal
- Medullary reticulospinal
- Pontine reticulospinal

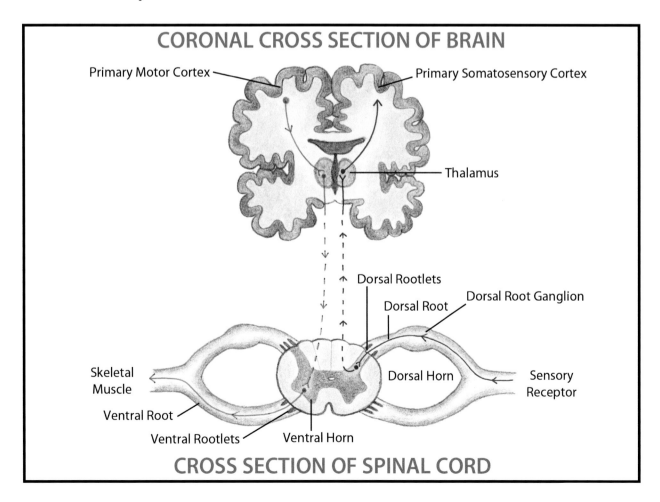

CORONAL CROSS SECTION OF BRAIN

CROSS SECTION OF SPINAL CORD

Ascending Sensory Spinal Cord Tracts

Dorsal Columns (also called *Medial Lemniscus* or *Posterior Columns*)[1-5]

- Believed to be a newer tract phylogenetically.

Function

- Carries conscious sensory information to the cortex regarding the following:
  - Discriminative touch
  - Pressure
  - Vibration
  - Proprioception
  - Kinesthesia

Origin

- Fasciculus gracilis and fasciculus cuneatus (in the dorsal root)

Decussation (Where the Tracts Cross)

- Caudal medulla level

Destination

- Postcentral gyrus (primary somatosensory area [SS1])

Pathway

- Skin receptors in the PNS send sensory information along the peripheral spinal nerves.
- The sensory spinal nerves travel through the dorsal root and rootlets (still in the PNS) (first order neuron).
- The spinal nerves then synapse on an interneuron in the dorsal horn of the SC (in the CNS).
- The interneuron then synapses on the cell bodies of the dorsal horn and ascends through the fasciculus gracilis and cuneatus in the dorsal columns (second order neuron).
- The dorsal column tract is considered to originate when the interneuron reaches the caudal medulla and synapses with the nucleus gracilis and cuneatus. At this point, the dorsal column tract decussates across the midline of the caudal medulla to the medial lemniscus.
- The tract ascends through the SC, brainstem, thalamus, and internal capsule and synapses in the postcentral gyrus (third order neuron).

Lesions

- Complete severance of the SC
  - *Bilateral loss of sensation*: discriminative touch, pressure, vibration, proprioception, and kinesthesia (below the severed cord level)
- A hemilesion (on one side of the SC) below the decussation
  - Ipsilateral loss
  - Example: If the right SC is severed at T1, right-sided sensory loss results.
- A hemilesion in the brainstem (above the medulla level)
  - Contralateral sensory loss
- A lesion in the cortex
  - Contralateral sensory loss

DORSAL COLUMNS

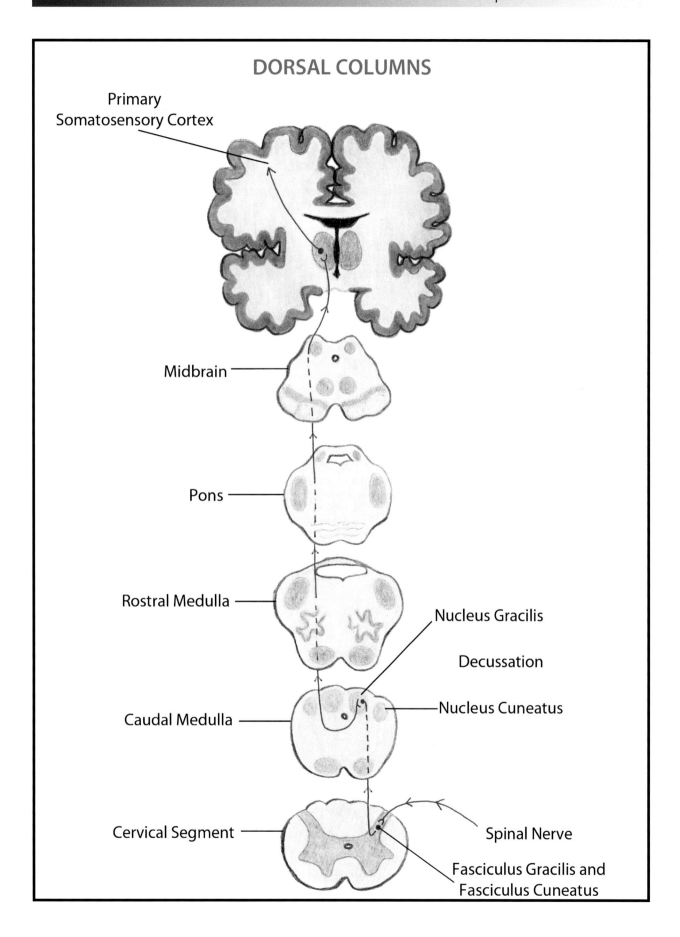

Primary Somatosensory Cortex

Midbrain

Pons

Rostral Medulla

Nucleus Gracilis

Decussation

Caudal Medulla

Nucleus Cuneatus

Cervical Segment

Spinal Nerve

Fasciculus Gracilis and Fasciculus Cuneatus

Lateral Spinothalamic Tract[1-5]

- Joins the dorsal column at the level of the pons

Function

- Carries conscious sensory information to the cortex regarding pain and temperature

Origin

- Nucleus proprius (in the dorsal horn)

Decussation

- SC level (crosses as soon as the spinal nerve enters the cord and synapses on the tract)

Destination

- Postcentral gyrus (SS1)

Pathway

- Skin receptors in the PNS send sensory information along peripheral sensory spinal nerves.
- The sensory spinal nerves travel through the dorsal root and rootlets (in the PNS) and enter the dorsal horn (in the CNS) (first order neuron).
- Once in the dorsal horn, the spinal nerves synapse on an interneuron that joins to the cell bodies of the lateral spinothalamic tract. This occurs in the nucleus proprius of the dorsal horn (second order neuron).
- The lateral spinothalamic tract crosses the midline as soon as it synapses in the dorsal horn. The tract then travels to the anterior white funiculus.
- From the anterior white funiculus, the tract travels to the lateral white funiculus and ascends up the SC.
- The tract joins the dorsal column in the pons and continues to ascend to the thalamus and internal capsule, and finally synapses in the postcentral gyrus in the cortex (third order neuron).

Lesions

- Complete severance of the SC
  - *Bilateral loss of sensation*: pain and temperature (below the severed cord level)
- A hemilesion (on one side of the cord) in the SC
  - *At the lesion level*: bilateral sensory loss
  - *Below the lesion level*: contralateral sensory loss
- A hemilesion (on one side) of the brainstem
  - Contralateral sensory loss
- A unilateral lesion in the postcentral gyrus
  - Contralateral sensory loss

LATERAL SPINOTHALAMIC TRACT

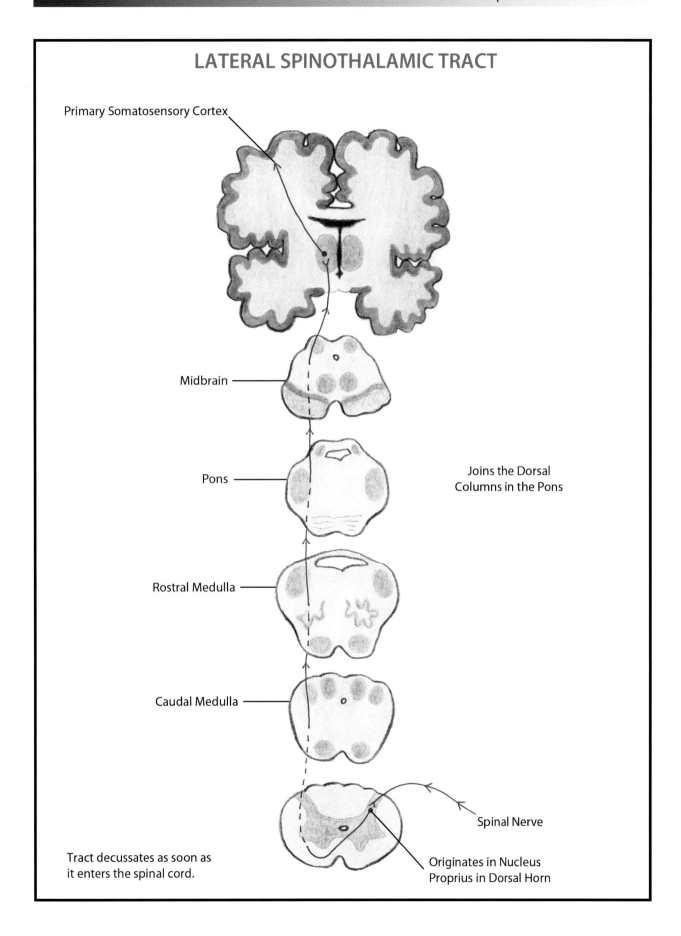

Primary Somatosensory Cortex

Midbrain

Pons

Joins the Dorsal
Columns in the Pons

Rostral Medulla

Caudal Medulla

Spinal Nerve

Tract decussates as soon as
it enters the spinal cord.

Originates in Nucleus
Proprius in Dorsal Horn

Anterior Spinothalamic Tract[1-5]

Function

- Carries conscious sensory information to the cortex regarding the following:
  - Crude touch, light touch
  - Some researchers believe that this tract may carry pain and temperature if the lateral spinothalamic tract is damaged.

Origin

- Nucleus proprius (in the dorsal horn)

Decussation

- SC level
- The tract crosses the midline as soon as spinal nerves have synapsed on its cell bodies in the dorsal horn.

Destination

- Postcentral gyrus (SS1)

Pathway

- Skin receptors in the PNS send sensory messages along the ascending sensory spinal nerves to the dorsal root and rootlets (first order neuron).
- The sensory spinal nerves synapse on an interneuron in the dorsal horn (specifically in the nucleus proprius) (second order neuron).
- The interneuron then synapses on the cell bodies of the ascending spinothalamic tract.
- At this time, the tract crosses the midline of the SC, travels to the ventral white funiculus, and begins to ascend.
- As it ascends, the tract travels through the posterolateral funiculus and eventually joins the lateral spinothalamic tract in the medulla.
- The tract ascends through the brainstem, thalamus, and internal capsule to the SS1 (third order neuron).

Lesions

- Complete severance of the SC
  - *Bilateral loss of sensation*: crude and light touch (below the severed cord level)
- A hemilesion (on one side) of the SC
  - *At the lesion level*: bilateral sensory loss
  - *Below the lesion level*: contralateral sensory loss
- A hemilesion (on one side) of the brainstem
  - Contralateral sensory loss
- A unilateral lesion in the postcentral gyrus
  - Contralateral sensory loss

ANTERIOR SPINOTHALAMIC TRACT

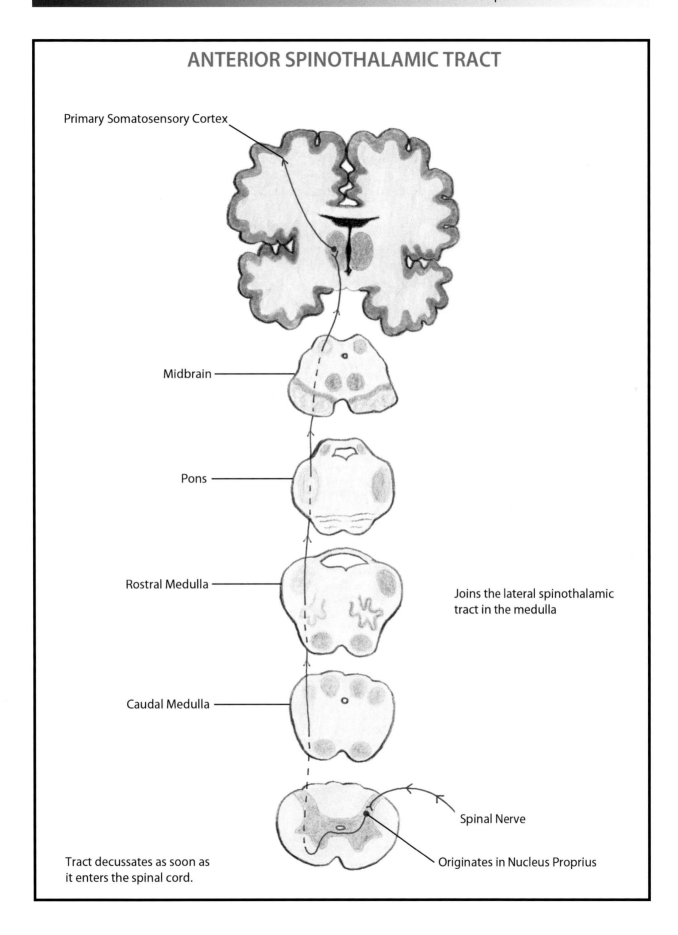

Primary Somatosensory Cortex

Midbrain

Pons

Rostral Medulla

Joins the lateral spinothalamic tract in the medulla

Caudal Medulla

Spinal Nerve

Originates in Nucleus Proprius

Tract decussates as soon as it enters the spinal cord.

Posterior Spinocerebellar Tract[1-5]

Function

- Carries unconscious sensory information from the lower extremities to the cerebellum regarding the following:
  - Proprioception:
    - Pressure and tension of skeletal muscles
    - Coordination of motoric movement of individual muscles
- Carries sensory information from the muscle spindles (MS), Golgi tendon organs (GTO), and joint receptors in the PNS.
- This information never reaches the cortex for conscious detection and interpretation.

Origin

- Clarke column in the dorsal horn in SC levels T6 and below (because this tract serves the lower extremities)
- The Clarke column contains the lower extremity proprioceptive and kinesthetic inputs.

Decussation

- None. This is an ipsilateral tract that does not cross.

Destination

- Cerebellum

Pathway

- The MSs, GTOs, and joint receptors in the PNS send proprioceptive information along the ascending sensory spinal nerves to the dorsal root and rootlets (first order neuron).
- The sensory spinal nerves then synapse on an interneuron in the dorsal horn (specifically in the Clarke column) (second order neuron).
- The interneuron joins to the cell bodies of the posterior spinocerebellar tract in the dorsal horn, and the tract begins to ascend up the posterolateral funiculus on the ipsilateral side.
- The tract ascends through the medulla to the inferior cerebellar peduncle.
- From the inferior cerebellar peduncle, the tract synapses in the cerebellum.

Lesions

- All lesions are ipsilateral because the tract does not decussate.

POSTERIOR SPINOCEREBELLAR TRACT

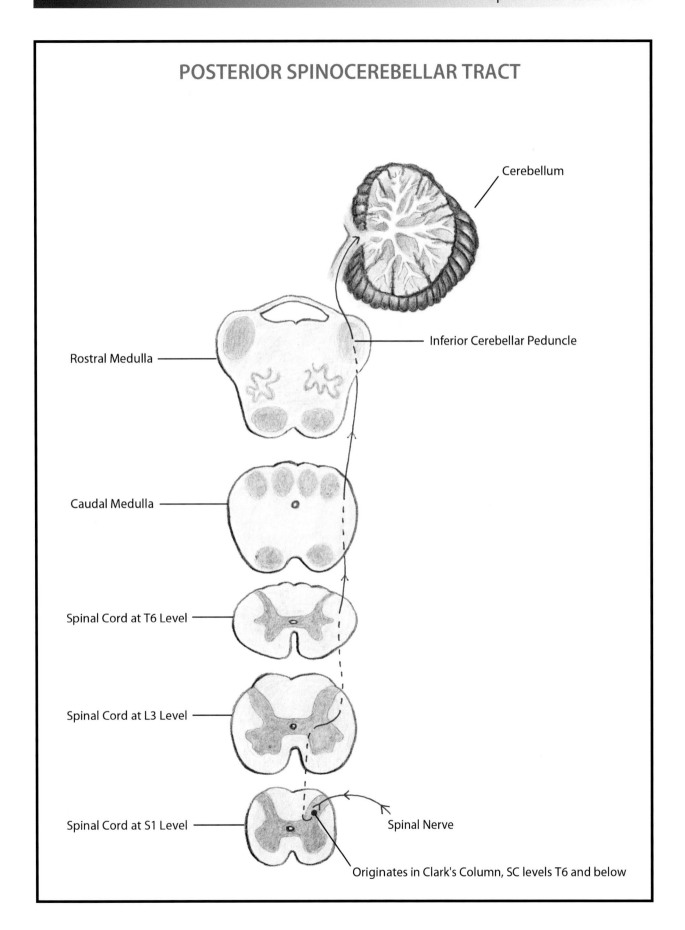

Cerebellum

Inferior Cerebellar Peduncle

Rostral Medulla

Caudal Medulla

Spinal Cord at T6 Level

Spinal Cord at L3 Level

Spinal Cord at S1 Level

Spinal Nerve

Originates in Clark's Column, SC levels T6 and below

Anterior Spinocerebellar Tract[1-5]

Function

- Carries unconscious sensory information from the lower extremities to the cerebellum regarding the following:
  - Proprioception:
    - ◆ Pressure and tension of skeletal muscles
    - ◆ Coordination of posture and movement of limbs (not individual muscles, as in the posterior spinocerebellar tract)
- Carries sensory information from the MSs, GTOs, and joint receptors to the cerebellum

Origin

- Nucleus proprius in the dorsal horn of the lumbar sections (because the tract serves the lower extremities)

Decussation

- SC level in the lumbar sections
- The tract decussates as soon as the spinal nerves synapse on the cell bodies of the anterior spinocerebellar tract.

Destination

- Cerebellum

Pathway

- The MSs, GTOs, and joint receptors in the PNS send proprioceptive information along the ascending sensory spinal nerves to the dorsal root and rootlets.
- The sensory spinal nerves synapse on an interneuron in the dorsal horn (specifically the nucleus proprius) (first order neuron).
- The interneuron then synapses on the cell bodies of the anterior spinocerebellar tract in the dorsal horn, and the tract then decussates across the midline to the anterior white funiculus (second order neuron).
- The tract begins to ascend in the lateral white funiculus and travels to the superior cerebellar peduncle in the pons.
- From the superior cerebellar peduncle, the tract synapses in the cerebellum. Most fibers cross back to the ipsilateral cerebellum.

Lesions

- Complete severance of the SC
  - *Bilateral loss of proprioception*: from the lower extremities
- A hemilesion (on one side) of the SC
  - *At the lesion level*: bilateral proprioceptive loss
  - *Below the lesion level*: contralateral proprioceptive loss
- A lesion in the superior cerebellar peduncle
  - Contralateral proprioceptive loss
- A lesion in one hemisphere of the cerebellum
  - Ipsilateral proprioceptive loss

ANTERIOR SPINOCEREBELLAR TRACT

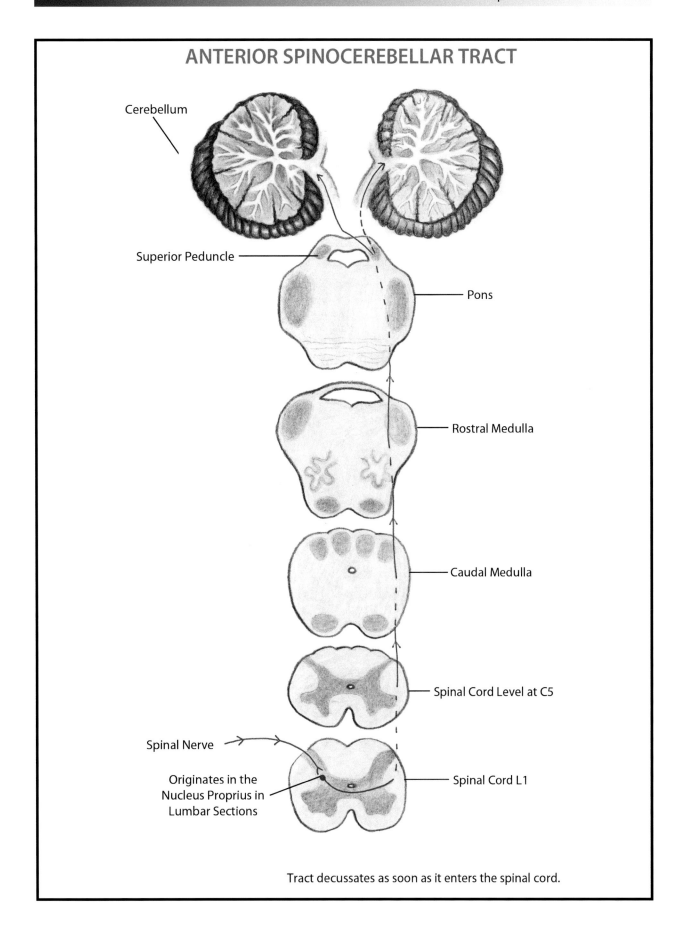

Cerebellum

Superior Peduncle

Pons

Rostral Medulla

Caudal Medulla

Spinal Cord Level at C5

Spinal Nerve

Originates in the
Nucleus Proprius in
Lumbar Sections

Spinal Cord L1

Tract decussates as soon as it enters the spinal cord.

Cuneocerebellar Tract[1-5]

Function

- Carries unconscious sensory information from the trunk and upper extremities to the cerebellum regarding the following:
  - Proprioception:
    - Pressure and tension of skeletal muscles
    - Coordination of motoric movement of individual muscles
- Carries sensory information from the MSs, GTOs, and the joint receptors to the cerebellum.

Origin

- Nucleus cuneatus in the dorsal horn of the SC of T6 and above (because the tract serves the upper extremities)

Decussation

- None. This is an ipsilateral tract that does not cross.

Destination

- Cerebellum

Pathway

- The MSs, GTOs, and joint receptors in the PNS send proprioceptive information along the ascending sensory spinal nerves to the dorsal root and rootlets of T6 and above (first order neuron).
- The sensory spinal nerves synapse on an interneuron in the dorsal horn (specifically in the nucleus cuneatus).
- The interneuron then synapses with the cell bodies of the cuneocerebellar tract in the dorsal horn (second order neuron).
- The tract begins to ascend in the posterolateral white funiculus and travels to the inferior cerebellar peduncle in the medulla.
- From the inferior cerebellar peduncle, the tract synapses in the cerebellum.

Lesions

- All lesions are ipsilateral because the tract does not decussate.

Bilateral Representation of Unconscious Proprioception

- The below 2 sets of tracts provide bilateral representation of unconscious proprioceptive information to the cerebellum.
  1. Proprioception from the lower extremities:
     - Posterior spinocerebellar
     - Anterior spinocerebellar
  2. Proprioception from the trunk and upper extremities:
     - Cuneocerebellar
     - Rostral cerebellar
- If one tract of each set is lost, the other will still send proprioceptive information to the cerebellum. An individual will not lose unconscious proprioceptive information from the upper or lower extremities unless both tracts within a set are lost.

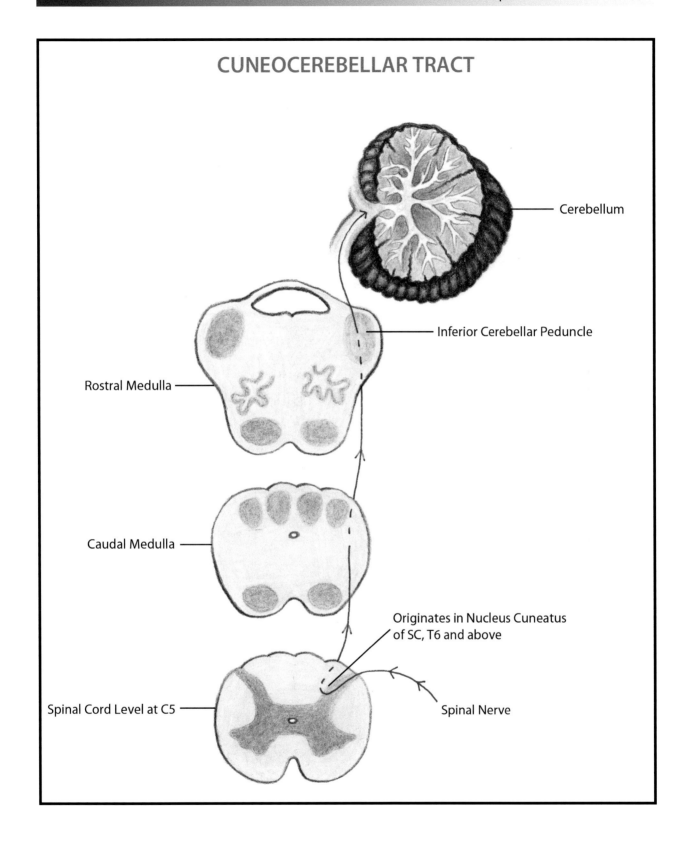

CUNEOCEREBELLAR TRACT

Cerebellum

Inferior Cerebellar Peduncle

Rostral Medulla

Caudal Medulla

Originates in Nucleus Cuneatus
of SC, T6 and above

Spinal Cord Level at C5

Spinal Nerve

Rostral Spinocerebellar Tract[1-5]

Function

- Carries unconscious sensory information from the trunk and upper extremities to the cerebellum regarding the following:
  ○ Proprioception:
    ◆ Pressure and tension of skeletal muscles
    ◆ Coordination of posture and movements of limbs
- Carries sensory information from the MSs, GTOs, and joint receptors to the cerebellum

Origin

- Ventrolateral gray of the SC in the cervical levels (because the tract serves the upper extremities)

Decussation

- None. This is an ipsilateral tract that does not cross.

Destination

- Cerebellum

Pathway

- The MSs, GTOs, and joint receptors in the PNS send proprioceptive information along the ascending sensory spinal nerves to the dorsal root and rootlets of the cervical levels (first order neuron).
- The sensory spinal nerves enter the dorsal horn of the SC and synapse in the ventrolateral gray on an interneuron.
- The interneuron then synapses on the cell bodies of the rostral spinocerebellar tract, and the tract begins to ascend up the lateral white funiculus (second order neuron).
- The tract joins the anterior spinocerebellar tract in the lateral white funiculus.
- The tract then ascends to either the inferior cerebellar peduncle or the superior cerebellar peduncle.
- From one of these peduncles, the tract then synapses in the cerebellum.

Lesions

- All lesions are ipsilateral.

ROSTRAL SPINOCEREBELLAR TRACT

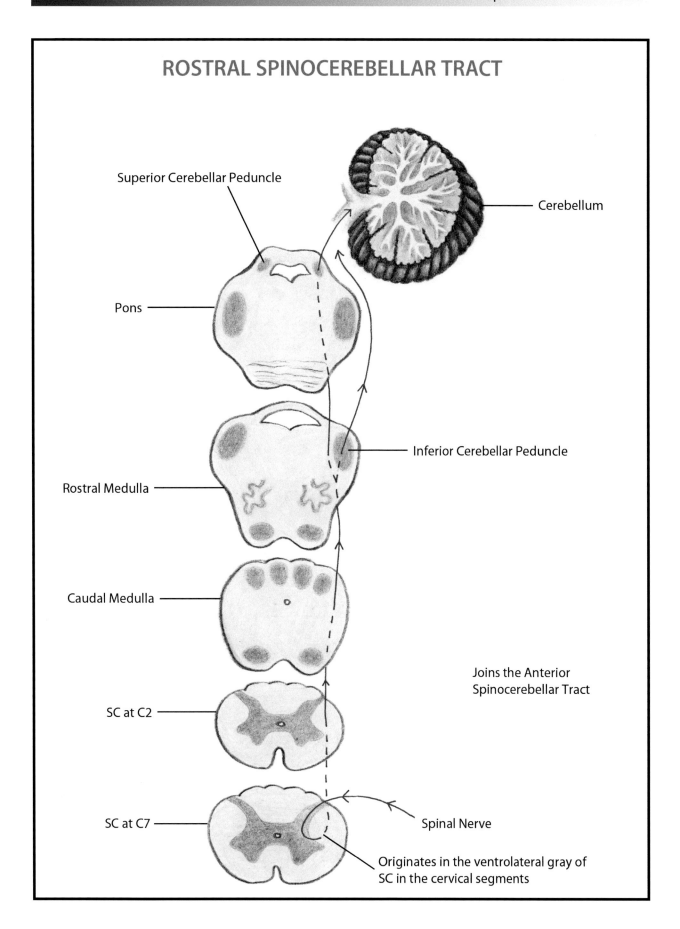

Superior Cerebellar Peduncle

Cerebellum

Pons

Inferior Cerebellar Peduncle

Rostral Medulla

Caudal Medulla

Joins the Anterior
Spinocerebellar Tract

SC at C2

SC at C7

Spinal Nerve

Originates in the ventrolateral gray of
SC in the cervical segments

CORTICALLY ORIGINATED DESCENDING MOTOR TRACTS

Lateral and Anterior Corticospinal Tracts[1-5]

Part of the Pyramidal System

- The lateral and anterior corticospinal tracts are descending motor tracts that travel through the pyramids of the medulla.
- The lateral corticospinal tract decussates at the pyramidal decussation; the anterior corticospinal tract remains ipsilateral and descends through the pyramids.
- These tracts are considered to be upper motor neurons (UMNs) in the CNS.

Function

- Carry conscious/voluntary motor information from the precentral gyrus (primary motor area [M1]) up to, but not including, the ventral horn.
- The tracts then synapse on motor spinal nerves (in the ventral horn) that innervate skeletal muscles.

Origin

- Precentral gyrus (M1)

Decussation

- *Lateral corticospinal tract*: Decussates in the pyramidal decussation of the medulla
- *Anterior corticospinal tract*: Does not decussate

Destination

- Synapses on an interneuron in the ventral horn.
- This interneuron then synapses on the motor neurons of the motor spinal nerves that innervate skeletal muscles in the PNS.

Pathway

- The cell bodies of the tract are located in the precentral gyrus. They send descending motor signals through the internal capsule, thalamus, and brainstem (first order neuron).
- In the brainstem (at the medulla level), the tract separates into the lateral and anterior corticospinal tracts (second order neuron).
- The lateral corticospinal tract (90% of the original tract before separation) decussates in the pyramidal decussation in the medulla.
- The anterior corticospinal tract (10% of the original tract before separation) remains ipsilateral and continues to descend through the pyramids.
- When the tract is ready to exit the cord, it synapses on an interneuron in the ventrolateral gray of the SC (third order neuron).
- The interneuron then synapses on a motor neuron (in the ventral horn) that innervates a descending motor spinal nerve.
- The motor spinal nerve then exits through the ventral rootlets and root and travels to a target skeletal muscle in the PNS.

Lesions

- A lesion in M1 (in one hemisphere)
  - Contralateral loss of voluntary muscle movement (because 90% of the tract decussates)
  - Spasticity of the distal musculature below the lesion level (UMN damage)
  - Hyperactive reflexes
- A lesion in the internal capsule
  - Contralateral spastic paralysis
  - Hyperactive reflexes
- A unilateral lesion in the brainstem above the decussation
  - Contralateral spastic paralysis

LATERAL AND ANTERIOR CORTICOSPINAL TRACTS

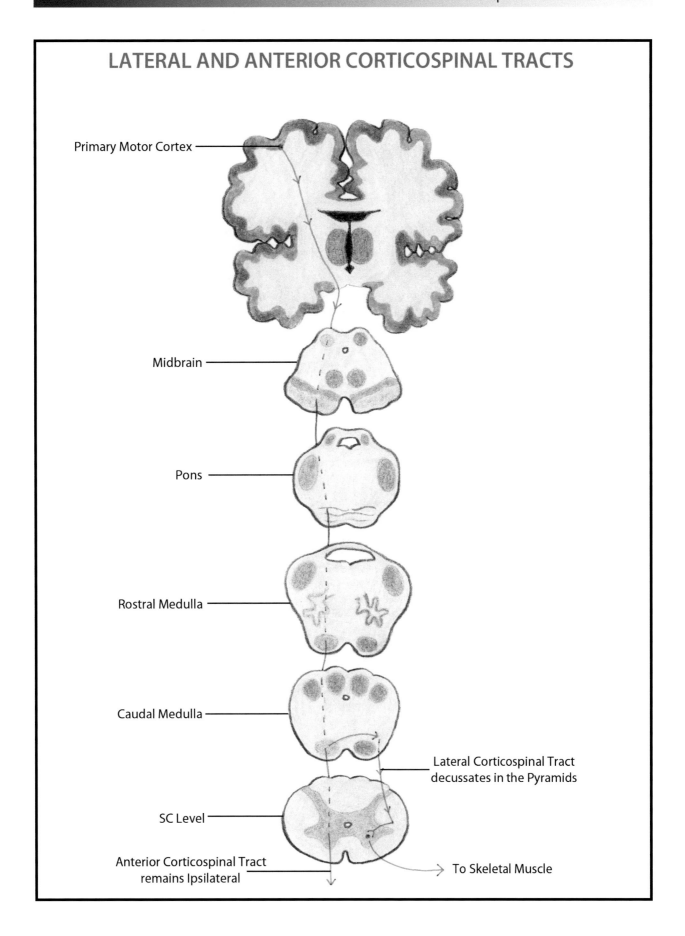

Primary Motor Cortex

Midbrain

Pons

Rostral Medulla

Caudal Medulla

Lateral Corticospinal Tract decussates in the Pyramids

SC Level

Anterior Corticospinal Tract remains Ipsilateral

To Skeletal Muscle

- A unilateral lesion in the SC below the decussation
  - Ipsilateral loss of voluntary motor control
  - Spasticity in the distal musculature (below the lesion level)
  - Flaccidity (at the lesion level)
  - Hyperactive reflexes
- A complete severance of the SC below the decussation
  - Bilateral loss of voluntary motor control
  - Spasticity below the lesion level
  - Flaccidity at the lesion level

Decorticate Rigidity

- Damage to the corticospinal tracts will result in decorticate rigidity.
- In decorticate rigidity:
  - The upper extremities are in a spastic flexed position.
  - The lower extremities are in a spastic extended position.
- Decorticate rigidity occurs because the corticospinal tracts fire without modification from the cortex.
- The rigidity that presents is more accurately described as spasticity, as it is derived from dysfunction of the pyramidal system and is characterized by increased tone on only one side of the joint rather than both.

Corticobulbar Tract

Pathway

- The corticobulbar tract descends from the corticospinal tract and projects to certain cranial nerve (CN) nuclei that have a motor component:
  - In the midbrain, the corticobulbar tract projects to CN nuclei 3, 4, and 6 (the extraocular CNs).
  - In the pons, the corticobulbar tract projects to CN nuclei 5 and 7 (for facial muscle innervation).
  - In the medulla, the corticobulbar tract projects to CN nuclei 9, 10, 11, and 12 (muscles for swallowing, eating, and speaking).

Function

- The corticobulbar tracts control CN lower motor neurons.

Lesions

- Lesions involve the previously listed CN nuclei.
- Lesions result in flaccidity of the anatomy innervated by these CNs.

CORTICOBULBAR TRACT

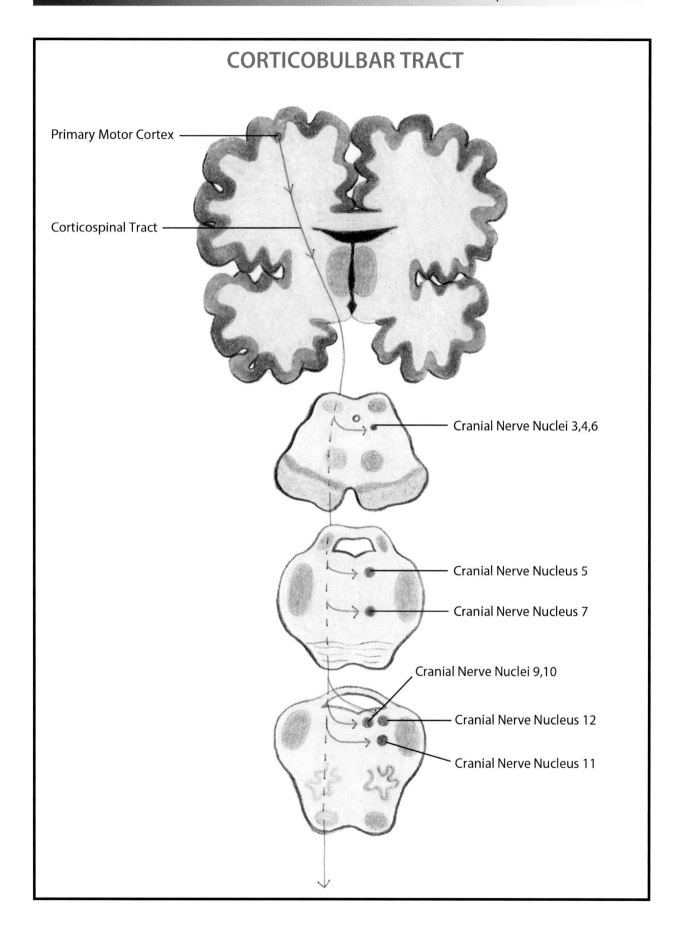

Primary Motor Cortex

Corticospinal Tract

Cranial Nerve Nuclei 3,4,6

Cranial Nerve Nucleus 5

Cranial Nerve Nucleus 7

Cranial Nerve Nuclei 9,10

Cranial Nerve Nucleus 12

Cranial Nerve Nucleus 11

Mixed Pathways Originating From the Brainstem

Medial Longitudinal Fasciculus[1-5]

- The MLF is a fiber bundle situated near the midline of the brainstem.
- The tract is composed of ascending and descending fibers.
- The MLF is part of the UMN system.

Descending Fibers of the Medial Longitudinal Fasciculus

Function

- The MLF exerts an inhibitory effect on the motor neurons of the ventral horn in the cervical SC.
- This inhibitory effect allows for the coordination of head and neck movements.

Origin

- Vestibular nuclei (in the medulla)

Decussation

- None. This is an ipsilateral tract that does not cross.

Destination

- From the cervical segments of the SC, the tract projects to spinal nerves in the PNS that innervate head and neck musculature.

Pathway

- The vestibular nuclei in the medulla (the origin of the tract) receive information from the following:
  - Superior colliculi in the midbrain
  - Oculomotor nuclei in the midbrain
  - Pontine reticular formation
- The tract then descends through the anterior white funiculus of the SC.
- When the tract is ready to exit the cord, it synapses on an interneuron in the ventral horn of the cervical cord segments.
- The interneuron then synapses on motor neurons (in the ventral horn) of descending motor spinal nerves that innervate head and neck musculature in the periphery.

Ascending Fibers of the Medial Longitudinal Fasciculus

Function

- The ascending fibers of the MLF are responsible for the visual tracking of a moving object through the coordinated movements of the eyes, head, and neck.
- The ascending fibers of the MLF are responsible for the refinement of extraocular eye movements.

Origin

- Vestibular nuclei (in the medulla)

Decussation

- None. This is an ipsilateral tract that does not cross.

Destination

- Oculomotor nerve nuclei
- Trochlear nerve nuclei
- Abducens nerve nuclei

Pathway

- The tract begins in the vestibular nuclei in the medulla and terminates on CN nuclei 3, 4, and 6.

MEDIAL LONGITUDINAL FASCICULUS: ASCENDING AND DESCENDING FIBERS

Superior Colliculus

Cranial Nerve Nucleus 3

Rostral Midbrain

Pontine Reticular Nucleus

Cranial Nerve Nucleus 4

Caudal Midbrain

Cranial Nerve Nucleus 6

Pons

Vestibular Nucleus

Vestibular Nucleus

Rostral Medulla

Caudal Medulla

Cervical Spinal Cord Level

DESCENDING MOTOR PATHWAYS ORIGINATING IN THE BRAINSTEM

Vestibulospinal Tract[1-5]

Extrapyramidal Tract

- The vestibular tract does not travel through the pyramids and is thus considered to be an extrapyramidal tract.

Function

- Facilitation of antigravity (extensor) muscles
- Facilitation of muscles responsible for posture and stance

Origin

- Vestibular nuclei (in the medulla)

Decussation

- None. The tract remains ipsilateral.

Destination

- The vestibulospinal tract innervates extensor muscle groups in the PNS.

Pathway

- The vestibular nuclei in the medulla (the tract's origin) receive messages from the following:
  - Vestibular apparatus in the inner ear via the vestibulocochlear nerve
  - Cerebellum
- From the vestibular nuclei, the tract then travels to the anterolateral white funiculus of the SC (first order neuron).
- When the tract is ready to exit the cord, it synapses on an interneuron that joins with a motor neuron in the ventral horn.
- The motor neuron synapses on a descending motor spinal nerve that innervates a target extensor muscle (second order neuron).

Decerebrate Rigidity

- Damage to any of the tracts that originate in the brainstem, including the vestibulospinal tract, result in decerebrate rigidity.
- When damage occurs to the brainstem, the vestibulospinal tract fires without modification from the brainstem and cortex, causing decerebrate rigidity.
- Decerebrate rigidity involves spastic extension of both the upper and lower extremities.
- The rigidity in decerebrate rigidity is more accurately described as spasticity (as it emerges from the extrapyramidal system and involves increased muscle tone on one side of the joint rather than both).
- The occurrence of decerebrate rigidity indicates a much poorer prognosis than does decorticate rigidity (because it signifies severe damage of the brainstem).

VESTIBULOSPINAL TRACT

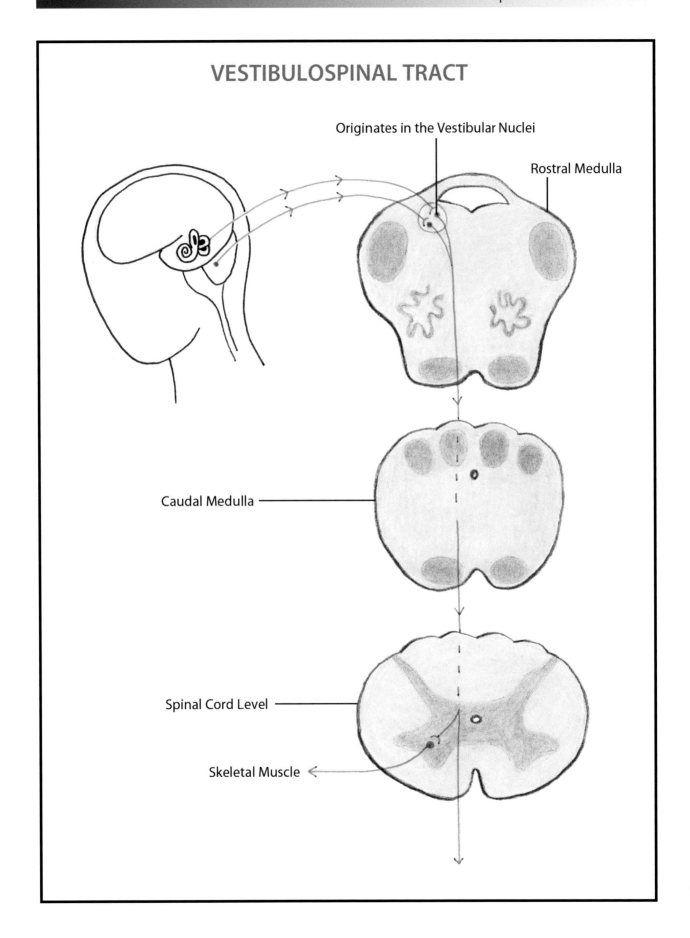

Originates in the Vestibular Nuclei

Rostral Medulla

Caudal Medulla

Spinal Cord Level

Skeletal Muscle

Rubrospinal Tract[1-5]

Extrapyramidal Tract

- The rubrospinal tract does not travel through the pyramids and is thus considered to be an extrapyramidal tract.

Function

- The rubrospinal tract facilitates the antagonist of antigravity muscles (mostly in the limbs) causing facilitation of flexor muscle groups.
- Activity of the rubrospinal tract is modified by the cerebellum and the cortex.
- The cerebellum and cortex modify the activity of the red nucleus in the midbrain, the origin of the rubrospinal tract.

Origin

- Red nucleus (in the midbrain)

Decussation

- Occurs at the midbrain level

Destination

- The rubrospinal tract innervates flexor muscles in the limbs.

Pathway

- The tract begins in the red nucleus of the midbrain (first order neuron).
- In the midbrain, the tract crosses the midline and enters the crus cerebri.
- Once the tract decussates, it begins to descend to the SC.
- The rubrospinal tract travels very close to the corticospinal tract as it descends in the SC (second order neuron).
- When the tract is ready to exit the cord, it synapses with an interneuron in the ventral horn.
- The interneuron joins with a descending motor spinal nerve that innervates flexor muscles in the PNS.

Decerebrate Rigidity

- A lesion to the rubrospinal tract results in decerebrate rigidity (involves spastic extension of the upper and lower extremities).
- If the rubrospinal tract is lost, the antagonists of the antigravity muscles are gone; in other words, the flexors are lost.
- The upper and lower extremities present with increased extensor tone.

RUBROSPINAL TRACT

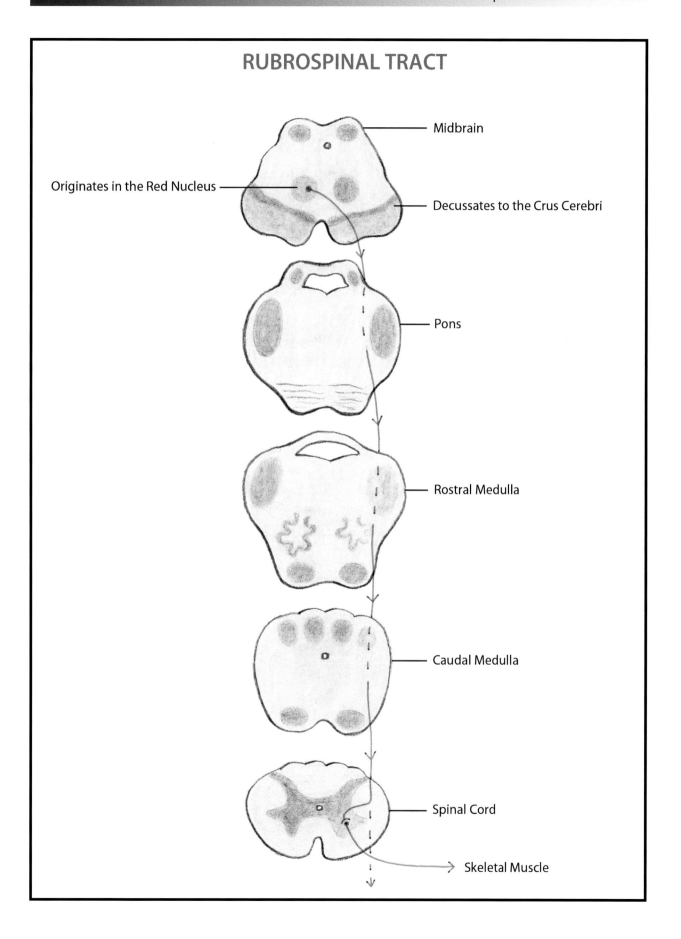

Midbrain

Originates in the Red Nucleus

Decussates to the Crus Cerebri

Pons

Rostral Medulla

Caudal Medulla

Spinal Cord

Skeletal Muscle

Medullary Reticulospinal Tract[1-5]

Extrapyramidal Tract
- The medullary reticulospinal tract does not travel through the pyramids and is thus considered to be an extrapyramidal tract.

Function
- Inhibits antigravity muscles; inhibits extensor tone.
- This tract also depresses cardiovascular responses (blood pressure, heart rate) and the inspiratory phase of respiration.
- The tract receives substantial modification from the corticospinal tracts.

Origin
- Medullary reticular formation (in the medulla)

Decussation
- Most of the fibers of this tract remain uncrossed.

Destination
- The medullary reticulospinal tract modifies antigravity or extensor muscles in the PNS.

Pathway
- This tract begins in the medullary reticular formation in the medulla (first order neuron).
- It descends through the anterior white funiculus.
- When this tract is ready to exit the cord, it synapses on an interneuron in the ventral horn (second order neuron).
- The interneuron then synapses on a motor spinal nerve that travels to an extensor muscle in the PNS.

Decerebrate Rigidity
- When the medullary reticulospinal tract is damaged, the tract that inhibits extensor tone is lost.
- This causes an increase in extensor tone or decerebrate rigidity (spastic extension of the upper and lower extremities).

MEDULLARY RETICULOSPINAL TRACT

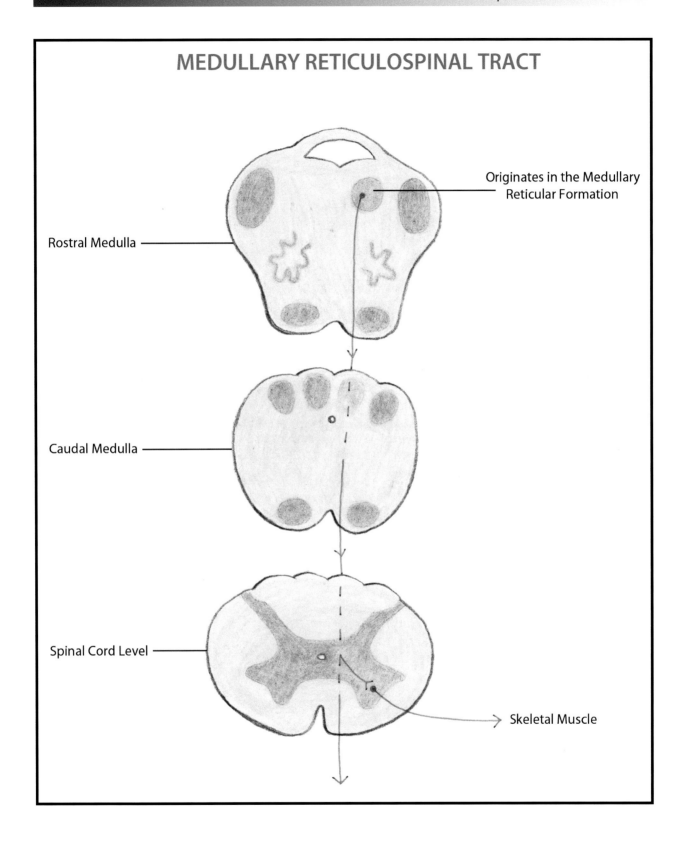

Rostral Medulla

Originates in the Medullary Reticular Formation

Caudal Medulla

Spinal Cord Level

Skeletal Muscle

Pontine Reticulospinal Tract[1-5]

Extrapyramidal Tract

- The pontine reticulospinal tract does not travel through the pyramids and is thus considered to be an extrapyramidal tract.

Function

- Facilitates antigravity muscles; facilitates extensor tone
- This tract receives substantial modification from the corticospinal tracts.

Origin

- Pontine reticular formation (in the pons)

Decussation

- None. This is an ipsilateral tract.

Destination

- The pontine reticulospinal tract innervates extensor muscles.

Pathway

- The tract begins in the pontine reticular formation (first order neuron).
- It descends through the anterior white funiculus of the SC.
- When this tract is ready to exit the cord, it synapses on an interneuron in the ventral horn (second order neuron).
- The interneuron then synapses with a motor spinal nerve that innervates an extensor muscle in the PNS.

Decerebrate Rigidity

- Damage to this tract results in decerebrate rigidity (spastic extension of the upper and lower extremities).
- Usually, damage to this tract is less important than damage to the tracts and neural regions surrounding it.
- If cortical or brainstem damage has occurred, then nothing modifies this tract's firing rate. Consequently, the tract fires without higher center modification, leading to increased extensor tone.

PONTINE RETICULOSPINAL TRACT

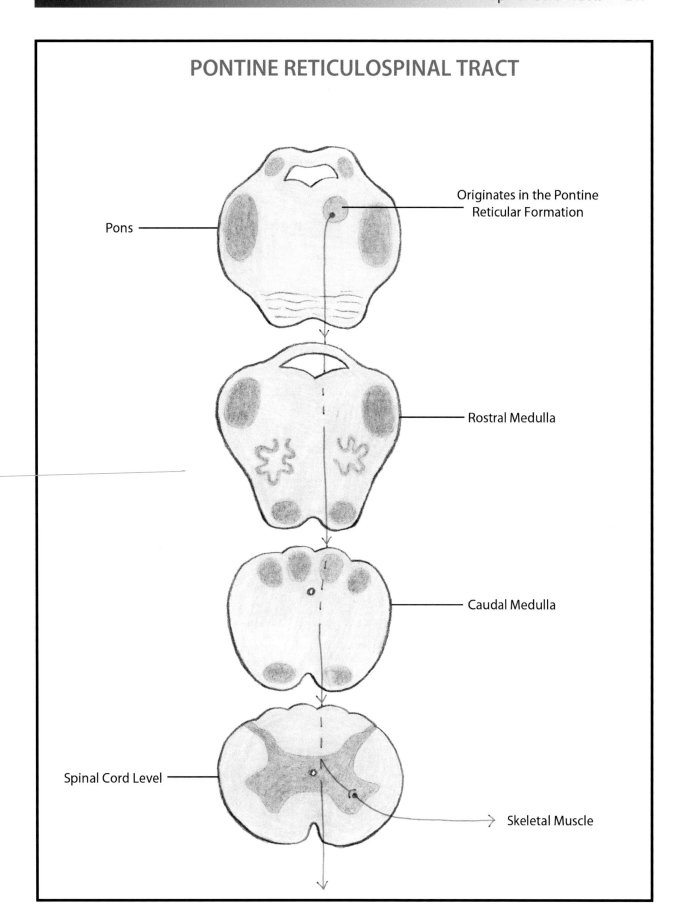

Pons

Originates in the Pontine Reticular Formation

Rostral Medulla

Caudal Medulla

Spinal Cord Level

Skeletal Muscle

Decorticate Rigidity. Results from a lesion to the corticospinal tracts. The upper extremities are in spastic flexion: head and neck are flexed; scapulae are elevated and retracted; shoulders are internally rotated and adducted; forearms are pronated; elbows, wrists, and fingers are flexed; wrists are ulnarly deviated. The lower extremities are in spastic extension: hips are rotated and adducted; feet are plantar flexed and inverted.

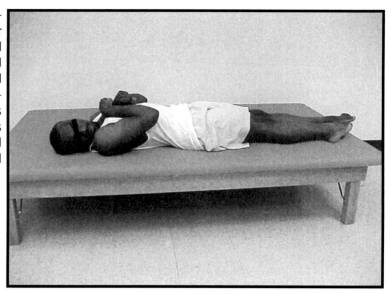

Decerebrate Rigidity. Results from a lesion to the extrapyramidal spinal cord tracts. Both the upper and lower extremities are in spastic extension. Head and neck are in hyperextension; jaws are clenched; scapulae are elevated and retracted; shoulders are internally rotated and adducted; elbows are extended; forearms are pronated; wrists are flexed and ulnarly deviated; fingers are flexed and adducted; hips and knees are extended; hips are internally rotated and adducted; feet are plantar flexed and inverted.

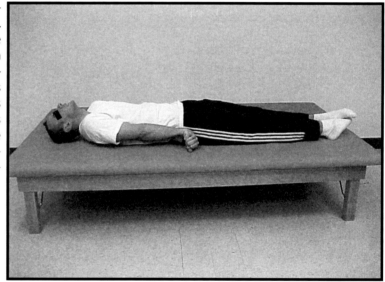

REFERENCES

1. Haines DE. *Neuroanatomy in Clinical Context: An Atlas of Structures, Sections, and Systems.* 9th ed. Philadelphia, PA: Lippincott, Williams, and Wilkins; 2014.

2. Notle J. *The Human Brain: An Introduction to Its Functional Anatomy.* 6th ed. St. Louis, MO: Mosby; 2008.

3. Woosley TA, Hanaway J, Gado MH. *The Brain Atlas: A Visual Guide to the Human Central Nervous System.* 3rd ed. New York, NY: Wiley; 2007.

4. Hendelman W. *Atlas of Functional Neuroanatomy.* 3rd ed. Boca Raton, FL: CRC Press; 2015.

5. Felten DL, Shetty A. *Netter's Atlas of Neuroscience.* 2nd ed. Philadelphia, PA: Saunders; 2010.

Spinal Cord Injury and Disease

INCOMPLETE VS COMPLETE SPINAL CORD INJURY

Complete Spinal Cord Injury

- A complete spinal cord injury (SCI) involves the absence of sensory and motor functions below the lesion level.
- Return of function of the last preserved spinal cord (SC) level may be enhanced by the administration of the corticosteroid methylprednisolone (stabilizes cell membranes, decreases inflammation, increases nerve impulse generation, and improves blood flow to the damaged area). Methylprednisolone must be administered in the first 3 to 8 hours after injury for optimal effectiveness.[1]

Incomplete Spinal Cord Injury

- An incomplete SCI involves partial preservation of sensory and motor functions below the lesion level.
- The prognosis is better than that of a complete SC injury, as a result of preserved axon function.
- Return of some function may be enhanced by the administration of methylprednisolone.
- Incomplete SCIs occur more frequently than complete severances.[2]

COMMON CAUSES OF SPINAL CORD INJURY/DISEASE

Transection

- A transection is a complete severance of the cord and involves interruption of all sensory and motor information at and below the lesion level.
- Transections can result from traumatic injury including auto accidents, knife wounds, gunshot wounds, and diving accidents.[3]

Compression

- Compression involves impingement of the cord; symptoms depend on the severity of the injury.
- Compressions can result from trauma, tumor, or vertebral degenerative joint disease.[4]

Infection

- Infection may compromise the integrity of the cord.
- An example is polio, which involves damage to the cell bodies in the ventral horn, causing lower motor neuron (LMN) loss.[5]

Degenerative Disorders

- Degenerative diseases can damage the motor SC tracts.
- One example is amyotrophic lateral sclerosis (ALS), which results in bilateral degeneration of the ventral horn and pyramidal tracts.
- Degenerative disorders affecting the SC involve both LMN and upper motor neuron (UMN) damage.[6]

Gutman SA. *Quick Reference Neuroscience for Rehabilitation Professionals: The Essential Neurologic Principles Underlying Rehabilitation Practice, Third Edition* (pp 220-234). © 2017 Taylor & Francis Group.

Five Most Important Tracts to Clinically Evaluate

1. *Lateral corticospinal tracts*: Responsible for voluntary motor control on the contralateral side
2. *Dorsal columns*: Responsible for conscious discriminative touch, pressure, vibration, and proprioception on the contralateral side
3. *Lateral spinothalamic tracts*: Responsible for conscious pain and temperature on the contralateral side
4. *Spinocerebellar tracts*: Responsible for unconscious proprioception
5. *Vestibulospinal tracts*: Responsible for facilitation of extensor tone (important to assess in neurologic injury)

UPPER MOTOR NEURON VS LOWER MOTOR NEURON LESIONS

Definition of Upper Motor Neuron

- An UMN is a motor neuron (MN) that carries motor information from the cortex or subcortical regions to either of the following:
  - The cranial nerve (CN) nuclei in the brainstem. The CN nuclei are considered to be part of the UMN system. The CN fibers that travel to target muscles are considered to be within the LMN system.
  - Interneurons that synapse with motor cell bodies in the ventral horn. An UMN travels up to but does not enter the ventral horn. The ventral horn is considered to be part of the LMN system.
- An UMN lesion includes all SC injuries and diseases that affect the cord between the levels of C1 and T12.[7]

Definition of Lower Motor Neuron

- A LMN is an MN that carries information from the motor cell bodies in the ventral horn to skeletal muscles.
- LMNs include the following:
  - CNs
  - Conus medullaris (at L1-L2 vertebrae)
  - Cauda equina
- Thus, cord lesions at the L1 vertebra area and lower are considered LMN injuries.
- All lesions to the peripheral nerves are also considered to be LMN conditions.[8]

SIGNS AND SYMPTOMS OF UPPER AND LOWER MOTOR NEURON LESIONS

Upper Motor Neuron Lesion Signs

Below the Lesion Level

- *Spasticity*[9]:
  - Spasticity is an increase in muscle tone with an associated inability to voluntarily control the muscle.
  - Spasticity involves difficulty actively and passively moving the muscles on one side of the joint, but not both sides.
  - Either the flexors or the extensors are spastic, but not both. (If both the flexors and the extensors display increased tone, rigidity is occurring. Rigidity usually results from basal ganglia dysfunction rather than SCI.)
  - Spasticity is velocity dependent; that is, spasticity can be elicited by passively moving an affected limb quickly. The same passive movement of the limb performed slowly may not elicit spasticity. Rigidity is velocity independent; that is, increased muscle tone exists whether an affected limb is passively moved slowly or quickly.
- *Hyperactive reflexes*[10]
- *Clonus*[11]:
  - Clonus is a sustained series of rhythmic jerks in a muscle.
  - It is usually caused by a quick stretch of the spastic muscle group.

At the Lesion Level

- *Flaccidity*: loss of muscle tone[12]

Lower Motor Neuron Lesion Signs

- Flaccidity[12]
- Hyporeflexia[13]
- Within a few weeks of LMN injury, muscles begin to atrophy.
- Muscles undergoing the early stages of atrophy may display the following:
  - *Fibrillations*: fine twitches of single muscle fibers that usually cannot be detected on clinical examination but can be identified on an electromyogram[14]
  - *Fasciculations*: brief contractions of motor units, which can be observed in skeletal muscle and detected on clinical examination[15]

SPINAL CORD DISEASE

Dorsal Column Disease (also called *Posterior Cord Syndrome* or *Tabes Dorsalis*)

Etiology

- Seen in patients with neurosyphilis[16]

Pathology

- Dorsal columns are lost bilaterally[16]

Symptomatology

- Causes a bilateral loss of the following[16]:
  - Tactile discrimination
  - Vibration
  - Pressure
  - Proprioception (often accompanied by ataxia)

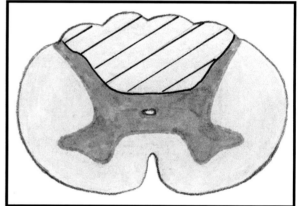

Brown-Séquard Syndrome

Etiology

- Multiple sclerosis
- Stab wound
- Tumor[17]

Pathology

- Brown-Séquard syndrome is a SC hemisection.[17]

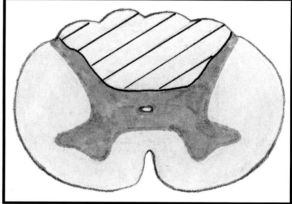

Symptomatology

- The lateral corticospinal tract is lost ipsilaterally.
  - Because the injury occurs in the SC, the patient presents with an ipsilateral loss of motor control and spasticity below the lesion level.
  - The patient presents with ipsilateral flaccidity at the lesion level.
- The dorsal column is lost ipsilaterally.
  - Because the decussation of this tract occurs at the caudal medulla level, the patient presents with an ipsilateral loss of discriminative touch, pressure, vibration, and proprioception.
- The spinothalamic tract is lost contralaterally.
  - Because the spinothalamic tracts decussate as soon as they enter the cord, pain and temperature sensation will be lost on the contralateral side (below the lesion level).
  - At the lesion level, the patient experiences bilateral loss of pain and temperature sensation.[17]

Anterior Cord Syndrome

Etiology

- Infarct
- Ischemia
- Trauma[18]

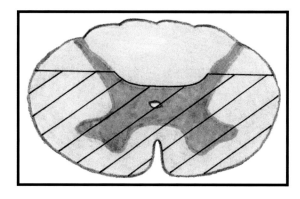

Pathology

- Anterior cord syndrome occurs when two-thirds of the anterior cord is lost.[18]

Symptomatology

- The dorsal columns are spared.
  - Discriminative touch, vibration, pressure, and proprioception are spared.
- The lateral corticospinal tracts are lost.
  - Because the lateral corticospinal tracts descend down the lateral white funiculus, they are lost.
  - This results in bilateral spastic paralysis.
  - The patient loses bilateral voluntary motor control below the level of the lesion.
- The ventral horn is lost.
  - The MNs in the ventral horn are part of the LMN system.
  - Because the ventral horn MNs are lost, the patient presents with flaccidity at and below the lesion level.
- The spinothalamic tracts are lost.
  - Because the spinothalamic tracts synapse in the dorsal horn and decussate across the anterior white funiculus as soon as they enter the cord, the patient presents with bilateral loss of pain and temperature sensation.[18]

Central Cord Syndrome (also called *Syringomyelia*)

Etiology

- Unknown
- More commonly occurs in elderly persons who have narrowing, or stenotic, changes in the spinal canal related to arthritis.
- Damage may also occur in people with congenital stenosis.[19]

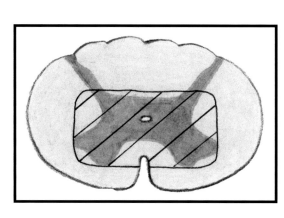

Pathology

- Central cord syndrome involves a cavitation of the central cord in the cervical segments.[19]

Symptomatology

- The spinothalamic tracts are the first to be lost
  - Because the spinothalamic tracts synapse in the dorsal horn and decussate to the anterior white funiculus as soon as they enter the cord, the spinothalamic tracts are lost.
  - This results in bilateral loss of pain and temperature.
- The ventral horn is lost
  - This results in flaccidity of the upper extremities because the disease occurs in the cervical regions of the SC.[19]

Posterolateral Cord Syndrome

Etiology

- Degeneration of the SC from severe vitamin B_{12} deficiency, pernicious anemia, or AIDS[16]

Pathology

- Affects the posterior and posterolateral white funiculi of the SC[16]

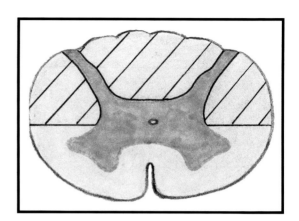

Symptomatology

- The dorsal columns are lost bilaterally.
  - Results in bilateral loss of discriminative touch, pressure, vibration, and proprioception
- The lateral corticospinal tracts are lost bilaterally.
  - Because the lateral corticospinal tracts descend in the lateral white funiculus, they are lost.
  - Results in bilateral spastic paralysis
- The spinocerebellar tracts are lost.
  - This results in bilateral ataxia.[16]

Anterior Horn Cell Syndrome (also called *Ventral Horn Syndrome*)

Etiology

- Disease process that destroys the MNs in the ventral horn[20]

Pathology

- Anterior horn cell syndrome involves LMN damage.[20]

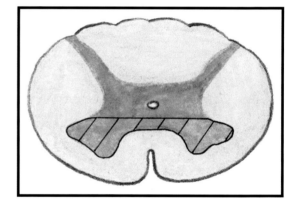

Symptomatology

- Results in bilateral flaccidity in the muscles innervated by the affected SC levels.
- An example is poliomyelitis, an acute viral disease affecting the ventral horn motor cell bodies.[20]

Spinal Shock

- Spinal shock is a state of areflexia that occurs immediately after SCI and involves the loss of all spinal reflexes below the lesion level.
- Because the motor pathways below the lesion level are also lost, the patient experiences the following:
  - Flaccid paralysis (because no spinal reflex arcs are firing)
  - Loss of tendon reflexes
  - Loss of autonomic function
- Spinal shock can last for hours, days, or weeks.
- Upon resolution, spinal reflex activity returns.
- Frequently, the severity of spinal shock increases as the level of injury increases.[21]

Autonomic Dysreflexia in Spinal Cord Injury

- Autonomic dysreflexia involves an acute episode of exaggerated sympathetic reflex responses in SCI that occurs because higher center reflex regulation is lost.
- Autonomic dysreflexia occurs only after spinal shock has resolved and autonomic reflexes return.
- It is characterized by the following:
  - Severe hypertension
  - Bradycardia
  - Severe headache
  - Vasodilation
  - Flushed skin
  - Profuse sweating above the lesion level
- Patients can experience one or several of these symptoms in one episode. Autonomic dysreflexia can initially occur or recur at any time during the patient's lifespan.
- Usually associated with SCIs at T6 and above.
- Common causes include the following:
  - Full bladder or rectum (frequent cause; catheter should be checked for overfill)
  - Stimulation of pain receptors (as occurs with pressure ulcers)
  - Ingrown toenails
  - Dressing changes
  - Visceral contractions (eg, ejaculation, bladder spasms, uterine contractions)
- Autonomic dysreflexia is a clinical emergency requiring immediate treatment.
- Convulsions, loss of consciousness, and even death may occur if autonomic dysreflexia is unattended.[22]

Orthostatic Hypotension in Spinal Cord Injury

- This is also called *postural hypotension*.
- Orthostatic hypotension usually occurs in patients with injuries at T6 and above.
- This occurs when sympathetic outflow to blood vessels in the extremities and abdomen is interrupted.
- There is a decrease in cardiac output when the patient is placed in an upright position. Venous return to the heart is impaired, and pooling of blood in the feet occurs.
- Blood pressure can drop precipitously.
- Signs of orthostatic hypotension include the following:
  ◦ Dizziness
  ◦ Pallor in the face (blood has shifted away from the head to the feet)
  ◦ Excessive sweating above the lesion level
  ◦ Blurred vision
  ◦ Possible fainting (syncope)
- Orthostatic hypotension can often be prevented by helping the patient to assume an upright position in a gradual and slow manner.[23]

Body Temperature Dysregulation in Spinal Cord Injury

- Body temperature is regulated by the sympathetic nervous system.
- The mechanisms for body temperature regulation are located largely in the hypothalamus.
- After SCI, communication between the hypothalamic temperature regulators and sympathetic function below the lesion level becomes disrupted.
- In other words, the body's ability to control blood vessel responses that conserve or dissipate heat is lost. Lost also are the abilities to sweat and shiver.
- Higher level injuries produce greater disturbances in temperature control.
- Poikilothermy is a condition in which the body takes on the temperature of its external environment. This commonly occurs in patients with injuries at T6 and above.[24]

Edema, Skin Breakdown, and Deep Vein Thrombosis in Spinal Cord Injury

Edema
- Edema is the presence of an abnormal accumulation of fluid in interstitial tissue.
- It can frequently occur in SCI as a result of immobility, causing increased venous pressure and abnormal pooling of blood in the abdomen, lower limbs, and upper extremities.[25]

Skin Breakdown
- The sympathetic nervous system influences skin integrity through the control of vasomotor and sweat gland activity.
- These functions ensure that the skin has adequate circulation, excretion of body fluids, and temperature regulation.
- SCI compromises skin integrity as a result of lost sensation and circulatory changes. Skin breakdown is a common but frequently preventable complication of SCI.[26]

Deep Vein Thrombosis
- Deep vein thrombosis is a clot in the venous system that may produce infarction. Such clots commonly originate in the legs and can travel to the lungs, causing pulmonary embolism.
- In SCI, deep vein thrombosis occurs as a result of impaired vasomotor tone, loss of muscle tone, trauma to the vein wall, immobility, and hypercoagulation.[27]

Disorders of Bladder and Bowel Function in Spinal Cord Injury

Bladder Function

- Bladder function is controlled by the sympathetic nerve fibers from T1 to L3. These allow for relaxation of the detrusor muscle during bladder filling, awareness of signals indicating bladder distention (S2 to S4), and relaxation of the external sphincter for bladder voiding.
- Patients with UMN lesions have a spastic bladder.
  - They lack awareness of bladder distension and have no voluntary control of voiding.
  - Involuntary voiding reflexes may be elicited during bladder filling, causing incontinence and an inability to completely empty the bladder.
- Patients with a LMN lesion have a flaccid bladder.
  - These patients lack an awareness of bladder distention and cannot void voluntarily or involuntarily.
  - Because there is no bladder function other than storage, retention (with overfill) and urine leakage occur.[28]

Bowel Function

- Bowel function is controlled by parasympathetic fibers from S2 to S4 that innervate the colon, rectum, and internal anal sphincter.
- Somatic innervation from S2 to S4 allow for voluntary control of the external anal sphincter.
- Defecation involves a reflex that increases peristaltic movements of the colon, rectum, and anus.
- Patients with SCI above S2 to S4 have a spastic defecation reflex and lose voluntary control of the external anal sphincter.
- Patients with SCI directly at the S2 to S4 level have a flaccid defecation reflex and lose anal sphincter tone. Without the defecation reflex, peristaltic movements cannot evacuate the stool.[29]

Sexual Function in Spinal Cord Injury

- Sexual function is mediated by the S2 to S4 segments of the SC.[30]
- The T11 to L2 cord segments are responsible for sexual arousal due to mental stimulation (referred to as the *psychogenic response*). This is the area where autonomic nerve pathways, in communication with the cortex, leave the cord and innervate the genitalia.
- The S2-S4 cord segments are responsible for sexual arousal due to touch (referred to as the *reflexogenic response*).[30]
- In patients with a T12/L1 or higher SCI (UMN injury):
  - Sexual arousal from touch remains intact, although the patient cannot feel the erection or vaginal lubrication.
  - Sexual arousal from mental stimulation is lost.
- In patients with a cord injury from L2 to S1 (LMN injury):
  - Sexual arousal from touch is possible, but the patient cannot feel the erection or vaginal lubrication.
  - Sexual arousal from mental stimulation is possible.

Level of Spinal Cord Injury and Functional Ability

SCI Level	Preserved Sensorimotor Function	Activities of Daily Living Function
C1 to C3	Head and neck sensation Some neck control Respirator dependent	Dependent in activities of daily living (ADL)
C4	Good head and neck sensation and motor control Scapular elevation Diaphragmatic movement (respiration)	Requires maximum assistance with all ADL
C5	Full head and neck control and sensation Some shoulder strength Shoulder external rotation Shoulder abduction to 90 degrees Elbow flexion and supination	Self-feeding with adaptive equipment Limited upper extremity dressing with adaptive equipment Limited self-care with adaptive equipment (brushing teeth, grooming)
C6	Fully innervated shoulder movement Forearm pronation Wrist extension Tenodesis	Self-feeding with adaptive equipment Upper and lower extremity dressing with adaptive equipment Requires greater assistance with lower extremity dressing Self-care with adaptive equipment
C7	Elbow extension Wrist flexion Finger extension	Independent in self-feeding, dressing, and grooming with adaptive equipment Independent bed mobility and transfers Meal preparation with adaptive equipment Can drive with hand controls
C8 to T1	All upper extremity muscles are innervated Fine motor coordination present Full grasp available	Independent in all self-care, grooming, and meal preparation with adaptive equipment Can drive with hand controls
T1 to T6	Top half of intercostal muscles are innervated, allowing increased respiratory reserve Long muscles of back are innervated, allowing for improved trunk control	Standing is possible with assistance but is not practical for dynamic ADL Independent self-catheterization
T6 to T12	All intercostal muscles and lower abdominals are innervated, providing improved trunk control and endurance	Limited ambulation is possible with lower extremity orthotics and assistive devices
T12 to L4	Hip flexion Hip adduction Knee extension	Functional ambulation is possible with bilateral lower extremity orthotics and assistive devices Wheelchair is used for energy conservation
L4 to L5	Knee extension is present but weak Ankle dorsiflexion	Functional ambulation is possible with bilateral lower extremity orthotics Wheelchair is used for energy conservation

REFERENCES

1. Fehlings MG, Wilson JR, Cho N. Methylprednisolone for the treatment of acute spinal cord injury: counterpoint. *Neurosurgery.* 2014;61:36-42. doi:10.1227/NEU.0000000000000412.

2. Harkema SJ, Schmidt-Read M, Lorenz DJ, Edgerton VR, Behrman AL. Balance and ambulation improvements in individuals with chronic incomplete spinal cord injury using locomotor training–based rehabilitation. *Arch Phys Med Rehabil.* 2012;93(9):1508-1517. doi:10.1016/j.apmr.2011.01.024.

3. Gao M, Lu P, Bednark B, et al. Templated agarose scaffolds for the support of motor axon regeneration into sites of complete spinal cord transection. *Biomaterials.* 2013;34(5):1529-1536. doi:10.1016/j.biomaterials.2012.10.070.

4. Savage P, Sharkey R, Kua T, et al. Malignant spinal cord compression: NICE guidance, improvements and challenges. *Q J Med.* 2014;107(4):277-282. doi:10.1093/qjmed/hct244.

5. Darouiche RO. Spinal epidural abscess. *N Engl J Med.* 2006;355(19):2012-2020. doi:10.1056/NEJMra055111.

6. Roh JS, Teng AL, Yoo JU, Davis J, Furey C, Bohlman HH. Degenerative disorders of the lumbar and cervical spine. *Orthop Clin North Am.* 2005;36(3):255-262. doi:10.1016/j.ocl.2005.01.007.

7 Douglass CP, Kandler RH, Shaw PJ, McDermott CJ. An evaluation of neurophysiological criteria used in the diagnosis of motor neuron disease. *J Neurol Neurosurg Psychiatry.* 2010;81(6):646-649. doi:10.1136/jnnp.2009.197434.

8. Pestronk A, Chaudhry V, Feldman EL, et al. Lower motor neuron syndromes defined by patterns of weakness, nerve conduction abnormalities, and high titers of antiglycolipid antibodies. *Ann Neurol.* 1990;27(3):316-326. doi:10.1002/ana.410270314.

9. Ivanhoe CB, Reistetter TA. Spasticity: the misunderstood part of the upper motor neuron syndrome. *Am J Phys Med Rehabil.* 2004;83(10):S3-S9.

10. Liu J, Xu D, Ren Y, Zhang LQ. Evaluations of neuromuscular dynamics of hyperactive reflexes poststroke. *J Rehabil Res Dev.* 2011;48(5):577-586. doi:10.1682/JRRD.2010.04.0065.

11. Wallace DM, Ross BH, Thomas CK. Characteristics of lower extremity clonus after human cervical spinal cord injury. *J Neurotrauma.* 2012;29(5):915-924. doi:10.1089/neu.2010.1549.

12. Formisano R, Pantano P, Buzzi MG, et al. Late motor recovery is influenced by muscle tone changes after stroke. *Arch Phys Med Rehabil.* 2005;86(2):308-311. doi:10.1016/j.apmr.2004.08.001.

13. Wu MN, Guo YC, Lai CL, Shen JT, Liou LM. Poststroke detrusor hyporeflexia in a patient with left medial pontine infarction. *Neurologist.* 2012;18(2):73-75. doi:10.1097/NRL.0b013e318247b9d9.

14. Alfen NV, Nienhuis M, Zwarts MJ, Pillen S. Detection of fibrillations using muscle ultrasound: diagnostic accuracy and identification of pitfalls. *Muscle Nerve.* 2011;43(2):178-182. doi:10.1002/mus.21863.

15. Fermont J, Arts IM, Overeem S, Kleine BU, Schelhaas HJ, Zwarts MJ. Prevalence and distribution of fasciculations in healthy adults: effect of age, caffeine consumption and exercise. *Amyotroph Lateral Scler.* 2010;11(1-2):181-186. doi:10.3109/17482960903062137.

16. McKinley W, Santos K, Meade M, Brooke K. Incidence and outcomes of spinal cord injury clinical syndromes. *J Spinal Cord Med.* 2007;30(3):215.

17. Amendola L, Corghi A, Cappuccio M, De Iure F. Two cases of Brown Sequard syndrome in penetrating spinal cord injuries. *Eur Rev Med Pharmacol Sci.* 2014;18(1):2-7.

18. Schneider GS. Anterior spinal cord syndrome after initiation of treatment with atenolol. *J Emerg Med.* 2010;38(5):e49-e52. doi:10.1016/j.jemermed.2007.08.061.

19. Aarabi B, Hadley MN, Dhall SS, et al. Management of acute traumatic central cord syndrome (ATCCS). *Neurosurgery.* 2013;72:195-204. doi:10.1227/NEU.0b013e318276f64b.

20. De Carvalho M, Swash M. Fasciculation-cramp syndrome preceding anterior horn cell disease: an intermediate syndrome? *J Neurol Neurosurg Psychiatry* 2011;82(4):459-61. doi:10.1136/jnnp.2009.194019

21. Boland RA, Lin CSY, Engel S, Kiernan MC. Adaptation of motor function after spinal cord injury: novel insights into spinal shock. *Brain.* 2011;134(2):495-505. doi:10.1093/brain/awq289.

22. Zhang Y, Guan Z, Reader B, et al. Autonomic dysreflexia causes chronic immune suppression after spinal cord injury. *J Neurosci.* 2013;33(32):12970-12981. doi:10.1523/JNEUROSCI.1974-13.2013.

23. Helmi M, Lima A, Gommers D, Van Bommel J, Bakker J. Inflatable external leg compression prevents orthostatic hypotension in a patient with a traumatic cervical spinal cord injury. *Future Cardiol.* 2013;9(5):645-648. doi:10.2217/fca.13.60.

24. Karlsson AK, Krassioukov A, Alexander MS, Donovan W, Biering-Sørensen F. International spinal cord injury skin and thermoregulation function basic data set. *Spinal Cord.* 2012;50(7):512-516. doi:10.1038/sc.2011.167.

25. Leonard AV, Thornton E, Vink R. The relative contribution of edema and hemorrhage to raised intrathecal pressure after traumatic spinal cord injury. *J Neurotrauma.* 2015;32(6):397-402. doi:10.1089/neu.2014.3543.

26. de Leon MP. Teamwork approach to prevention and treatment of skin breakdown in spinal cord patients. *Continuum (Minneap Minn).* 2015;21(1):206-210. doi: 10.1212/01.CON.0000461095.84186.a0.

27. Chung WS, Lin CL, Chang SN, Chung HA, Sung FC, Kao CH. Increased risk of deep vein thrombosis and pulmonary thromboembolism in patients with spinal cord injury: a nationwide cohort prospective study. *Thromb Res.* 2014;133(4):579-584. doi:10.1016/j.thromres.2014.01.008.

28. Horst M, Heutschi J, Van Den Brand R, et al. Multisystem neuroprosthetic training improves bladder function after severe spinal cord injury. *J Urol.* 2013;189(2):747-753. doi:10.1016/j.juro.2012.08.200.

29. Burns AS, St-Germain D, Connolly M. Phenomenological study of neurogenic bowel from the perspective of individuals living with spinal cord injury. *Arch Phys Med Rehabil.* 2015;96(1):49-55. doi:10.1016/j.apmr.2014.07.417.

30. Alexander MS, Biering-Sørensen F, Elliott S, Kreuter M, Sønksen J. International spinal cord injury male sexual function basic data set. *Spinal Cord.* 2011;49(7):795-798. doi:10.1038/sc.2010.192.

CLINICAL TEST QUESTIONS

Sections 18 to 19

1. After Alex's spinal cord injury, he can no longer feel sensation (discriminative touch, pressure, vibration, proprioception, and kinesthesia) at or below his injury level at T10. Which spinal cord tract is responsible for discriminative touch, pressure, vibration, proprioception, and kinesthesia?
   a. dorsal columns
   b. lateral spinothalamic
   c. anterior spinothalamic
   d. cuneocerebellar

2. Alex, in the above question, has also lost his bilateral sense of pain and temperature at and below the lesion level. Which spinal cord tract is responsible for the sensation of pain and temperature?
   a. dorsal columns
   b. lateral spinothalamic
   c. posterior spinocerebellar
   d. rostral spinocerebellar

3. Alex has no voluntary movement below T10. His lower extremity muscles are spastic; all reflexes in the lower extremities are hyperreflexive. Which spinal cord tract is responsible for voluntary movement?
   a. medial longitudinal fasciculus
   b. vestibulospinal
   c. spinocerebellar
   d. corticospinal

4. After his auto vehicle accident, Lorenzo lies in a coma with his upper and lower extremities in spastic extension. This condition is called _____ and results from a lesion to the _____.
   a. decorticate rigidity; corticospinal tracts
   b. decerebrate rigidity; corticospinal tracts
   c. decorticate rigidity; extrapyramidal spinal cord tracts in the brainstem
   d. decerebrate rigidity; extrapyramidal spinal cord tracts in the brainstem

5. Mr. Kim had a complete spinal cord injury at L2. He experiences flaccidity in his lower extremities and hyporesponsive reflexes below the lesion level. Mr. Kim's spinal cord injury involved:
   a. lower motor neurons
   b. upper motor neurons

6. Manuel has just been admitted to the emergency unit after a spinal cord injury. He is currently in a state of areflexia involving flaccid paralysis below the lesion level, loss of reflexes below the lesion level, and loss of autonomic function. This state is referred to as _____, occurs immediately after SCI, and can last anywhere from hours to weeks after a SCI. When this state resolves, all spinal reflex activity returns.
   a. autonomic dysreflexia
   b. orthostatic hypotension
   c. spinal shock (neurogenic shock)
   d. poikilothermy

7. Laura's SCI occurred at T2. One day, when her therapist is helping her to sit upright, Laura experiences significantly decreased blood pressure, dizziness, excessive sweating above the lesion level, and blurred vision. Although she feels faint, she does not lose consciousness. The condition resolves after her therapist declines her position and allows her to rest. This condition is called:
   a. spinal shock (neurogenic shock)
   b. poikilothermy
   c. orthostatic hypertension
   d. autonomic dysreflexia

8. Jackson's SCI occurred at C4. After injury, Jackson is unable to sweat, shiver, and regulate his body temperature. His body's ability to control blood vessel responses that conserve or dissipate heat is lost. As a result, Jackson's body takes on the temperature of the environment, and he is in danger of becoming too hot or cold. This condition is known as:

   a. spinal shock (neurogenic shock)
   b. poikilothermy
   c. orthostatic hypertension
   d. autonomic dysreflexia

9. Adam had a SCI 6 months ago. He is independent in self-feeding, dressing, and grooming with adaptive equipment and set-up. He is independent in bed mobility and transfers and can perform meal preparation with adaptive equipment and set-up. Adam is learning to drive an adapted vehicle with hand controls. His injury level is likely at which of the following?

   a. C3
   b. C7
   c. T4
   d. L2

10. Samantha, whose SCI is at level C8, is experiencing an acute episode of sympathetic reflex responses characterized by severe hypertension, increased heart rate, headache, vasodilation, and profuse sweating above the lesion level. This condition is considered to be a clinical emergency and can result in convulsions, loss of consciousness, and even death if not addressed. The condition is known as:

   a. spinal shock (neurogenic shock)
   b. poikilothermy
   c. orthostatic hypertension
   d. autonomic dysreflexia

Answers

1. a
2. b
3. d
4. d
5. a
6. c
7. c
8. b
9. b
10. d

Proprioception

- Sherrington named the term *proprioception* and defined it as the sixth sense: "The sense by which the body knows itself, judges with perfect, automatic, instantaneous precision the position and motion of all of its movable parts, their relations to one another, and their alignment in space."[1]
- Proprioception is the ability to sense one's body position in space.
- The Latin root *proprius* means to "own oneself" or to feel one's body as one's own.
- Proprioception occurs mostly on an unconscious level because it is primarily mediated by the cerebellum.
- The term *kinesthesia* refers to the ability to sense one's body movement in space.

THE ABILITY TO SENSE ONE'S BODY IN SPACE IS BASED ON THREE SYSTEMS

Visual System

- Humans use visual cues to negotiate the environment.[2]

Vestibular System

- The labyrinthine system in the inner ear—the semicircular canals—contains continuously moving liquid that is constantly monitored by the vestibular system to provide feedback regarding the head's position in space.
- The vestibular system also has neural connections to the cerebellum to provide feedback about the head's position in space.[3]

Proprioceptive System

- The proprioceptive system is a feedback/feedforward loop between the muscle spindles (MS), Golgi tendon organs, joint receptors, and the cerebellum.
- Together, these provide constant information about the body's position in space.[4]

MUSCLE SPINDLE

- MSs are proprioceptors located in skeletal muscle.
- MSs are sensory receptors that provide a constant flow of information regarding length, tension, and load on the muscles.
- MSs detect when a muscle has been stretched and initiate a reflex that resists the stretch.[5]

Extrafusal Muscle Fibers

- Extrafusal muscle fibers are the bulk of the muscle.[6]

Intrafusal Muscle Fibers

- Intrafusal muscle fibers are the MSs that sit within the bulk of the muscle.
- The intrafusal muscle fibers are attached to the extrafusal muscle fibers.[6]

Density of Muscle Spindles in an Extrafusal Muscle Fiber

- The more MSs in an extrafusal muscle fiber, the greater the muscle's precision control.
- Muscles with the highest density of MSs are small muscles designed for fine motor control.[7]

Gutman SA. *Quick Reference Neuroscience for Rehabilitation Professionals: The Essential Neurologic Principles Underlying Rehabilitation Practice, Third Edition* (pp 236-245).
© 2017 Taylor & Francis Group.

Nuclear Chain Fibers and Nuclear Bag Fibers

- The nuclear chain and nuclear bag are structures within the MS.

Nuclear Bag

- The nuclear bag is responsive to changes in muscle length.
- When the length of the muscle changes, the nuclear bag fires.
- The nuclear bag also detects the velocity of the muscular stretch, or how quickly the muscle stretched.[8]

Nuclear Chain

- The nuclear chain only fires in response to a new muscle length; it does not respond to velocity, like the nuclear bag.[8]

Properties of the Equatorial Regions of the Nuclear Bag and Chain

- The equatorial region of the bag is elastic and phasic (quick responding).
- The equatorial region of the chain is elastic and tonic (slow responding).[8]

Properties of the Polar Regions of the Nuclear Bag and Chain

- The polar regions of the bag are contractile and tonic (slow responding).
- The polar regions of the chain are contractile and phasic (quick responding).[8]

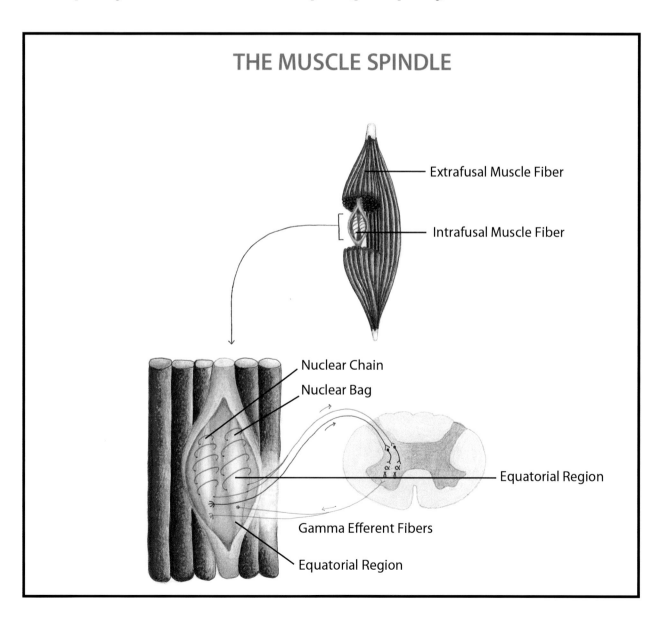

THE MUSCLE SPINDLE

The Muscle Spindles Use Two Types of Sensory Fibers to Send Information to the Ventral Horn

Ia (Primary Ending)

- The Ia sensory fibers are large and heavily myelinated.
- They are fast conducting.
- The Ia fibers wrap around the equatorial region of both the bag and chain.
- The Ia fibers respond to the rate of muscle stretch (velocity) and to changes in muscle length.
- The Ia fibers are fast adapting (phasic).[9]

II (Secondary Ending)

- II fibers are medium-size fibers.
- They terminate on the equatorial region of the chain only.
- II fibers are predominantly located on the chain.
- II fibers respond to changes in the length of the MS (the rate of the stretch is not involved).
- II fibers are slow adapting (tonic).[9]

Muscle Spindle Sequence of Events

- The extrafusal muscle fiber stretches.
- This causes the MS (the intrafusal muscle fibers) to stretch.
- The equatorial region of the bag stretches right away because the equatorial region of the bag is elastic and responds more to stretch than does the polar region. (If the stretch is a sustained stretch, the equatorial region of the chain will also stretch.)
- Stretching of the MS causes the Ia fibers to fire.
- The Ia fibers will fire in response to a quick or phasic response because the Ia fibers from the bag are phasic.
- The Ia fibers will also fire in response to a tonic or sustained and slow response because the Ia fibers from the chain are tonic.
- The secondary fibers, the II fibers, then fire.
- The II fibers are attached only to the chain, and the chain only detects length and position changes.
- The II fibers are tonic and respond to a slow, sustained stretch.[7]

Proprioceptive Information From the Muscle Spindles Travels to Four Places

- Proprioceptive information from the MS travels along the Ia and II fibers to the dorsal horn.
- In the dorsal horn, the fibers synapse on an interneuron and connect to alpha motor *neurons* (MNs) in the ventral horn.
- Information from the MS travels to the following[7]:
  - *An alpha MN of the same muscle (the agonist)*: for facilitation of that muscle. Referred to as *autogenic excitation*
  - *An alpha MN of the antagonist muscle*: for inhibition of the antagonist. Referred to as *reciprocal inhibition*; every time an alpha turns on an agonist, an alpha turns off the antagonist.
  - *Renshaw cells (special interneurons that modify the action of synergy muscles)*: a Renshaw cell is a short axon that connects motor nerve fibers with each other to produce refined motor movement. Referred to as *recurrent inhibition*; every time an alpha turns on an agonist, an alpha also modifies (usually inhibits) the action of the synergy muscles.
  - *The cerebellum*: MSs send proprioceptive signals to inform the cerebellum of all changes in muscle position and length.

Information from the muscle spindle travels to four primary neuroanatomical structures.

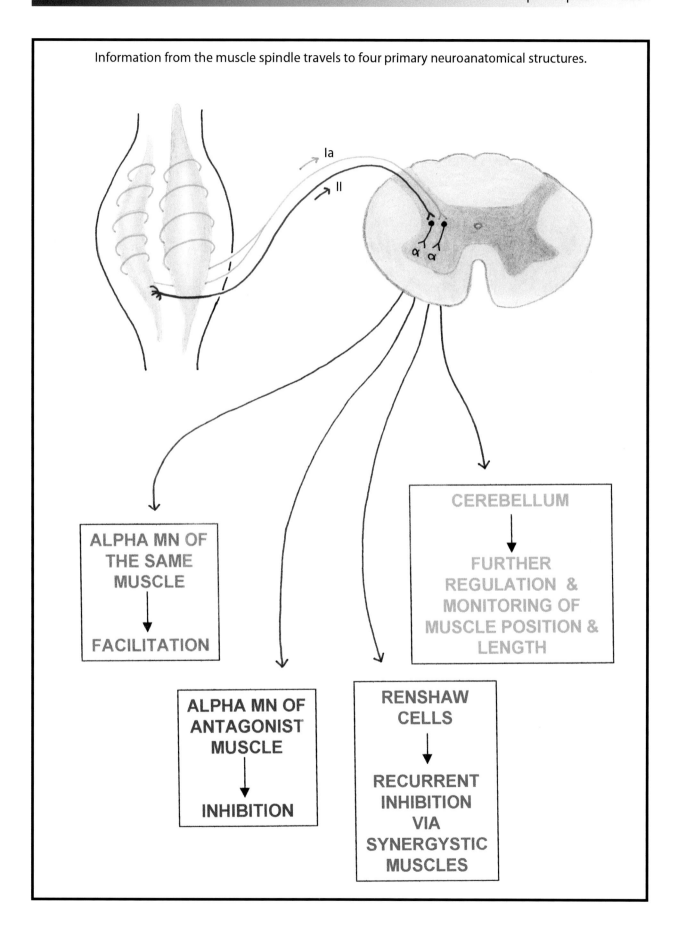

THE GAMMA MOTOR NEURON SYSTEM

- The gamma motor neurons (MNs) are also located in the ventral horn, along with the alpha MNs.
- The gamma MNs send proprioceptive information from the ventral horn back to the MS.
- Gamma MNs are fast conducting because they are heavily myelinated and large.
- Gamma MNs innervate the MSs.
- Alpha MNs innervate the extrafusal muscle fibers (the muscle bulk).[10,11]

Two Types of Gamma Motor Neurons

Gamma 1 Fibers

- Gamma 1 fibers have plate endings and terminate on the polar regions of the nuclear bag.[10,11]

Gamma 2 Fibers

- Gamma 2 fibers have trail (or multi-branching) endings and terminate predominately on the nuclear chain, adjacent to the equatorial region.[10,11]

Gamma Motor Neuron Stimulation

- When the gamma MNs in the ventral horn are stimulated, they fire, causing the polar regions of the bag and chain to contract.
- This causes the equatorial regions to stretch (or distort).
- The Ia fibers then fire, causing the alpha MNs in the ventral horn to fire.
- An alpha MN in the ventral horn innervates the agonist, causing the extrafusal muscle fiber to contract.[10,11]

Fusimotor System

- The fusimotor system allows the central nervous system (CNS) to influence muscle spindle sensitivity.
- Fusimotor neurons consist of beta and gamma MNs.
- Beta MNs innervate both extra- and intrafusal muscle fibers.
- Two types of beta MNs exist:
  1. Static beta MNs innervate nuclear chain fibers.
  2. Dynamic beta MNs innervate nuclear bag fibers.
- Gamma MNs are efferent; that is, they send proprioceptive signals away from the CNS.
- Muscle spindles are afferent; that is, they send proprioceptive signals to the CNS.[11,12]

GOLGI TENDON ORGANS

Location

- The Golgi tendon organs (GTOs) are embedded in the tendons, close to the skeletal muscle insertions.[13,14]

Function

- The GTOs are proprioceptors that detect tension in the tendon of a contracting muscle.[13,14]

Golgi Tendon Organs Use Ib Afferent Neurons

- The GTOs use Ib afferent (or sensory) neurons to send proprioceptive information to the dorsal horn.
- The Ib fibers synapse on interneurons in the ventral horn.
- In the ventral horn, the interneurons synapse on alpha MNs.[13,14]

Autogenic Inhibition

- Activation of the GTOs causes a contracting muscle to be inhibited; in other words, it relaxes.
- This is a protective function. If the GTOs did not become activated in response to a muscle's stretch, an individual could easily tear his or her muscles.[13,14]

Sequence of Golgi Tendon Organs Events

- The agonist muscle contracts.
- This activates the GTOs (which are embedded in the contracting muscle).
- The GTOs send proprioceptive information along the Ib sensory fibers to the dorsal horn.
- In the dorsal horn, the Ib fibers synapse with an interneuron.
- The interneuron connects with an alpha MN in the ventral horn.
- Information from the GTOs travels to 3 places[13,14]:
    1. An alpha MN to inhibit the contracting agonist muscle. Referred to as *autogenic inhibition*
    2. An alpha MN to facilitate the antagonist of the contracting muscle
    3. The cerebellum for further proprioceptive feedback

GOLGI TENDON ORGAN FUNCTIONAL IMPLICATIONS

- The GTOs help to control the speed of a contraction for coordinated, fine, precision movements.[13,14]
- Protective mechanism; humans need the action of the GTOs to protect against muscle tears and pulls.
- The GTOs help to reduce muscle cramps.
    - When an individual has a cramp in a muscle group (eg, when the plantar flexors are cramping), placing a sustained stretch on that muscle group will activate the GTOs to reduce the cramp. In other words, position the plantarflexors in a sustained stretch (ie, pull the plantar flexors into dorsiflexion for a sustained stretch).
    - The GTOs in the agonist become activated and inhibit the cramping agonist (the plantar flexors).
- The GTOs can help to reduce clasp knife phenomenon.
    - Clasp knife phenomenon occurs when a muscle group is hypertonic (involves severe spasticity at a joint).
    - To reduce spasticity, perform a sustained stretch on the contracting spastic muscle.
    - This will activate the GTOs and relax the spastic muscle.

Information from the Golgi tendon organ travels to three primary neuroanatomical structures.

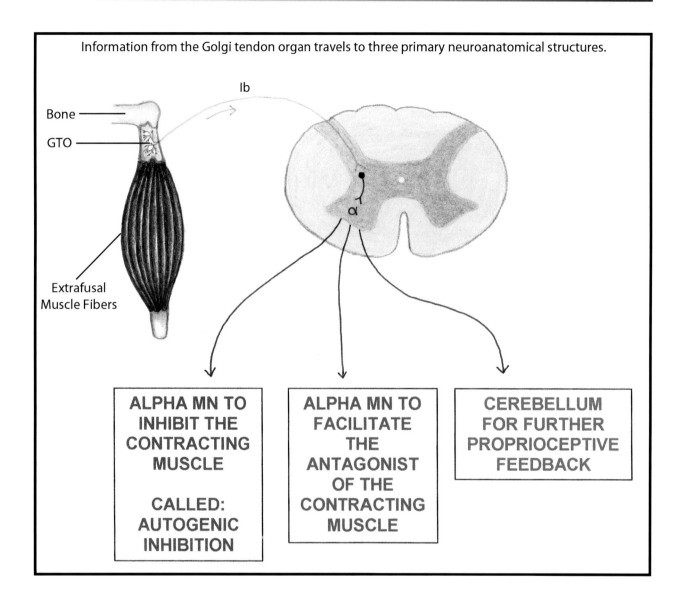

Neurologic Concepts Underlying the Basis of Many Therapeutic Techniques

- Slow sustained stretch will reduce spasticity in a muscle group by activating the GTOs. The GTOs will inhibit the contracting spastic agonist and facilitate the antagonist.[15]
- Splinting a spastic muscle group essentially positions the spastic limb in a sustained stretch. The GTOs become activated and inhibit the spastic contracting muscle groups (agonists) while also facilitating the antagonists.[16]
- Serial casting also places a spastic contracting muscle group (agonists) on a sustained stretch. This activates the GTOs, causing inhibition of the spastic muscle group and facilitation of the antagonists.[17]
- *Seating and positioning techniques* are also used to place a spastic contracting muscle group on a sustained stretch. Again, the GTOs will become activated, causing a reduction in the spastic muscle groups and facilitating the antagonist muscle groups.[18]

Muscle Spindles and Gamma Motor Neurons Work Together in a Feedback/Feedforward Loop

Sequence of Events

- Some change occurs in the extrafusal muscle fiber (eg, a muscle stretch).
- The intrafusal muscle fibers (the nuclear bag and chain of the MS) then stretch.
- The bag and chain send proprioceptive information to the alpha MNs in the ventral horn via the Ia and II fibers.
- This proprioceptive information from the MS travels to 4 places:
  1. *An alpha MN of the same muscle (the agonist)*: for facilitation of that muscle. Referred to as *autogenic excitation*.
  2. *An alpha MN of the antagonist muscle*: for inhibition of the antagonist. Referred to as *reciprocal inhibition*.
  3. *Renshaw cells*: for modification (usually inhibition) of synergy muscles. Referred to as *recurrent inhibition*.
  4. *The cerebellum*: for further monitoring and modification of that muscle group's movement. The cerebellum uses this proprioceptive information for the fine tuning of precision, coordinated movement.
- Alpha excitation also stimulates the gamma MNs in the ventral horn.
- Gamma MNs fire and send proprioceptive information along gamma 1 and 2 fibers to the MSs.
- This causes the intrafusal muscle fibers (the MSs) to contract.
- The MSs send their proprioceptive information to the ventral horn via the Ia and II fibers.
- The feedback/feedforward system begins over again, sending information to the 4 places described previously.[7,13,14]

Gamma Biasing

- The function of the gamma MNs is to make the MS more sensitive and keep the muscles primed, or ready for action.
- Gamma biasing raises the level of firing of the MS.
- When activation of the gamma MNs raises the level of MS firing, it causes the muscle to prepare, or set, for an anticipated activity.[19]

Examples of Gamma Biasing

- A person begins walking up a set of steps in which the step height is not uniform. She raises her foot upward to meet the next higher step level. However, because the step is lower than anticipated, she places her foot down too heavily.
- A person lifts a box of supplies that he believes is much heavier than it actually is. He lifts the box too quickly and too high as a result of anticipating the box to be heavier. His muscles were primed, by gamma biasing, to lift a heavier box.

Three Events Cause the Gammas to Fire

1. *Stimulation of the supraspinal motor centers*: the supraspinal motor centers include the basal ganglia, vestibular nuclei, and the reticular formation. These motor centers send projections to the gammas in the ventral horn through descending pathways; that is, the vestibulospinal and reticulospinal tracts.
2. *Cutaneous stimulation*: sensory information from the skin is sent to the dorsal horn. This information synapses on interneurons and excites the gamma MNs.
3. *Alpha and gamma coactivation*: every time an alpha MN is activated, a gamma MN is coactivated.[13,14]

Joint Receptors

Location

- Joint receptors are located in the connective tissue of a joint capsule.[20,21]

Function

- Joint receptors respond to mechanical deformation occurring in the joint capsule and ligaments.
- Joint receptors send this proprioceptive information to the cerebellum and to the ventral horn.[20,21]

What Stimulates the Joint Receptors?

Ruffini Endings

- Ruffini endings are located in the joint capsule.
- These sensory receptors are active both during rest and joint movement.
- Activation of Ruffini endings signals static joint position, dynamic joint movement, and the direction and velocity of joint movement.[20,21]

Paciniform Corpuscles

- Paciniform corpuscles are located in the joint capsule.
- These sensory nerve endings only respond to dynamic movement; that is, when the joint is moving.
- Paciniform corpuscles signal dynamic joint movement onset and termination, and joint movement velocity.[20,21]

Ligament Receptors

- Ligament receptors are similar in function to GTOs.
- These sensory nerve endings are located in the ligaments of a joint capsule and become active at the end of joint range.
- Ligament receptors respond to tension in the joint capsule.[20,21]

Free Nerve Endings

- Free nerve endings are located in the joint capsule.
- These sensory nerve endings are most often stimulated by inflammation and irritation.
- When these sensory nerve endings fire, they signal the detection of pain in a joint.[20,21]

Joint Receptors Use Several Different Sensory Fibers to Send Proprioceptive Information to the Cerebellum and Ventral Horn

- Ligament receptors use Ib sensory fibers.
- Ruffini endings and paciniform corpuscles use II sensory fibers.
- Free nerve endings use delta A and C sensory fibers.[20,21]

Joint Receptor Pathway

- The joint receptors use sensory fibers to send proprioceptive information to the dorsal horn.
- Here, the messages synapse on an interneuron.
- The interneuron connects with a MN in the ventral horn and sends proprioceptive messages back to the muscles surrounding the joint.
- An alpha MN in the ventral horn also sends joint receptor information to the cerebellum for constant feedback about joint position and movement.[20,21]

Joint Receptors and Proprioception

- While MSs, GTOs, and joint receptors are critical for normal proprioception, joint receptors alone may not be essential for proprioception.
- This is suggested because patients with joint replacements still retain good proprioception in joint midrange.[20,21]

REFERENCES

1. Sacks O. *The Man Who Mistook His Wife for a Hat*. New York, NY: Simon and Schuster; 1986.

2. Brown LE, Marlin MC, Morrow S. On the contributions of vision and proprioception to the representation of hand-near targets. *J Neurophysiology*. 2015;113(2):409-419. doi:10.1152/jn.00005.2014.

3. Cutfield NJ, Scott G, Waldman AD, Sharp DJ, Bronstein AM. Visual and proprioceptive interaction in patients with bilateral vestibular loss. *Neuroimage Clin*. 2014;4:274-282. doi:10.1016/j.nicl.2013.12.013.

4. Hillier S, Immink M, Thewlis D. Assessing proprioception: a systematic review of possibilities. *Neurorehabil Neural Repair*. 2015;29(10):933-49. doi:10.1177/1545968315573055.

5. Proske U. The role of muscle proprioceptors in human limb position sense: a hypothesis. *J Anat*. 2015;227(2):178-183. doi:10.1111/joa.12289.

6. Dimitriou M. Human muscle spindle sensitivity reflects the balance of activity between antagonistic muscles. *J Neurosci*. 2014;34(41):13644-13655. doi:10.1523/JNEUROSCI.2611-14.2014.

7. Mileusnic MP, Brown IE, Lan N, Loeb GE. Mathematical models of proprioceptors. I. Control and transduction in the muscle spindle. *J Neurophysiol*. 2006;96(4):1772-1788. doi:10.1152/jn.00868.2005.

8. Liu JX, Eriksson PO, Thornell LE, Pedrosa-Domellöf F. Fiber content and myosin heavy chain composition of muscle spindles in aged human biceps brachii. *J Histochem Cytochem*. 2005;53(4):445-454. doi:10.1369/jhc.4A6257.2005.

9. Arber S, Ladle DR, Lin JH, Frank E, Jessell TM. ETS gene Er81 controls the formation of functional connections between group Ia sensory afferents and motor neurons. *Cell*. 2000;101(5):485-498. doi:10.1016/S0092-8674(00)80859-4.

10. Enjin A, Leão KE, Mikulovic S, Le Merre P, Tourtellotte WG, Kullander K. Sensorimotor function is modulated by the serotonin receptor 1d, a novel marker for gamma motor neurons. *Mol Cell Neurosci*. 2012;49(3):322-332. doi:10.1016/j.mcn.2012.01.003.

11. Ellaway PH, Taylor A, Durbaba R. Muscle spindle and fusimotor activity in locomotion. *J Anat*. 2015;227(2):157-166. doi:10.1111/joa.12299.

12. Matthews PB. Where anatomy led, physiology followed: a survey of our developing understanding of the muscle spindle, what it does and how it works. *J Anat*. 2015;227(2):104-114. doi:10.1111/joa.12345.

13. Miller KC, Burne JA. Golgi tendon organ reflex inhibition following manually applied acute static stretching. *J Sports Sci*. 2014;32(15):1491-1497. doi:10.1080/02640414.2014.899708.

14. Kistemaker DA, Van Soest AJK, Wong JD, Kurtzer I, Gribble PL. Control of position and movement is simplified by combined muscle spindle and Golgi tendon organ feedback. *J Neurophysiol*. 2013;109(4):1126-1139. doi:10.1152/jn.00751.2012.

15. Gracies JM. Pathophysiology of impairment in patients with spasticity and use of stretch as a treatment of spastic hypertonia. *Phys Med Rehabil Clin North Am*. 2001;12(4):747-68.

16. Pizzi A, Carlucci G, Falsini C, Verdesca S, Grippo A. Application of a volar static splint in poststroke spasticity of the upper limb. *Arch Phys Med Rehabil*. 2005;86(9):1855-1859. doi:10.1016/j.apmr.2005.03.032.

17. Yasar E, Tok F, Safaz I, Balaban B, Yilmaz B, Alaca R. The efficacy of serial casting after botulinum toxin type A injection in improving equinovarus deformity in patients with chronic stroke. *Brain Inj*. 2010;24(5):736-739.

18. Kirkwood CA, Bardsley GI. Seating and positioning. In: Barnes MP, Johnson GR, eds. *Upper Motor Neurone Syndrome and Spasticity: Clinical Management and Neurophysiology*. New York, NY: Cambridge University Press; 2008:99.

19. Fuentes CT, Bastian AJ. Where is your arm? Variations in proprioception across space and tasks. *J Neurophysiol*. 2010;103(1):164-171. doi:10.1152/jn.00494.2009.

20. Proske U, Gandevia SC. The kinaesthetic senses. *J Physiol*. 2009;587(17):4139-4146. doi:10.1113/jphysiol.2009.175372.

21. Riemann BL, Lephart SM. The sensorimotor system, part I: the physiologic basis of functional joint stability. *J Athl Train*. 2002;37(1):71-79.

Disorders of Muscle Tone

MUSCLE TONE

- Muscle tone is a continuous state of muscle contraction at rest that helps to maintain posture.
- Tone is an unconscious phenomenon; humans cannot consciously will muscles to increase or decrease in tone.[1]

PRIMARY MECHANISMS THAT MEDIATE TONE

Extrapyramidal Structures (Part of the Upper Motor Neuron System)

- The extrapyramidal structures are motor centers and pathways located outside the pyramidal system.
- These include brainstem centers such as the vestibular nuclei and the reticular nuclei.
- The extrapyramidal structures also include extrapyramidal motor tracts such as the vestibulospinal, rubrospinal, and reticulospinal pathways.[2]

Basal Ganglia

- The basal ganglia consist of the caudate, putamen, and globus pallidus (of the upper motor neuron [UMN] system).
- These nuclei also include the substantia nigra and the subthalamic nuclei.[2,3]

Pyramidal Structures

- The pyramidal structures include the corticospinal tracts (of the UMN system).[4]

Cerebellum

- The cerebellum works in a feedback/feedforward loop with the (a) brainstem, basal ganglia, and extrapyramidal structures; and (b) the muscle spindles (MSs), Golgi tendon organs (GTOs), and joint receptors.
- The cerebellum also mediates tone through the afferent sensory tracts that travel to the cerebellum: posterior and anterior spinocerebellar tracts, cuneocerebellar tracts, and rostral spinocerebellar tracts.[4]

Motor Neurons of the Ventral Horn (of the Lower Motor Neuron System)

- The alpha and gamma motor neurons (MNs) of the ventral horn mediate tone.[5]

Peripheral Nerves That Innervate Skeletal Muscle (of the Lower Motor Neuron System)

- The peripheral nerves that innervate the skeletal muscles also mediate tone.[6]

CLASSIFICATIONS OF TONE

Hypotonicity

- Hypotonicity is an abnormal decrease in muscle tone (eg, hypotonicity can be observed in floppy babies and individuals with spinal cord injury [SCI] below L1).

Gutman SA. *Quick Reference Neuroscience for Rehabilitation Professionals: The Essential Neurologic Principles Underlying Rehabilitation Practice, Third Edition* (pp 246-255).

- Hypotonicity is caused by lower motor neuron (LMN) lesions[7]:
  - Damage to the MNs in the ventral horn
  - Damage to the spinal nerves in the periphery
- Lesions to the posterior cerebellar lobe (neocerebellar lobe) produce hypotonicity and hyporeflexia.[8]

Hypertonicity

- Hypertonicity is an abnormal increase in muscle tone accompanied by resistance to active and passive movement.
- Hypertonicity is caused by UMN damage.
- Lesions to the anterior cerebellar lobe (paleocerebellar lobe) also produce hypertonicity and hyperactive reflexes.[9]

Spasticity

- Spasticity is a form of hypertonicity.
- Spasticity involves difficulty actively and passively moving the spastic muscle groups on one side of a joint.
- Either the flexors or extensors are spastic, but not both.
- Spasticity is velocity dependent; that is, spasticity can be elicited by passively moving an affected limb quickly. The same passive movement of the limb performed slowly may not elicit spasticity.
- Spasticity is associated with such disorders as SCI (T12 and above), head injury, cerebrovascular accident, and cerebral palsy.[4,10]

Rigidity

- Rigidity is a form of hypertonicity and involves difficulty actively and passively moving the muscle groups on both sides of a joint.
- Rigidity is velocity independent; that is, increased muscle tone exists whether an affected limb is passively moved slowly or quickly.
- Rigidity is associated with such disorders as Parkinson disease.[11]

Clasp Knife Phenomenon

- Clasp knife phenomenon involves severe spasticity at a joint.
- A sustained stretch will relax the muscle group, and the spasticity will suddenly give way.[12]

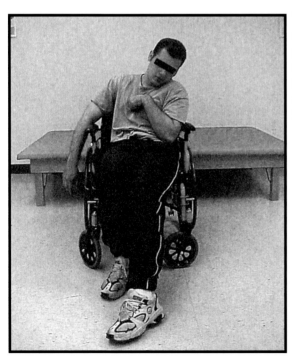

Typical posture of an individual with left hemiplegia. Increased tone on the contralateral side of the body. Head and neck are flexed; scapula is retracted and depressed; shoulder is adducted and internally rotated; elbow, wrist, and fingers are flexed; forearm is pronated; wrist is ulnarly deviated; fingers are adducted; hip, leg, knee, and ankle are extended; pelvis is posteriorly tilted; thigh is internally rotated; foot is inverted.

Cogwheel Rigidity

- Cogwheel rigidity occurs when increased muscle tone results in jerky, alternating resistance to passive movement as muscles contract and relax.
- In cogwheel rigidity, the resistance is jerky and characterized by a pattern of release/resistance in a quick jerky movement.
- This is often seen in Parkinson disease.[13]

Lead Pipe Rigidity

- Lead pipe rigidity occurs when increased muscle tone results in continuous and sustained resistance to passive movement through a limb's entire range of motion.
- Lead pipe rigidity is characterized by a uniform and continuous resistance to passive movement as the extremity is moved through its range of motion (in all planes).[14]

Clonus

- Clonus is an uncontrolled oscillation of a muscle that occurs in a spastic muscle group (results from UMN lesions).[15]

THEORIES OF SPASTICITY (ETIOLOGY)

Hyperactive Reflex Arcs

- The reflex arc is firing without modification from the cortex.
- This occurs in an UMN SCI when the corticospinal tracts are lost.
- Below the lesion level, the corticospinal tracts are lost; however, the reflex arc remains intact and fires without modification from the higher centers.
- This results in spasticity.[10]

Reduced Reciprocal Inhibition of the Antagonist and Synergy Muscles

- When lesions cause a reduction in the ability of the alpha MNs to inhibit the activity of antagonist and synergy muscle groups, the agonist fires without modification.
- This can result in spasticity.[4,10]

Loss of the Cortical Modification of the Alpha Motor Neurons in the Ventral Horn

- When lesions to the brainstem and subcortical motor center occur, cortical inhibition of these motor centers is lost.
- This causes the alpha and gamma MNs to fire without modification from the cortex.
- This can result in increased tone.[4,10]

Damage to the Primary Motor Area

- When damage to the primary motor area occurs, the corticospinal tracts fire without cortical modification, causing spasticity.[4,10]

Damage to the Brainstem Regions That Contain the Supraspinal Motor Centers

- The supraspinal motor centers include the vestibular nuclei, reticular nuclei, and pontine nuclei.
- When these are damaged, severe spasticity can occur in the form of extensor tone.[4,10]

THERAPEUTIC TECHNIQUES TO INFLUENCE TONE

Sustained Stretch on the Agonist

- Any sustained stretch on an agonist (of a spastic contracting muscle group) will activate the GTOs, located in the spastic agonist.
- The GTOs serve to inhibit the spasticity of the agonist and facilitate the antagonist muscle group.
- Example: If the biceps are spastic, place the elbow joint on a sustained stretch (in extension). This will activate the GTOs; the GTOs will inhibit the spastic contracting agonist and facilitate the antagonist muscle groups.[16,17]

Quick Stretch on the Agonist

- A quick stretch on the agonist activates the MS.
- The MS sends messages to the alpha MNs in the ventral horn to continue innervating the agonist.
- Example: In a floppy baby, quick stretches on the biceps may increase tone in the biceps for functional upper extremity use.[16,17]

Placing Pressure on the Tendon of the Agonist

- Placing pressure on the tendon of the agonist of a spastic muscle group will activate the GTOs.
- The GTOs will inhibit the spastic contracting agonist and facilitate the antagonist.
- Example: If the biceps are spastic, place sustained pressure on the tendons of the biceps to activate the GTOs. This will relax the spasticity in the biceps and facilitate activity in the triceps.
- Never place pressure on the muscle belly of the contracting spastic muscle. This will activate the MS and continue to increase spasticity in the spastic muscle.[12]

Splinting

- Splinting works on the premise of positioning the spastic muscle group on a sustained stretch to reduce tone in the agonist.
- Example: Spasticity in the wrist flexors
- Use a resting pan splint to place the wrist flexors on a sustained stretch in extension.
- The GTOs will become activated and will serve to reduce the spasticity in the agonist and facilitate activity in the antagonist (the wrist extensors).
- It is very important to make sure that the splint is well-fitting, or the cutaneous receptors will activate the gamma MNs. The gamma MNs will send signals to the MS to fire, thus facilitating spasticity in the agonist (the wrist flexors).[18]

Serial Casting

- Serial casting involves placing the spastic muscle groups around a joint in a cast to increase range of motion (ROM) over time.
- Example: Elbow flexors are spastic.
- In the initial cast, the therapist pulls the elbow flexors into slightly greater extension and places a cast on the elbow joint in this position.
- Essentially, the cast places the elbow flexors on a prolonged sustained stretch.

- The GTOs become activated and reduce the spasticity in the elbow flexors.
- Every few days or once per week, the therapist places a new cast on the spastic joint.
- With each successive cast, the elbow joint is positioned in greater extension to gradually increase ROM.
- A common problem with serial casting is skin breakdown. If skin breakdown occurs, the cast must be removed and the skin must heal until any further casting can be done. Unfortunately, while the skin is healing, the patient's spastic muscle group will often resume its initial degree of spasticity. Any ROM that has been gained as a result of serial casting is often lost.[19]

Reducing Clonus Through Sustained Stretching

- Clonus is an uncontrolled oscillation of a muscle that occurs in a spastic muscle group.
- Clonus can frequently be observed in the ankle joint of individuals with quadriplegia.
- When the therapist places the patient's foot on the wheelchair footplate, the therapist is essentially giving a quick stretch to the plantarflexors.
- This quick stretch activates the MS and causes the plantarflexors to contract uncontrollably.
- To reduce clonus[20]:
  ◦ Position the plantarflexors on a sustained stretch; in other words, pull the foot into dorsiflexion on a sustained stretch.
  ◦ This will activate the GTOs. The spastic muscle group (the plantarflexors) will relax.

Modified Ashworth Scale: Used to Evaluate Tone

0 No increase in muscle tone
1 Slight increase in tone manifested by a catch and release or by minimal resistance at the end of the ROM when the affected joint is flexed or extended
−1 Slight increase in muscle tone manifested by a catch followed by minimal resistance throughout the remainder (less than half) of the ROM
2 More marked increase in muscle tone through most of the ROM, but the affected joint is easily moved
3 Considerable increase in muscle tone, making passive movement difficult
4 Affected joint is rigid in flexion or extension[21]

Synergy Patterns of the Upper and Lower Extremities

- A synergy pattern is a stereotyped set of movements that occur in response to a stimulus or voluntary movement.
- Synergy patterns involve pathology of muscle tone that affects joint position after neurologic damage, such as traumatic brain injury (TBI) and cerebrovascular accident (CVA).
- Synergies are described as patterns because the involved joint positions occur consistently as a result of specific neurologic damage.
- Specific flexor and extensor synergies can be observed in the upper and lower extremities.
- Synergy patterns can change as the patient experiences stages of recovery, or they may continue if recovery of damaged brain structures cannot occur.[22]

Joint	Flexor Synergy Pattern	Extensor Synergy Pattern
Scapula	Elevation and retraction	Protraction and depression
Shoulder	Abduction and external rotation	Horizontal adduction and internal rotation
Elbow	Flexion	Extension and pronation
Forearm	Supination	Pronation
Wrist	Flexion and ulnar deviation	Extension
Fingers	Flexion and adduction	Flexion and adduction
Thumb	Flexion and adduction	Flexion and adduction
Hip	Flexion, abduction, and external rotation	Extension, adduction, and internal rotation
Knee	Flexion	Extension
Ankle	Dorsiflexion and inversion	Plantarflexion and inversion
Toes	Dorsiflexion	Plantarflexion

Associated Reactions

- Associated reactions are stereotyped movements in which effortful use of one extremity influences the posture and tone of another extremity (usually the opposite extremity). In other words, voluntary movements of one extremity produce unintentional movements in another extremity.
- Associated reactions can occur in normal movement as a result of reflex stimulation. For example, yawning, sneezing, coughing, and stretching all involve unintentional movements.
- Associated reactions can also occur as a result of pathology. Example: A patient several days post-stroke has a right upper extremity flexor synergy pattern. When she uses her uninvolved left limb to brush her hair, her affected right upper extremity becomes more flexed and abducted.
- Associated reactions can also occur during voluntary strenuous movement. Example: A patient with a right upper extremity flexor synergy pattern is attempting to ambulate. As he ambulates, a marked increase in spasticity can be observed in his right upper extremity.
- Associated reactions result from an overflow of activity into the opposite limb. This occurs because of an inability to selectively inhibit the interneurons that synapse with the motor cell bodies of the opposite limb.[23,24]

REFERENCES

1. Gurfinkel V, Cacciatore TW, Cordo P, Horak F, Nutt J, Skoss R. Postural muscle tone in the body axis of healthy humans. *J Neurophysiol.* 2006;96(5):2678-2687. doi:10.1152/jn.00406.2006.

2. Takakusaki K, Habaguchi T, Ohtinata-Sugimoto J, Saitoh K, Sakamoto T. Basal ganglia efferents to the brainstem centers controlling postural muscle tone and locomotion: a new concept for understanding motor disorders in basal ganglia dysfunction. *Neuroscience.* 2003;119(1):293-308. doi:10.1016/S0306-4522(03)00095-2.

3. DeLong MR, Georgopoulos AP. Motor functions of the basal ganglia. In: *Comprehensive Physiology.* Published online 2011. doi:10.1002/cphy.cp010221.

4. Ivanhoe CB, Reistetter TA. Spasticity: the misunderstood part of the upper motor neuron syndrome. *Am J Phys Med Rehabil.* 2004;83(10):S3-S9.

5. Lai YY, Kodama T, Siegel JM. Changes in monoamine release in the ventral horn and hypoglossal nucleus linked to pontine inhibition of muscle tone: an in vivo microdialysis study. *J Neurosci.* 2001;21(18):7384-7391.

6. Dietz V, Sinkjaer T. Spastic movement disorder: impaired reflex function and altered muscle mechanics. *Lancet Neurol.* 2007;6(8):725-733. doi:10.1016/S1474-4422(07)70193-X.

7. Richer LP, Shevell MI, Miller SP. Diagnostic profile of neonatal hypotonia: an 11-year study. *Pediatr Neurol.* 2001;25(1): 32-37. doi:10.1016/S0887-8994(01)00277-6.

8. Wassmer E, Davies P, Whitehouse WP, Green SH. Clinical spectrum associated with cerebellar hypoplasia. *Pediatr Neurol.* 2003;28(5):347-351. doi:10.1016/S0887-8994(03)00016-X.

9. Sanger TD, Delgado MR, Gaebler-Spira D, Hallett M, Mink JW. Classification and definition of disorders causing hypertonia in childhood. *Pediatrics.* 2003;111(1):e89-97. doi:10.1542/peds.111.1.e89.

10. Sheean G. The pathophysiology of spasticity. *Eur J Neurol.* 2002;9(Suppl 1):3-9. doi:10.1046/j.1468-1331.2002.0090s1003.x.

11. Levin J, Krafczyk S, Valkovič P, Eggert T, Claassen J, Bötzel K. Objective measurement of muscle rigidity in Parkinsonian patients treated with subthalamic stimulation. *Mov Disord.* 2009;24(1):57-63. doi:10.1002/mds.22291.

12. Kheder A, Nair KPS. Spasticity: pathophysiology, evaluation and management. *Pract Neurol.* 2012;12(5):289-298. doi:10.1136/practneurol-2011-000155.

13. Ghiglione P, Mutani R, Chiò A. Cogwheel rigidity. *Arch Neurol.* 2005;62(5):828-830. doi:10.1001/archneur.62.5.828.

14. Endo T, Okuno R, Yokoe M, Akazawa K, Sakoda S. A novel method for systematic analysis of rigidity in Parkinson's disease. *Mov Disord.* 2009;24(15):2218-2224. doi:10.1002/mds.22752.

15. Wallace DM, Ross BH, Thomas CK. Characteristics of lower extremity clonus after human cervical spinal cord injury. *J Neurotrauma.* 2012;29(5):915-924. doi:10.1089/neu.2010.1549.

16. Gracies JM. Pathophysiology of impairment in patients with spasticity and use of stretch as a treatment of spastic hypertonia. *Phys Med Rehabil Clin North Am.* 2001;12(4):747-68.

17. Cooper A, Musa IM, Van Deursen R, Wiles CM. Electromyography characterization of stretch responses in hemiparetic stroke patients and their relationship with the Modified Ashworth Scale. *Clin Rehabil.* 2005;19(7):760-766. doi:10.1191/0269215505cr888oa.

18. Pizzi A, Carlucci G, Falsini C, Verdesca S, Grippo A. Application of a volar static splint in poststroke spasticity of the upper limb. *Arch Phys Med Rehabil.* 2005;86(9):1855-1859. doi:10.1016/j.apmr.2005.03.032.

19. Yasar E, Tok F, Safaz I, Balaban B, Yilmaz B, Alaca R. The efficacy of serial casting after botulinum toxin type A injection in improving equinovarus deformity in patients with chronic stroke. *Brain Inj.* 2010;24(5):736-739.

20. Sheean G, McGuire JR. (2009). Spastic hypertonia and movement disorders: pathophysiology, clinical presentation, and quantification. *Phys Med Rehabil.* 2009;1(9):827-833. doi:10.1016/j.pmrj.2009.08.002.

21. Bohannon RW, Smith MB. Interrater reliability of a Modified Ashworth Scale of Muscle Spasticity. *Phys Ther.* 1987;67(2):206-207.

22. Cheung VC, Turolla A, Agostini M. Muscle synergy patterns as physiological markers of motor cortical damage. *Proc Natl Acad Sci U S A.* 2012;109(36):14652-14656. doi: 10.1073/pnas.1212056109.

23. Bhakta BB, Cozens JA, Chamberlain MA, Bamford JM. Quantifying associated reactions in the paretic arm in stroke and their relationship to spasticity. *Clinical Rehabil.* 2001;15(2):195-206. doi:10.1191/026921501671342614.

24. Bhakta BB, O'Connor RJ, Cozens AJ. Associated reactions after stroke: a randomized controlled trial of the effect of botulinum toxin type A. *J Rehabil Med.* 2008;40(1):36-41. doi:10.2340/16501977-0120.

CLINICAL TEST QUESTIONS

Sections 20 to 21

1. Since her head injury causing cerebellar damage, Mrs. Johnson has difficulty understanding where her limbs are in relation to each other and where her body is in space. Which neurological system is responsible for the recognition of an organism's position in relationship to the environment?
   a. vestibular system
   b. proprioceptive system
   c. basal ganglia system
   d. ventricular system

2. After her stroke, Mrs. Williams's occupational therapist fabricated a wrist cock-up splint for her spastic right wrist and hand. Splinting is a therapeutic technique that works on which of the following principles?
   a. A quick stretch of a spastic muscle group facilitates the Golgi tendon organs, which inhibit the spastic muscles.
   b. Placing pressure on the muscle belly of a spastic muscle group facilitates the Golgi tendon organs, which inhibit the spastic muscles.
   c. A sustained stretch of a muscle group facilitates the Golgi tendon organs, which inhibit the spastic muscles.

3. Mr. Tomlinson had a right hemisphere stroke 2 weeks ago. When his therapist passively moves his left elbow joint into extension, the elbow joint is initially highly spastic and cannot be moved. With sustained stretched on the elbow flexors, the spasticity suddenly gives way and the elbow joint can be moved into extension. This type of spasticity is referred to as:
   a. cogwheel rigidity
   b. lead pipe rigidity
   c. clonus
   d. clasp knife phenomenon

4. Mr. Okonjo has been diagnosed with Parkinson disease. When the therapist attempts to range his elbow joint, the joint resistance is jerky and characterized by a pattern of release/resistance. This type of rigidity is known as:
   a. cogwheel rigidity
   b. lead pipe rigidity
   c. clonus
   d. clasp knife phenomenon

5. Mandeep's SCI occurred at level T6, and he uses a wheelchair for mobility. When his wife attempts to move his foot onto the footplate of the wheelchair, his ankle flexor muscles uncontrollably oscillate, causing his lower extremity to rhythmically jerk and spasm. This phenomenon is called _____ and can be reduced by _____.
   1. cogwheel rigidity
   2. clonus
   3. placing the spastic muscle (ankle flexors) on a sustained stretch, thereby facilitating the Golgi tendon organs
   4. performing a quick stretch of the spastic muscles (ankle flexors) to facilitate the muscle spindles
   a. 1, 3
   b. 2, 3
   c. 1, 4
   d. 2, 4

6. Mrs. Goldstein has been diagnosed with Parkinson disease. When the therapist attempts to passively range her elbow joint, the movement is characterized by a uniform and continuous resistance to passive movement. This form of hypertonicity is known as:
   a. cogwheel rigidity
   b. clasp knife phenomenon
   c. clonus
   d. lead pipe rigidity

7. After his stroke, Mr. Nakai is observed to exhibit scapular elevation and retraction, shoulder abduction and external rotation, elbow flexion, forearm supination, and wrist and finger flexion. This upper extremity pattern is a stereotyped set of movements that occur in response to neurological damage and may be further promoted by an environmental stimulus or by the patient's voluntary movement. This movement pattern is known as:
   a. an associated reaction
   b. decerebrate rigidity
   c. a synergy pattern

8. After Mrs. Perloff's stroke, she demonstrates increased spasticity in her right upper extremity when she brushes her hair or engages in any effortful movement using her left arm. This phenomenon is called _____ and results from an inability to selectively inhibit the interneurons that synapse on motor cell bodies of the opposing limb.
   a. an associated reaction
   b. a synergy pattern
   c. decorticate rigidity

9. Mackenzie is a 3-year-old child with low muscle tone. To increase tone in her upper extremities and trunk, her occupational therapist is likely to use which of the following techniques?
   a. placing pressure on the muscle belly of Mackenzie's hypotonic muscles
   b. performing sustained stretches of Mackenzie's hypotonic muscles
   c. performing quick stretches of Mackenzie's hypotonic muscles

10. Mr. Kronberger is in a progressed stage of Parkinson disease. He has the type of hypertonicity in which his muscles are resistant to passive stretch on both sides of a joint and the resistance is not velocity dependent. This type of hypertonicity is called _____ and is caused by _____ motor neuron damage.
    1. spasticity
    2. rigidity
    3. upper
    4. lower
   a. 1, 3
   b. 1, 4
   c. 2, 3
   d. 2, 4

Answers

1. b
2. c
3. d
4. a
5. b
6. d
7. c
8. a
9. c
10. c

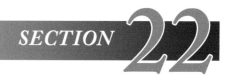

Motor Functions and Dysfunctions of the Central Nervous System
Cortex, Basal Ganglia, Cerebellum

CEREBRAL CORTEX

Cortical Mapping of the Brain

- The first neuroanatomist to attempt brain mapping was Brodmann, who numbered each area of the cortex.
- In 1909, Brodmann mapped 52 brain areas.
- Brodmann believed that each numbered area corresponded to a precise brain function.
- The boundaries between each area were often imprecise.
- Today, we know that the correlation between Brodmann's areas and a specific function is not precise.
- Positron emission tomography (PET) and magnetic resonance imaging (MRI) scans are used to more precisely map brain areas today.[1]

Functional Divisions of the Cerebrum

Archicortex

- The archicortex is the core of the brain and is believed to be phylogenetically old.
- The archicortex is composed of the hippocampal formation, which is located deep in the brain and is involved in learning and memory.[2]

Paleocortex

- The palcocortex is the outer layer that sits over the core. It includes the piriform cortex and the parahippocampal gyrus.
- The parahippocampal gyrus is a region of the limbic system that is adjacent to the hippocampus.
- The piriform cortex is part of the rhinencephalon and functions in olfaction.
- The parahippocampal gyrus and piriform cortex relay information between the hippocampus and other brain regions.[3]

Neocortex

- The neocortex is considered to be the newest part of the brain phylogenetically.
- It is composed of the most superficial layers of the brain and includes the primary motor cortex, the primary sensory cortex, and the association cortices.
- The neocortex is found only in mammals and makes up 50% to 80% of the brain's total volume.[4]

Gutman SA. *Quick Reference Neuroscience for Rehabilitation Professionals:*
The Essential Neurologic Principles Underlying Rehabilitation Practice,
Third Edition (pp 256-280).
© 2017 Taylor & Francis Group.

The Cerebrum's Role in Motor Control

Primary Motor Area

- The primary motor area (M1) is located in the precentral gyrus. This is where voluntary/conscious movement is initiated.
- The corticospinal tracts originate here, and it is the site of the motor homunculus.
- The primary motor cortex works interactively with other motor areas (the supplementary motor area, the premotor cortex, frontal eye fields, and motor association areas) to plan and implement movement.[5]

Motor Homunculus

- The motor homunculus is the map that denotes each body part's cortical representation for voluntary movement.
- The face and mouth have a large amount of cortical representation for the purpose of speech and eating.
- The hands also have a large cortical representation for the fine motor control necessary to explore the environment.
- The cortical representation for the lower extremities is located in the medial longitudinal fissure.[6]

Organization of the Motor Homunculus

- The organization of the motor homunculus is not permanent.
- Individuals need to use each body part, or the cortical representation for that body part disappears, as with amputees over time.[6]

Lesion to the Primary Motor Area

- A lesion to M1 causes a loss of voluntary movement of the contralateral body part.
- The loss of voluntary movement in a body part corresponds to the area of the motor homunculus that was damaged.
- A lesion to M1 may also result in a loss of the ability to implement a specific motor plan.[7]

Premotor Area

- The premotor area is located just anterior to M1.
- The premotor area has a role in motor planning, or *praxis*.[7]

Lesion to the Premotor Area

- A lesion to the premotor area causes apraxia, or *motor planning difficulties*.
- Apraxia involves either the inability to understand the demands of the task or the inability to access the appropriate motor plan.[7]

Motto of the Brain: "Use It or Lose It"

- Cortical representations of each body part on the sensory and motor homunculi are use-dependent.
- In other words, each body part must be consistently used, or it will lose its place on the topographical map of the homunculi.
- The cortical representation for a specific body region can be rapidly appropriated by other body regions if that specific body part loses its function due to pathology (eg, amputation, peripheral nerve injury, orthopedic injury causing prolonged inactivity of a limb).
- Once a cortical area representing a specific body region is gone from the topographical map, the person must recreate it through new experiences. For example, if a patient has lost hand function from a peripheral nerve injury lasting several months, the patient must recreate the hand area on the cortical map through use of the hand as the muscles become reinnervated.[8]

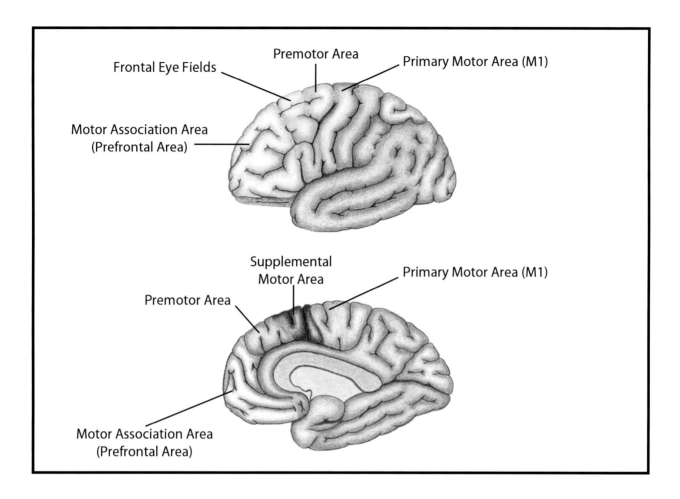

Motor Association Area

- The motor association area is also called the *prefrontal area* and is located in the anterior frontal lobe.
- The motor association area has a role in the cognitive planning of movement.[9]

Lesion to the Motor Association Area

- A lesion to the motor association area causes the storage of specific motor plans to be lost.
- This involves an inability to cognitively understand how to carry out a motor task that was once known before injury/disease.
- The premotor area may be able to take over and compensate for damage to the motor association area.[9]

Supplementary Motor Area

- The supplementary motor area is part of the premotor area and is located inside the medial longitudinal fissure.
- The supplementary motor area has a role in the bilateral control of posture.[10]

Lesion to the Supplementary Motor Area

- A lesion to the supplementary area may result in loss of bilateral control of posture.
- Other areas may take over and compensate for this loss; for example, the cerebellum or vestibular system.[10]

Frontal Eye Field

- The frontal eye fields are located in the middle frontal gyrus, anterior to the premotor area, and are responsible for visual saccades.[11]

Lesion to the Frontal Eye Field

- A lesion to the frontal eye field results in deviation of the eyes to the same side of the lesion.[11]

Praxis Involves Three Processes

Ideational Praxis
- Ideational praxis is the ability to cognitively understand the motor demands of the task.
- For example, when shown a shirt, the patient must be able to understand that this is an article of clothing that is worn on the trunk and upper extremities. The patient must also understand the motor plans needed to don a shirt.
- Ideational praxis is largely a function of the motor association area.[12]

Ideomotor Planning I
- Ideomotor planning I is the ability to access the appropriate motor plan. For example, the ability to sort through all stored motor plans and identify the specific one for shirt donning involves ideomotor planning I.
- Such motor plans are commonly stored in the premotor area.[12]

Ideomotor Planning II
- Ideomotor planning II is the ability to execute the appropriate motor plan, or put it into action. For example, after identifying the appropriate motor plan for donning a shirt, the patient must put that plan into action.
- Implementing motor plans commonly involves M1.[12]
- Pathology can occur in any of these 3 stages of motor planning.

Emergence of Primitive Reflexes as a Result of Neurologic Damage

- When serious neurologic damage occurs to the cortex, internal capsule, diencephalon, brainstem, and/or basal ganglia, often as a result of stroke or traumatic brain injury, it is common for primitive reflexes to re-emerge.
- Primitive reflexes develop during gestation and infancy and become integrated by the *central nervous system* (CNS) in the first months or years of life.
- These reflexes facilitate normal movement.
- The re-emergence of these reflexes in an adult with neurologic damage indicates severe CNS pathology. Volitional movement is compromised by the presence of such reflexes.
- There are 2 primary types of primitive reflexes[13]:
    1. Spinal level (or elemental) reflexes
    2. Brainstem level reflexes

Spinal Level Reflexes

Flexor withdrawal	When the sole of the foot is stimulated, the toes extend, the foot dorsiflexes, and the leg flexes. In an adult with neurologic damage, this often interferes with attempts to stand.	Develops at 28 weeks of gestation Integrated at 1 to 2 months
Crossed extension	When an extended leg is passively flexed, the opposite leg extends. In an adult with neurologic damage, this can interfere with attempts to assume a seated position, such as returning to a seated position in a wheelchair. It can also interfere with transfer training.	Develops at 28 weeks of gestation Integrated at 1 to 2 months
Extensor thrust	When the ball of the foot of a flexed leg is stimulated, that leg extends. In an adult with neurologic damage, this can interfere with attempts to assume a seated position, such as returning to a seated position in a wheelchair. It can also interfere with transfer training.	Develops between birth and 2 months Integrated at 1 to 2 months

(continued)

Emergence of Primitive Reflexes as a Result of Neurologic Damage

(continued)

Brainstem Level Reflexes

Asymmetrical tonic neck	When the head is rotated to one side, the opposite shoulder and elbow flex in a bow and arrow position. In an adult with neurologic damage, this interferes with volitional use of the upper extremities.	Develops at birth Integrated at 4 to 6 months
Symmetrical tonic neck	When the head flexes, the arms flex and the legs extend. When the head extends, the arms extend and the legs flex. In an adult with neurologic damage, this interferes with volitional movement of the upper and lower extremities.	Develops at 4 to 6 months Integrated at 8 to 12 months
Symmetrical tonic labyrinthine	When placed in a prone position, the patient's arms and legs flex. When placed in a supine position, the arms and legs extend. In an adult with neurologic damage, this interferes with learning to transfer from bed to wheelchair.	Develops at birth Integrated at 6 months
Positive support reaction	When the ball of the foot makes contact with the floor (in a standing position), the legs experience rigid extensor tone. In an adult with neurologic damage, this interferes with relearning to walk.	Develops at birth Integrated at 6 months
Associated reactions	In response to effortful, voluntary movement (in any limb), the patient experiences involuntary movement usually in the opposite limb. In an adult with neurologic damage, this interferes with volitional movement.	Develops between birth and 3 months Integrated at 8 to 9 years

Babinski Sign

- The Babinski sign is a superficial cutaneous reflex that is elicited by stroking the outer border of the plantar surface of the foot.
- The reflex is caused by a brief contraction of muscles that are innervated by the same spinal segments that respond to the cutaneous stimulation.
- A positive Babinski sign is indicated by extension of the first toe accompanied by fanning of the other toes.
- A positive Babinski sign in an adult with neurologic damage is always indicative of damage to the corticospinal tracts (or to CNS damage involving the corticospinal tracts, such as damage to the internal capsule, thalamus, and brainstem).[14]

Hoffman Sign

- Hoffman sign is another superficial cutaneous reflex.
- This reflex can be elicited by flicking the nail of the patient's third finger.
- A positive Hoffman sign is indicated by prompt adduction of the thumb and flexion of the index finger.
- The presence of Hoffman sign in an adult with neurologic damage is indicative of damage to the corticospinal tracts (or to CNS damage involving the corticospinal tracts, such as damage to the internal capsule, thalamus, and brainstem).[15]

Absence of Higher-Level Reactions as a Result of Neurologic Damage

- Higher-level reactions are reflexes that develop during infancy or early childhood and remain throughout the lifespan.
- These types of reactions are controlled by centers in the midbrain, basal ganglia, and cortex:
  - Righting reactions
  - Equilibrium reactions
  - Protective extension
- Higher-level reactions are important for normal postural control and movement.
- When neurologic damage occurs in an adult, higher-level reactions typically disappear.
- Their absence leads to postural instability, balance problems, and an inability to protect oneself when falling.[16]

Midbrain Level Reactions

Righting Reactions

Neck righting on body	When the head is passively rotated to one side (in supine), the body also rotates as a whole (log rolls) to align with the head.	Develops at 4 to 6 months Integrated at 5 years
Body righting on body	When the upper or lower trunk is passively rotated (in supine) as an isolated segment, the other segment also rotates to become aligned.	Develops at 4 to 6 months Integrated at 5 years
Labyrinthine head righting	When the body is tipped in different positions (with vision occluded), the head orients to a vertical position. When this reaction is lost, the ability to maintain the head in a vertical position for orientation is lost.	Develops between birth and 2 years Persists throughout life

Basal Ganglial Level Reactions

Protective extension (PE)	When the patient's center of gravity is displaced, the arms and legs extend outward to protect the body when falling. Patients who lose protective extension are at an increased risk for injuring themselves when they lose their balance.	PE of the arms develops at 4 to 6 months; PE of the legs develops at 6 to 9 months Persists throughout life
Equilibrium reactions (tilting)	When the center of gravity is displaced by moving the support surface, the trunk will curve and the extremities will extend and abduct. The maintenance of balance and postural control is severely impaired when this reaction is lost.	Develops between 6 and 21 months Persists throughout life
Equilibrium reactions (postural fixation)	When the body is pushed, altering the center of gravity, the trunk will curve toward the external force. The extremities will extend and abduct. The maintenance of balance and postural control is severely impaired when this reaction is lost.	Develops between 6 and 21 months Persists throughout life

Cortical Level Reaction

Optic righting	When the body is repositioned by tipping it in different directions, the head orients to a vertical position.	Develops between birth to 2 months Persists throughout life

THE BASAL GANGLIA'S ROLE IN MOTOR CONTROL

Basal Ganglia

- The basal ganglia have a role in stereotypic and automated movement patterns (eg, walking, riding a bike, and writing).[17]
- The basal ganglia structures include the caudate, the putamen, and the globus pallidus. The subthalamic nucleus of the diencephalon, the substantia nigra of the midbrain, and the nucleus accumbens of the basal forebrain are also considered to be part of the basal ganglia.
- The axons of the substantia nigra form the nigrostriatal pathway, which supplies dopamine to the striatum. Dopamine is produced by the substantia nigra.
- While the basal ganglia have traditionally been thought of as a subcortical (and involuntary) motor system, recent research suggests that the basal ganglia may also function in cognitive and affective processes requiring precision timing, such as the ability to know when it is appropriate to contribute to social interaction or the ability to inhibit one's desire to act upon personal impulses.[18]
- Children with attention deficit hyperactivity disorder (ADHD) who display difficulty taking turns, refraining from calling out in class, and controlling the urge to physically move may experience such difficulty, in part, because of pathology in the basal ganglia's ability to balance inhibitory and excitatory actions.[19]
- Research also suggests that the basal ganglia may have roles in the cognitive processing of decisions regarding rewarding and addicting behaviors.[20]
- With regard to motor performance, the basal ganglia achieve precision control as a result of a balance between their inhibitory and excitatory effects.
- The basal ganglia are also modulated by 3 primary neurotransmitters: dopamine, γ-aminobutyric acid (GABA), and acetylcholine (ACh).
- The majority of basal ganglia neurons use the neurotransmitter GABA, which exerts inhibition of target areas and functions.[21]
- Generally, dopamine stimulates the basal ganglia pathways and, as a result, exerts an excitatory effect upon the cerebral cortex.
- Conversely, dopamine depletion, such as that found in Parkinson disease, causes a severe inhibitory effect upon movement.
- ACh works in opposition to dopamine.
- GABA, dopamine, and ACh work collaboratively to achieve a balanced inhibition and excitation of movement, which is necessary for precision and timed action.
- Motor disorders of the basal ganglia result in a disequilibrium between inhibitory and excitatory movement.

Divisions of the Basal Ganglia

Neostriatum

- The neostriatum is considered to be the newest region of the basal ganglia phylogenetically.
- It includes the caudate and putamen.
- The putamen is an excitatory structure.
- The caudate has a role in the inhibitory control of movement. The caudate acts like a brake on certain motor activities.
- When that brake is gone, hyperkinetic movement disorders can occur, like tics or Tourette syndrome.
- The caudate and putamen may also have roles in decision making regarding participation in activities that stimulate the reward centers of the brain.[22]

Paleostriatum

- The paleostriatum is considered to be the older part of the basal ganglia phylogenetically.
- It includes the globus pallidus, an inhibitory structure.[23]

Corpus Striatum

- The corpus striatum is the collective name for all 3 structures: the caudate, putamen, and globus pallidus.

BASIL GANGLIA AFFERENT PATHWAY

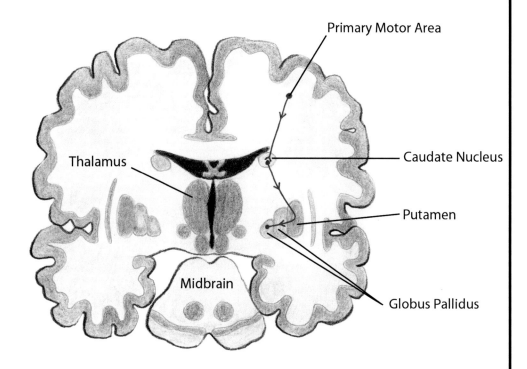

LENTICULAR FASCICULUS PATHWAY

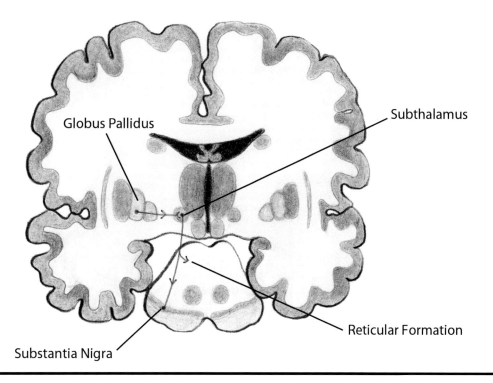

Collective Functions of the Basal Ganglia

Stereotypic Movement

- Stereotypic movements are motor patterns that are "hard-wired" (ie, do not have to be learned on a conscious level) and develop normally as the individual's nervous system matures (eg, stretching the arms during yawning, using a reciprocal arm swing when walking).[24]

Automated Movements

- Automated movements are movement patterns that used to be mediated by conscious cortical control but have been assumed by the basal ganglia structures once learned.
- This process underlies the saying, "Once you learn to ride a bike, you never forget," unless damage is sustained to the basal ganglia.
- Automated movements include driving, riding a bike, and writing.[25]

The Basal Ganglia Also Influence Tone

- The basal ganglia send input to the alpha and gamma motor neurons (MNs) in the ventral horn to influence muscle tone.[26]

Basal Ganglia Pathways

Afferent Basal Ganglia Pathways (Leading to the Basal Ganglia)

- The primary motor area and the premotor area send motor signals to the caudate, putamen, and globus pallidus.[27]

Lenticular Formation (Traveling From the Basal Ganglia)

- This pathway travels from the globus pallidus to the subthalamus, reticular formation, and substantia nigra.[27]

Ansa Lenticularis (Traveling From the Basal Ganglia)

- This pathway travels from the globus pallidus to the ventrolateral nucleus of the thalamus, M1, and the premotor area.[28]

Nigrostriatal Pathway (Feedback Circuit of the Basal Ganglia)

- This pathway travels from the substantia nigra to the globus pallidus and subthalamus.
- This circuit modifies the ansa lenticularis pathway.
- In Parkinson disease, the substantia nigra degenerates, and modification of the ansa lenticularis is lost.[29]

BASAL GANGLIA LESIONS

Symptoms

- Difficulty initiating, continuing, or stopping movement
- Problems with muscle tone (particularly rigidity)
- Increased involuntary, undesired movements (tremor, chorea)

Hemiballismus

- Hemiballismus is a lesion of the subthalamus and caudate causing a disinhibition of neuronal activity between the thalamus and the cortex.
- It results in violent thrashing of the contralateral extremity.
- Ballismus is the name of the disorder if the lesion is bilateral.[30]

Athetosis

- Athetosis involves a slow flailing of the upper and lower extremities and continuous movement.
- The disorder involves slow, aimless, purposeless movement, especially of the distal musculature.
- Movements often have a twisting or turning quality to them.
- Such movements are caused by continuous and prolonged contraction of agonist and antagonist muscle groups.
- Athetosis is caused by a lesion to the putamen and caudate with some cortical involvement.
- Athetosis is a slower movement than chorea.[31]

ANSA LENTICULARIS PATHWAY

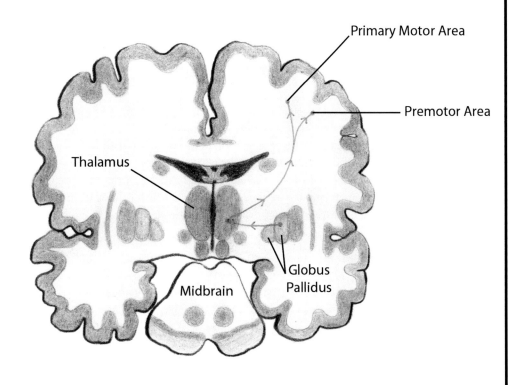

Primary Motor Area

Premotor Area

Thalamus

Globus Pallidus

Midbrain

NIGROSTRIATAL PATHWAY

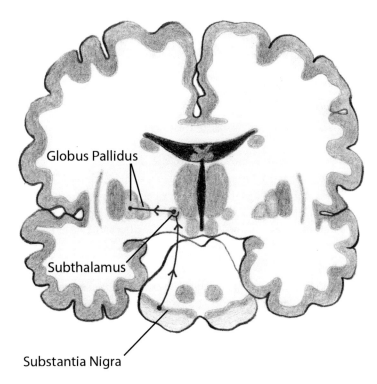

Globus Pallidus

Subthalamus

Substantia Nigra

Chorea

- Choreiform means to dance. Chorea is sudden, involuntary, jerky movements that appear dance-like in quality. Movement may appear as more coordinated and graceful than in athetoid conditions.
- The disorder usually involves axial and proximal limb areas: shoulder shrugs, moving hips, crossing and uncrossing the legs.
- Movements of the face may involve grimacing, eyebrow raising, eye rolling, and tongue protrusion.
- Chorea is caused by a lesion to the caudate and putamen.[32]

Huntington Chorea

- Huntington chorea is a chronic degenerative disorder that also involves a progressive dementia. The occurrence of dementia is likely related to the basal ganglia's role in cognition.
- It is an inherited disease that involves degeneration of the caudate nucleus and some areas of the cortex.
- GABA levels are diminished in the striatum and globus pallidus.
- GABA is a neurotransmitter that runs in the nigrostriatal pathway (from the striatum to the globus pallidus).
- GABA in this pathway modulates the outflow of dopamine, which runs in the nigrostriatal pathway.
- Increased dopamine in the basal ganglia is believed to cause Huntington disease.[33]

Dystonia

- Dystonia involves muscle contractions producing twisting movements that are repetitive and often result in abnormal postures.
- The sustained muscle contractions of dystonia can last from seconds to hours.
- Such postures often result from simultaneous opposing movements that produce paralysis.
- Dystonic muscle contractions that occur or recur over a length of time can eventually cause joint degeneration and permanent fixed postures.
- Dystonia can occur in the limbs, face, neck, and trunk.
- Experimental research has shown some evidence for the effectiveness of deep brain stimulation in the treatment of dystonia. This procedure involves placing electrodes in the globus pallidus, which are stimulated by a battery surgically implanted in the abdomen. It appears that continuous stimulation of the globus pallidus can shut it down, thereby alleviating the major symptoms of dystonia.[34]

Dyskinesia

- Dyskinesia involves rhythmic, repetitive movements that have an odd quality.
- It more frequently affects the face, mouth, jaw, and tongue (eg, grimacing, lip pursing, tongue protrusion, mouth opening and closing, jaw deviation) rather than the limbs.[35]

Tardive Dyskinesia

- Tardive dyskinesia is a movement disorder related to treatment with dopamine receptor antagonists (neuroleptics and antiemetics).
- The term *tardive* refers to the fact that this movement disorder occurs after chronic use of these drugs.
- It is characterized by choreiform movements, dystonia, tics, and/or myoclonus.
- Example: tongue protrusions (orobuccolingual movements), chewing-type movements, facial grimacing, blepharospasm, lip smacking
- Tardive dyskinesia is different from most disorders because the discontinuation of the causative agent (the neuroleptic) does not result in the amelioration of the movement disorder.[36]

Pathology of Tardive Dyskinesia

- The chronic use of neuroleptics results in a chronic blockage of dopamine receptors in the basal ganglia.
- The sensitivity of the dopamine receptors becomes severely decreased.
- Also suspected is a decrease in the neurotransmitter GABA in the basal ganglia.[36]

Parkinson Disease

- This results from damage to the nigrostriatal pathway between the substantia nigra and the basal ganglia. Dopamine is the neurotransmitter that uses this pathway.
- Parkinson disease is caused by cell death of the dopaminergic neurons of the substantia nigra; in other words, the substantia nigra degenerates.

Glossary of Terms of Idiopathic (no known origin) Torsion Dystonia

Involving the Eye
- *Blepharospasm*: eyes are involuntarily kept closed
- *Oculogyric crises*: attacks of forced deviation of gaze, often associated with a surge of Parkinsonism, catatonia, tics, and obsessiveness
- *Ophthalmoplegia*: paralysis of gaze

Involving the Throat, Jaw, Lips, or Tongue
- *Oromandibular dystonia*: involuntary opening and closing of the jaw, retraction or puckering of the lips
- *Lingual dystonia*: repetitive protrusion of the tongue or upward deflection of the tongue toward the hard palate
- *Laryngeal dystonia*: speech is tight, constricted, and forced. Smooth flow of speech is lost.
- *Pharyngeal dystonia*: Associated with dysphagia, dysphonia (hoarseness), and dysarthria (slurred words)

Involving the Neck
- *Torticollis*: dystonic contractions of the neck muscles
- *Retrocollis*: neck forced backward into hyperextension
- *Anterocollis*: neck forced forward into hyperflexion
- *Laterocollis*: neck forced laterally

Involving the Trunk
- *Truncal dystonia*: manifests as a lordosis, scoliosis, kyphosis, tortipelvis, opisthotonos (forced flexion of the head on the chest)

Involving the Legs
- *Crural dystonia*: Dystonic movement of the legs

Dystonia of Single or Multiple Body Parts
- *Focal dystonia*: dystonia in a single body part
- *Multifocal dystonia*: dystonia of more than one body part
- *Hemidystonia*: involvement of limbs on one side of the body (due to a space occupying lesion or infarction)
- *Generalized dystonia*: dystonia in a leg, the trunk, and one other body part; or both legs and the trunk
- As with most hyperkinetic movement disorders, the abnormal movements usually disappear during sleep and worsen with anxiety, fatigue, temperature changes, and pain.

- This leads to decreased levels of dopamine available for use by the basal ganglia.
- Depletion of dopamine then causes decreased modification of the ansa lenticularis pathway (the pathway that modifies the basal ganglia activity).
- Movement becomes disjointed and uncontrollable.
- As movement slows, mental processes also become delayed and halted. Problem solving drags, and language and communication become difficult.
- Half of all patients with Parkinson also experience depression and anxiety disorders. This likely occurs because dopamine also regulates mood and affective processes.
- One-third of patients with Parkinson develop dementia; again, this likely occurs because of the basal ganglia's collaborative role in cognition.[37,38]

Parkinson Symptoms
- Hypertonicity
- Cogwheel rigidity
- Bradykinesia (poverty of movement)
- Masklike face (facial muscles are affected by bradykinesia)
- Tremors at rest (pill-rolling)

- Cunctation-festinating gait: cunctation means to resist movement. Festination means to hurry. The individual experiences difficulty initiating and stopping movement.
- Loss of arm swing while walking
- Impaired postural reflexes (difficulty righting oneself and maintaining balance)
- Micrographia (handwriting becomes very small)[37]

Pharmacologic Treatment for Parkinson Disease

- L dopa
  - L dopa has been the most common treatment for Parkinson disease.
  - L dopa, or *levodopa*, is a precursor compound that the brain converts to dopamine.
  - Unlike dopamine, however, L dopa is able to cross the blood-brain barrier, the membrane that surrounds the brain and protects it from direct exposure to harmful substances.
  - When L dopa is used and crosses the blood-brain barrier, it is synthesized into dopamine.
  - With the increase in dopamine, the nigrostriatal pathway can run properly and modify the ansa lenticularis pathway.
  - While the initial effects of L dopa are accompanied by a return of fluid movement, patients generally become less responsive to such drugs over time.[39]
- Dopamine agonists
  - Dopamine agonists, another class of drugs, imitate the function of dopamine. These include bromocriptine, cabergoline, pramipexole, and ropinirole.
  - While initially such drugs are not as effective as L dopa, over time, their dosage in the body can be more accurately regulated.[40]

Kinesia Paradoxa in Parkinson Disease

- Kinesia paradoxa is the sudden total conversion of Parkinsonism to normality or to hyperkinesia due to pharmacologic treatment and/or visual and auditory cues from the environment.
- The cause of kinesia paradoxa is unknown, although some theoretical suggestions include the idea that visual and auditory cues activate different neural pathways and can bypass pathways damaged by the disease.
- For example, a person with Parkinson disease may be able to suddenly walk when brought to a floor surface having clear and distinct visual cues for depth.[41]
- Music has also been used to help people with Parkinson disease move more normally. People with the disease who have difficulty initiating movement may suddenly demonstrate the ability to move in response to music.[42]

Surgical Procedures for Parkinson Disease

- In the 1960s and 1970s, the only surgical option was pallidotomy, ablation of the globus pallidus.
- This was often a last resort treatment option and posed severe negative side effects.
- Today, deep brain stimulation (DBS) has become a more common procedure.
- DBS involves the implantation of electrodes into the basal ganglia or thalamic nuclei. A battery and controller implanted beneath the skin near the clavicle or abdomen send timed currents to the basal ganglia to improve motor performance.
- Patients often experience a significant reduction in Parkinsonian symptoms.
- DBS allows patients to decrease their drug intake and can provide improvement in motor function that can last for years.
- It does not, however, improve cognitive function or stop the progression of the disease.
- Undesirable side effects can include deafness and speech disorders.[43]

Stem Cell Research

- Stem cells are structurally fundamental cells that are able to mature into any type of cell.
- They can be found in embryonic as well as some adult tissue; for example, the subventricular midbrain and the hippocampus.
- Researchers are attempting to transform stem cells into dopamine-producing neurons via natural growth factors.
- Such cells would then be transplanted into patients in an effort to reverse Parkinsonian symptoms.[44]

Genetic Research

- Several researchers are involved in gene-based therapy, in which modified viruses are used to carry genes into the midbrain.
- The genes would then activate specific enzymes that could release or transport dopamine.
- While initial animal experiments have produced promising results, greater research is needed to better understand the benefits and risks of gene-based treatment.[45]

Tremor

- Tremor is involuntary oscillating movement resulting from alternating or synchronistic contractions of opposing muscles.
- There are different types of tremor.[46]

Essential Tremor

- Essential tremor is the most common form and is characterized by tremor upon movement (not a resting tremor, as in Parkinson disease).
- The fingers and hands are affected first.
- Tremor moves proximally to the head and neck.
- Essential tremor is a slow progressive disorder.[46]

Tics

- Tics are repetitive, brief, rapid, involuntary, and purposeless movements involving a single muscle or groups of muscles.
- Tics can also be fragments of movements or thoughts that are split off from more integrated behavior.
- People with tics describe an inner tension that builds. This inner tension can be relieved by the ticing behavior.
- Tics have a conscious component. The conscious experience of feeling compelled to make sound may imply that tics are a form of compulsion.
- Most people can suppress their tics for a brief period of time; however, suppression is often associated with a buildup of inner tension that causes the subsequent expression of tics to be more forceful than they would be otherwise.
- A tic can involve a brief, isolated movement like eye blinks, head jerks, or shoulder shrugs. Tics involving movement are referred to as *motor tics*.
- A tic can also be a variety of sounds such as throat clearing or grunting. Such tics are referred to as *phonic tics*.
- Tics can additionally be associated with intrusive thoughts that the individual feels compelled to express.
- Tics can be meaningful utterances:
  - Echolalia is an involuntary repetition of words just spoken by another person.
  - Palilalia is an involuntary repetition of words or sentences.
  - Coprolalia is an involuntary utterance of curse words.
- Tics frequently have a waxing and waning course. A specific tic can be present for weeks or even years. Other tics emerge and disappear with no predictable course.
- Tics will commonly increase during periods of stress and decrease during tasks requiring heightened concentration.
- While the long-term course of a tic disorder can be variable, most studies suggest that tics improve in late adolescence and early adulthood.
- Clinicians characterize tics by their anatomical location, number, frequency, intensity, and complexity.[47]

Etiology of Tics

- The dopamine system is a form of modifying and modulating movement.
- Increased sensitivity to dopamine in the basal ganglia causes severe tics.
- People with a normal response to dopamine have mild tics; this explains why normal people sometimes have tics or mild obsessional thoughts, especially with stress.
- With increased sensitivity to dopamine, the caudate (which normally acts like a brake on certain extraneous movements) cannot suppress movements like tics.[48]
- Pediatric autoimmune neuropsychiatric disorders associated with streptococcal infections (PANDAS) have been suggested as one possible cause for the childhood onset of tic disorders, in at least some percentage of children diagnosed with tics. In this subset of tic disorder, onset is abrupt, follows recovery from a streptococcal infection, occurs before puberty, and occurs in children with obsessive compulsive disorder (OCD) and motor hyperactivity.[49]

Treatment

- Non-neuroleptic drugs (eg, clonidine, guanfacine, baclofen, and clonazepam) are indicated for the suppression of mild tics.
- Neuroleptic drugs and dopamine receptor antagonists (eg, risperidone, olanzapine, ziprasidone, and quetiapine) are indicated for severe tic disorders.[50]

Tourette Syndrome

- Tourette syndrome is a type of movement disorder involving motor and vocal tics that begin during childhood; persist for more than 1 year; and fluctuate with regard to type, frequency, and anatomical distribution over time.
- Symptoms of the disorder commonly first appear in childhood and adolescence. Approximately 10% of children have some form of tic disorder; 1% are diagnosed with Tourette syndrome. Most tics fade by age 18 years; however, even when tics persist into adulthood, they tend to become less severe.
- The disorder is 3 times more common in boys than in girls.
- It also has a strong genetic component.[51]
- Seventy percent of people with Tourette syndrome also have OCD.
- OCD may represent an alternative expression of Tourette syndrome. Tourette has been suggested as part of the obsessive compulsive spectrum, a range of compulsions with simple tics at one end and complex rituals and obsessional thoughts at the other.[52]
- The cause of Tourette and OCD likely involves a dopamine and basal ganglia disorder. The orbitofrontal cortex, a center of judgment and decision making, has also been implicated, particularly in obsessions of thought.
- Sixty percent of people with Tourette have ADHD, involving short attention span, physical and mental restlessness, poor concentration, and diminished impulse control.
- A high percentage of people with Tourette have concomitant learning disabilities, aggressiveness, anxiety, panic disorder, depression, mania, conduct disorder, oppositional defiant disorder, phobias, dyslexia, and stuttering. These disorders have been found to be 5 to 20 times more common in people who have Tourette syndrome than in the general population.[53]
- Tourette also involves a defect in motor pattern generators. Motor pattern generators are found in the brainstem and cortex and produce a variety of hard-wired movements (eg, reaching, grasping, walking, standing upright).[54]
- These movement patterns are involved in all body postures and are present at birth; they are ready to mature as an infant begins to move.
- Increased sensitivity to dopamine causes faulty inhibition of motor pattern generators.
- The same drugs used to treat tic disorders (non-neuroleptic and neuroleptic drugs, as noted previously) are used to treat Tourette syndrome.

THE CEREBELLUM'S ROLE IN MOTOR CONTROL

Cerebellum

- The cerebellum has a role in the coordination of movement, the maintenance of posture, and equilibrium.
- While its major role is proprioception, the cerebellum has more recently been implicated in other functions: attention shifting, practice-related learning, spatial organization, and memory. The cerebellum also appears to work collaboratively with cortically based cognitive functions to predict and prepare functional responses to environmental demands.[55]
- With regard to motor performance, the cerebellum could be called an *error-correcting device* for the motor system. It receives proprioceptive information from the body and sends back information to modify muscle and joint activity for the achievement of precision motor control.[56]

Three Cerebellar Lobes

Archicerebellum (Flocculonodular Lobe)

- The flocculonodular lobe receives input from the vestibular nuclei through the inferior cerebellar peduncle.
- This cerebellar lobe has roles in balance and spatial orientation.
- Damage to this lobe results in balance and gait problems.[57]

Paleocerebellum (Anterior Lobe)

- The paleocerebellum receives the posterior and anterior spinocerebellar tracts.
- It influences muscle tone by sending efferent fibers to the vestibular nuclei and the reticular formation through the superior cerebellar peduncle.
- The anterior lobe has a role in precision movement of the body and limbs.[58]

Neocerebellum (Posterior Lobe)

- The neocerebellum receives information from the cerebral hemispheres.
- Information from the cortex descends to the pontine nuclei and then travels to the cerebellum through the middle cerebellar peduncle.
- The neocerebellum may have a role in planning anticipatory movement (movement about to occur) and some cognitive functions.[58]

CEREBELLAR LESIONS

Neocerebellar Lesions

Neocerebellar Lesions Present With the Following[59]

- *Ipsilateral ataxia*: the posterior lobe receives input from the cortex. The dorsal columns mediate conscious proprioception. Loss of this cortical input results in ataxia.
- Ipsilateral hypotonia and hyporeflexia
- *Dysmetria*: inability to judge distance. Past-pointing, over-shooting, or underestimating one's grasp of objects occurs. People with dysmetria use visual cues for the readjustment of imprecise movement.
- Hypermetria involves an overestimation of the distance needed to reach an object (overshooting).
- Hypometria involves an underestimation (undershooting).
- *Adiadochokinesia*: inability to perform rapid alternating movements. Dysdiadochokinesia involves an impaired ability. Rapid alternating movements involve the ability to switch back and forth between 2 joint positions, such as forearm supination and pronation. Drifting and lag commonly appear as the patient attempts to increase the speed of movement.
- *Movement decomposition*: the movement is performed in a sequence of isolated parts rather than as a smooth, singular motion. Also referred to as *dyssynergia*
- *Asthenia*: muscle weakness
- *Intention tremors*: these occur during movement, as opposed to resting tremors, which occur in Parkinson disease.
- *Rebound phenomenon*: inability to regulate reciprocal movements. Example: The therapist gives resistance to the patient's flexed arm. When the therapist releases his or her resistance, the patient has no control or regulation over his or her speed of movement, and the patient's hand hits his or her chest. This occurs because immediate proprioceptive feedback is lost; the individual cannot regulate the speed of his or her arm movement quickly enough to prevent it from hitting his or her body.
- *Ataxic gait*: the posterior lobe receives input from the cortex. The dorsal columns mediate conscious proprioception. Loss of this cortical input results in an ataxic gait.
- *Staccato voice*: broken speech. The modulation of speech is a proprioceptive function.

Paleocerebellar Lesions

- Lesions in the paleocerebellar, or anterior, lobe produce severe disturbances in extensor tone.
- This occurs because the paleocerebellar lobe receives the spinocerebellar tracts.
- When the spinocerebellar tracts are lost, an increase in extensor tone results.[60]

Archicerebellar Lesions

- Lesions of the archicerebellar, or *flocculonodular*, lobe result in uncoordinated trunk movements; ataxia.
- The flocculonodular lobe receives input from the vestibular nuclei, the cuneocerebellar tract, and the rostral cerebellar tract.
- Loss of this vestibular input results in balance deficits, particularly in the trunk and upper extremities.
- Nystagmus also occurs because the cerebellum has connections to the oculomotor system via the medial longitudinal fasciculus.[60]

MOTOR CONTROL AND MOTOR LEARNING

- Motor control is the coordination of (1) CNS and peripheral nervous system (PNS) sensory, motor, and proprioceptive information with (2) muscle and joint movements to perform a desired motor action.[61,62]
- Motor control involves the interpretation of and appropriate response to sensory information from the environment/PNS in order to select and execute a set of integrated muscle and joint movements.
- Motor control depends on the ability to use feedback to process sensory information, select a motor plan, execute the selected motor plan, assess the motor plan's effectiveness, and modify the motor plan to achieve a specific targeted motor goal.
- Closed loop motor control involves (1) a motoric response to sensory stimuli, (2) feedback from proprioceptors and the environment, and (3) modification of muscle and joint movement that is ongoing and required to achieve continuous movement, such as using one's legs and feet to progressively kick a soccer ball across a field in short, 3-foot strides.
- Feedforward motor control involves movement that occurs too quickly to integrate sensory stimuli on a conscious level. Open loop control involves a feedforward control mechanism in which rapid movement is executed and terminated before conscious processing (eg, ducking quickly to avoid being hit by a fast approaching object thrown in one's direction).
- Motor learning is the practice of normal movement to enhance the fluidity and accuracy of a targeted motor task.
- Motor learning involves the development of motor programs for specific motor tasks that can be stored, retrieved, and implemented by the CNS when needed.
- Motor learning is used with patients who are able to engage in repeated practice of desired skills and who can cognitively use feedback to modify movement errors.
- Motor learning relies heavily on actual practice, mental practice, and feedback.
- Motor learning is based on the theory that relearning motor skills is achieved best when practice takes place in real-life environments.
- Cues, guidance, and feedback are provided to help patients relearn normal movements as they are practiced in real-life activities.
- Feedback is critical for motor learning and involves a patient's detection and processing of sensory information in response to movement.
- Feedback often involves visual, proprioceptive, and vestibular information that allows patients to evaluate movement and make modifications to enhance accuracy and precision.
- Intrinsic and augmented feedback are used to help patients understand what normal movement feels like. Intrinsic feedback provides proprioceptive and tactile information about a patient's movement.
- Augmented feedback provides information about a patient's movements from external sources, such as verbal cues from the therapist and visual cues from observing one's own movement in a mirror.
- Constant practice involves a single motor skill that is rehearsed repeatedly until mastered. For example, a patient may practice palmar prehension with wrist extension to retrieve similarly sized food items presented on a plate.

- Variable practice involves the ability to modify motor patterns in accordance with the demands of a specific activity. Variable practice is a higher level skill than constant practice and should be addressed after constant practice has sufficiently been performed. For example, a patient is given a plate of food items having varied sizes and weights and is asked to retrieve each food item separately. The demands of this activity require the patient to modify grasp and prehension patterns in accordance with each food item as it varies in weight and size.
- Knowledge of performance is a type of augmented feedback that involves information from others about a patient's movement based on quality, speed, and accuracy. Rehabilitation therapists use knowledge of performance to help patients enhance their motor plans for specific activities. For example, a therapist may offer verbal feedback to a patient about his or her use of shoulder elevation to compensate for impaired shoulder flexion during reaching.
- Knowledge of results is another form of augmented feedback and involves feedback from others about the outcome of a patient's actions with regard to a targeted activity in the environment. For example, after repeated practice and feedback, a patient may be better able to spear food with decreased shoulder elevation and increased shoulder flexion.
- Mental practice is a form of practice in which the patient uses cognitive rehearsal to improve motor patterns, without actually attempting physical movement. For example, as a patient begins to practice desired movement patterns in therapy, the therapist may instruct the patient to spend 15 minutes in the afternoon and before bed mentally rehearsing the performance of reaching to retrieve a glass using shoulder stabilization without elevation.
- The type and amount of practice must be considered when using motor learning principles. Research has shown that variable practice (in which a patient is asked to make rapid skill modifications to meet the changing demands of a task or environment) is better able to facilitate generalization of learning when compared with constant practice (in which a patient is asked to repeatedly practice a single motor skill that does not change). Movement patterns should be practiced using varied positions, heights, and ranges that best simulate real-life activity demands.
- The use of massed practice (in which the amount of rest time is less than the total practice time) vs distributed practice (in which the amount of rest time is equal to or greater than the total practice time) must also be considered.

REFERENCES

1. Zilles K, Amunts K. Centenary of Brodmann's map—conception and fate. *Nat Rev Neurosci.* 2010;11(2):139-145. doi:10.1038/nrn2776.

2. Pakkenberg B, Pelvig D, Marner L, et al. Aging and the human neocortex. *Exper Gerontol.* 2003;38(1):95-99. doi:10.1016/S0531-5565(02)00151-1.

3. Soudry Y, Lemogne C, Malinvaud D, Consoli SM, Bonfils P. Olfactory system and emotion: common substrates. *Eur Ann Otorhinolaryngol Head Neck Dis.* 2011;128(1):18-23. doi:10.1016/j.anorl.2010.09.007.

4. Lui JH, Hansen DV, Kriegstein AR. Development and evolution of the human neocortex. *Cell.* 2011;146(1):18-36. doi:10.1016/j.cell.2011.06.030.

5. Calautti C, Jones PS, Naccarato M. The relationship between motor deficit and primary motor cortex hemispheric activation balance after stroke: longitudinal fMRI study. *J Neurol Neurosurg Psychiatry.* 2010;81(7):788-792. doi:10.1136/jnnp.2009.190512.

6. Kocak M, Ulmer JL, Sahin Ugurel M, Gaggl W, Prost RW. Motor homunculus: passive mapping in healthy volunteers by using functional MR imaging—Initial results 1. *Radiology.* 2009;251(2):485-492. doi:10.1148/radiol.2512080231.

7. Chouinard PA, Paus T. The primary motor and premotor areas of the human cerebral cortex. *Neuroscientist.* 2006;12(2):143-152. doi: 10.1177/1073858405284255.

8. Monfils MH, Plautz EJ, Kleim JA. In search of the motor engram: motor map plasticity as a mechanism for encoding motor experience. *Neuroscientist.* 2005;11(5):471-483. doi: 10.1177/1073858405278015.

9. Hanakawa T, Dimyan MA, Hallett M. Motor planning, imagery, and execution in the distributed motor network: a time-course study with functional MRI. *Cereb Cortex.* 2008;18(12):2775-2788. doi: 10.1093/cercor/bhn036.

10. Péran P, Catani S, Falletta Caravasso C, Nemmi F, Sabatini U, Formisano R. Supplementary motor area activation is impaired in severe traumatic brain injury Parkinsonism. *J Neurotrauma.* 2014;31(7):642-648. doi:10.1089/neu.2013.3103.

11. Jantz JJ, Watanabe M, Everling S, Munoz DP. Threshold mechanism for saccade initiation in frontal eye field and superior colliculus. *J Neurophysiol.* 2013;109(11):2767-2780. doi:10.1152/jn.00611.2012.

12. Chainay H, Humphreys GW. Ideomotor and ideational apraxia in corticobasal degeneration: a case study. *Neurocase.* 2003;9(2):177-186. doi:10.1076/neur.9.2.177.15073.

13. Wortzel HS, Frey KL, Anderson CA, Arciniegas DB. Subtle neurological signs predict the severity of subacute cognitive and functional impairments after traumatic brain injury. *J Neuropsychiatr Clin Neurosci.* 2009;21(4):463-466.

14. Jaramillo SPI, Uribe CSU, Jimenez FAG, Cornejo-Ochoa W, Restrepo JFÁ, Román GC. Accuracy of the Babinski sign in the identification of pyramidal tract dysfunction. *J Neurol Sci.* 2014;343(1):66-68. doi:10.1016/j.jns.2014.05.028.

15. Tejus MN, Singh V, Ramesh A, Kumar VR, Maurya VP, Madhugiri VS. An evaluation of the finger flexion, Hoffman's and plantar reflexes as markers of cervical spinal cord compression—a comparative clinical study. *Clin Neurol Neurosurg.* 2015;134:12-16. doi:10.1016/j.clineuro.2015.04.009.

16. Zafeiriou DI. Primitive reflexes and postural reactions in the neurodevelopmental examination. *Pediatr Neurol.* 2004;31(1):1-8. doi:10.1016/j.pediatrneurol.2004.01.012.

17. Nelson AB, Kreitzer AC. Reassessing models of basal ganglia function and dysfunction. *Annu Rev Neurosci.* 2014;37:117-135. doi:10.1146/annurev-neuro-071013-013916.

18. Wiecki TV, Frank MJ. A computational model of inhibitory control in frontal cortex and basal ganglia. *Psychol Rev.* 2013;120(2):329-355. doi:10.1037/a0031542.

19. Hart H, Radua J, Nakao T, Mataix-Cols D, Rubia K. Meta-analysis of functional magnetic resonance imaging studies of inhibition and attention in attention-deficit/hyperactivity disorder: exploring task-specific, stimulant medication, and age effects. *JAMA Psychiatry.* 2013;70(2):185-198. doi:10.1001/jamapsychiatry.2013.277.

20. Grueter BA, Rothwell PE, Malenka RC. Integrating synaptic plasticity and striatal circuit function in addiction. *Curr Opin Neurobiol.* 2012;22(3):545-551. doi:10.1016/j.conb.2011.09.009.

21. Saunders A, Oldenburg, IA, Berezovskii VK, et al. A direct GABAergic output from the basal ganglia to frontal cortex. *Nature.* 2015;521(7550):85-89. doi:10.1038/nature14179.

22. Bednark JG, Campbell ME, Cunnington R. Basal ganglia and cortical networks for sequential ordering and rhythm of complex movements. *Front Hum Neurosci.* 2015;9:421. doi:10.3389/fnhum.2015.00421.

23. Gittis AH, Berke JD, Bevan MD, et al. New roles for the external globus pallidus in basal ganglia circuits and behavior. *J Neurosci.* 2014;34(46):15178-15183. doi: 10.1523/JNEUROSCI.3252-14.2014.

24. Gao S, Singer HS. Complex motor stereotypies: an evolving neurobiological concept. *Future Neurol.* 2013;8(3):273-285. doi:10.2217/fnl.13.4.

25. Kim HF, Hikosaka O. Parallel basal ganglia circuits for voluntary and automatic behaviour to reach rewards. *Brain.* 2015;138(Pt 7):1776-1780. doi.org/10.1093/brain/awv134.

26. DeLong MR, Georgopoulos AP. Motor functions of the basal ganglia. In: *Comprehensive Physiology.* Published online 2011. doi:10.1002/cphy.cp010221.

27. Freeze BS, Kravitz AV, Hammack N, Berke JD, Kreitzer AC. Control of basal ganglia output by direct and indirect pathway projection neurons. *J Neurosci.* 2013;33(47):18531-18539. doi:10.1523/JNEUROSCI.1278-13.2013.

28. Saint-Cyr JA. Frontal-striatal circuit functions: context, sequence, and consequence. *J Int Neuropsychol Soc.* 2003;9(01): 103-128. doi:10.1017/S1355617703910125.

29. Jin X, Costa RM. Start/stop signals emerge in nigrostriatal circuits during sequence learning. *Nature.* 2010;466(7305): 457-462. doi:10.1038/nature09263.

30. Hawley JS, Weiner WJ. Hemiballismus: current concepts and review. *Parkinsonism Relat Disord.* 2012;18(2):125-129. doi:10.1016/j.parkreldis.2011.08.015.

31. Lanska DJ. Early controversies over athetosis: I. Clinical features, differentiation from other movement disorders, associated conditions, and pathology [published online ahead of print January 14, 2013]. *Tremor Other Hyperkinet Mov.* doi: 10.7916/D8TT4PPH.

32. de Gusmão CM, Berkowitz AL, Hung AY, Westover MB. Cerebrospinal fluid shunt-induced chorea: case report and review of the literature on shunt-related movement disorders. *Pract Neurol.* 2015;15(1):42-44. doi:10.1136/practneurol-2014-000913.

33. Wexler A. Stigma, history, and Huntington's disease. *Lancet.* 2010;376(9734):18-19. doi:10.1016/S0140-6736(10)60957-9.

34. Albanese A, Bhatia K, Bressman SB, et al. Phenomenology and classification of dystonia: a consensus update. *Mov Disord.* 2013;28(7):863-873. doi:10.1002/mds.25475.

35. Stannard WA, Chilvers MA, Rutman AR, Williams CD, O'Callaghan C. Diagnostic testing of patients suspected of primary ciliary dyskinesia. *Am J Respir Crit Care Med.* 2010;181(4):307-314. doi:10.1164/rccm.200903-0459OC.

36. Kim J, MacMaster E, Schwartz TL. Tardive dyskinesia in patients treated with atypical antipsychotics: case series and brief review of etiologic and treatment considerations. *Drugs Context.* 2014;3:212259. doi:10.7573/dic.212259.

37. Kordower JH, Olanow CW, Dodiya HB, et al. Disease duration and the integrity of the nigrostriatal system in Parkinson's disease. *Brain.* 2013;136(8):2419-2431. doi:10.1093/brain/awt192.

38. Irwin DJ, Lee VMY, Trojanowski JQ. Parkinson's disease dementia: convergence of [alpha]-synuclein, tau and amyloid-[beta] pathologies. *Nat Rev Neurosci.* 2013;14(9):626-636. doi:10.1038/nrn3549.

39. Belujon P, Grace AA. L-dopa treatment duration versus Parkinson's disease progression: the dorsal-ventral divide. *Mov Disord.* 2013;28(2):120-121. doi:10.1002/mds.25334.

40. Collins L, Cummins G, Barker RA. Parkinson's disease: diagnosis and current management. *Prescriber.* 2015;26(5):16-23. doi:10.1002/psb.1316.

41. Okuma Y. Freezing of gait in Parkinson's disease. *J Neurol.* 2006;253(7):vii27-vii32. doi:10.1007/s00415-006-7007-2.

42. Nombela C, Hughes LE, Owen AM, Grahn JA. Into the groove: can rhythm influence Parkinson's disease? *Neurosci Biobehav Rev.* 2013;37(10):2564-2570. doi:10.1016/j.neubiorev.2013.08.003.

43. Odekerken VJ, van Laar T, Staal MJ, et al. Subthalamic nucleus versus globus pallidus bilateral deep brain stimulation for advanced Parkinson's disease (NSTAPS study): a randomised controlled trial. *Lancet Neurol.* 2013;12(1):37-44. doi:10.1016/S1474-4422(12)70264-8.

44. Ambasudhan R, Dolatabadi N, Nutter A, Masliah E, Mckercher SR, Lipton SA. Potential for cell therapy in Parkinson's disease using genetically programmed human embryonic stem cell–derived neural progenitor cells. *J Compar Neurol.* 2014;522(12):2845-2856. doi:10.1002/cne.23617.

45. Olanow CW. Parkinson disease: Gene therapy for Parkinson disease—a hope, or a dream? *Nat Rev Neurol.* 2014;10(4): 186-187. doi:10.1038/nrneurol.2014.45.

46. Louis ED. Essential tremor. *Lancet Neurol.* 2005;4(2):100-110. doi:10.1016/S1474-4422(05)00991-9.

47. de Alvarenga PG, de Mathis MA, Dominguez Alves AC, et al. Clinical features of tic-related obsessive-compulsive disorder: results from a large multicenter study. *CNS Spectr.* 2012;17(02):87-93. doi:10.1017/S1092852912000491.

48. Dale RC, Merheb V, Pillai S, et al. Antibodies to surface dopamine-2 receptor in autoimmune movement and psychiatric disorders. *Brain.* 2012;135(Pt 11):3453-3468. doi:10.1093/brain/aws256.

49. Swedo SE, Leonard HL, Garvey M, et al. Pediatric autoimmune neuropsychiatric disorders associated with streptococcal infections. *FOCUS.* 2014;2(3):496-506. doi:10.1176/foc.2.3.496.

50. Thomas R, Cavanna AE. The pharmacology of Tourette syndrome. *J Neural Transm.* 2013;120(4):689-694. doi:10.1007/s00702-013-0979-z.

51. Leckman JF, Bloch MH, Smith ME, Larabi D, Hampson M. Neurobiological substrates of Tourette's disorder. *J Child Adolesc Psychopharmacol.* 2010;20(4):237-247. doi:10.1089/cap.2009.0118.

52. Lochner C, Fineberg NA, Zohar J, et al. Comorbidity in obsessive–compulsive disorder (OCD): a report from the International College of Obsessive-Compulsive Spectrum Disorders (ICOCS). *Compr Psychiatr.* 2014;55(7):1513-1519. doi:10.1016/j.comppsych.2014.05.020.

53. Kurlan R. Tourette's syndrome. *N Engl J Med.* 2010;363(24):2332-2338. doi:10.1056/NEJMcp1007805.

54. Albin RL, Mink JW. Recent advances in Tourette syndrome research. *Trends Neurosci.* 2006;29(3):175-182. doi:10.1016/j.tins.2006.01.001.

55. Chen SHA, Ho MHR, Desmond JE. A meta-analysis of cerebellar contributions to higher cognition from PET and fMRI studies. *Hum Brain Mapp.* 2014;35(2):593-615. doi:10.1002/hbm.22194.

56. Herzfeld DJ, Pastor D, Haith AM, Rossetti Y, Shadmehr R, O'Shea J. Contributions of the cerebellum and the motor cortex to acquisition and retention of motor memories. *Neuroimage.* 2014;98:147-158. doi:10.1016/j.neuroimage.2014.04.076.

57. Roostaei T, Nazeri A, Sahraian MA, Minagar A. The human cerebellum: a review of physiologic neuroanatomy. *Neurol Clin.* 2014;32(4):859-869. doi:10.1016/j.ncl.2014.07.013.

58. Stoodley CJ, Valera EM, Schmahmann JD. Functional topography of the cerebellum for motor and cognitive tasks: an fMRI study. *Neuroimage.* 2012;59(2):1560-1570. doi:10.1016/j.neuroimage.2011.08.065.

59. Bhanpuri NH, Okamura AM, Bastian AJ. Predicting and correcting ataxia using a model of cerebellar function. *Brain.* 2014;137(Pt 7):1931-1944. doi:10.1093/brain/awu115.

60. Strata P, Provini L, Redman S. On the concept of spinocerebellum. *Proc Natl Acad Sci U S A.* 2012;109(11):E622-E622. doi:10.1073/pnas.1121224109.

61. Shumway-Cook A, Woollacott MH. *Motor Control: Translating Research into Clinical Practice.* 4th ed. Philadelphia, PA: Lippincott, Williams, and Wilkins; 2011.

62. Magill R, Anderson D. *Motor Learning and Control: Concepts and Applications.* 10th ed. New York, NY: McGraw-Hill; 2010.

Clinical Test Questions

Section 22

1. Mr. Iwu has lost voluntary motor control of the right side of his body as a result of a brain injury. Mr. Iwu's brain injury is likely located in the _____ hemisphere and in the _____ motor area.
    1. left
    2. right
    3. primary
    4. premotor
   a. 1, 3
   b. 2, 3
   c. 1, 4
   d. 2, 4

2. As a result of his head injury, Jayson has difficulty implementing the correct motor plan for a specific task. For example, when given a shirt, he attempts to slip his head through the sleeve. This is referred to as _____ and results from injury to the _____ motor area.
    1. aphasia
    2. apraxia
    3. primary
    4. premotor
   a. 1, 3
   b. 2, 3
   c. 1, 4
   d. 2, 4

3. Toneal sustained a traumatic brain injury in a motorcycle accident. His physician flicks the nail of his third finger and in response, Toneal involuntarily exhibits thumb adduction and index finger flexion. This primitive reflex is called _____, and its re-emergence after neurological injury indicates damage to the _____.
    1. Babinski sign
    2. Hoffman sign
    3. cortex
    4. cerebellum
   a. 1, 3
   b. 1, 4
   c. 2, 3
   d. 2, 4

4. When the therapist displaces Toneal's center of gravity, he falls to the left instead of extending his arms and legs to prevent falling. The ability to extend the arms and legs to prevent falling when one's center of gravity is displaced is a higher level reaction called _____. When this reaction is lost, it is indicative of _____ damage and places the patient at risk for falls.
    1. protective extension
    2. equilibrium reaction
    3. brainstem
    4. basal ganglia
   a. 1, 3
   b. 1, 4
   c. 2, 3
   d. 2, 4

5. Mr. Bhandari, who was diagnosed with Parkinson disease 2 years ago, displays difficulty initiating, continuing, and stopping movement; muscular rigidity (eg, cogwheel and lead pipe rigidity); and resting tremors. Parkinson disease results from a lesion in the _____ and depletion of the neurotransmitter _____.
    1. cerebellum
    2. basal ganglia
    3. norepinephrine
    4. dopamine
    a. 1, 3
    b. 1, 4
    c. 2, 3
    d. 2, 4

6. Mr. Shaw has a neurological motor disorder in which he displays violent thrashing of his contralateral extremity. This condition is known as _____ and results from a lesion to the _____.
    1. hemiballismus
    2. chorea
    3. basal ganglia
    4. cerebellum
    a. 1, 3
    b. 2, 3
    c. 1, 4
    d. 2, 4

7. After taking neuroleptic medication all of her adult life for schizophrenia, April has developed tongue protrusions, facial grimacing, blepharospasm, and lip smacking. These involuntary movements are collectively called _____ and result from long-term treatment with dopamine receptor antagonists.
    a. tics
    b. chorea
    c. tardive dyskinesia
    d. idiopathic dystonia

8. Ms. Graham displays ataxia, intention tremors, broken speech, and nystagmus. Her physician suspects a lesion of the _____.
    a. basal ganglia
    b. brainstem
    c. cortex
    d. cerebellum

9. Sean commonly displays tics such as shoulder shrugging, throat clearing, eye blinks, and head jerks. Occasionally, he exhibits vocal tics and shouts out repetitive words or noises. Sean states that he feels compelled to engage in these repetitive motor and vocal tics and that although he is able to suppress these for a time, his compulsion builds until he can no longer control his urges. This condition is known as _____ and results from pathology of the _____.
    1. obsessive compulsive disorder
    2. Tourette syndrome
    3. dopamine system
    4. norepinephrine system
    a. 1, 3
    b. 2, 3
    c. 1, 4
    d. 2, 4

10. Henry is a 6-year-old child who, from birth, has displayed abnormal and repetitive movements caused by severe muscle contractions producing twisting postures. These muscle contractions can last up to several hours, disappear during sleep, and worsen with anxiety. For example, Henry experiences muscle contractions that force his neck into hyperextension (called *retrocollis*). Such abnormal twisting movements are collectively called _____ and result from _____ pathology.

    1. dystonia

    2. chorea

    3. cerebellar

    4. basal ganglia

  a. 1, 3

  b. 2, 3

  c. 1, 4

  d. 2, 4

Answers

1. a
2. d
3. c
4. b
5. d
6. a
7. c
8. d
9. b
10. c

Sensory Functions and Dysfunctions of the Central Nervous System

SOMATOSENSORY CORTEX

Postcentral Gyrus (also called *Primary Somatosensory Area*)

- The primary somatosensory area (SS1) is responsible for the detection of incoming sensory information from the periphery.
- This neural region is not responsible for the interpretation of sensory data.
- All sensory data travel through the thalamus before reaching the postcentral gyrus.
- SS1 is also the site of the sensory homunculus.[1]

Sensory Homunculus

- The sensory homunculus is the cortical representation of every body part's sensation and is located in the postcentral gyrus.
- It is the somatotopic organization of body sensation from the contralateral side of the body.
- The sensory homunculus is akin to the motor homunculus in the precentral gyrus.
- The face, hands, and mouth have a large amount of representation for exploration of the external world.
- Like the motor homunculus, the sensory homunculus does not have a permanent organization.
- There is a plasticity to the homunculi should injury or disease occur.
- For example, in people who read braille, the reading finger has a very large representation in the primary somatosensory cortex.
- In amputees, other body parts appropriate, or take over, the cortical representation or region that had been used for the amputated part.[1,2]

Lesions to the Primary Somatosensory Area

- Lesions to the primary somatosensory area result in a loss of sensation of the contralateral body part.
- The loss will depend on which part of the sensory homunculus was damaged.[1,2]

Secondary Somatosensory Area

- The secondary somatosensory area (SS2) is responsible for the interpretation of sensory information.
- This is the area where meaning is attached to incoming sensory data.
- SS2 is located just *posterior* to the postcentral gyrus.[3]

Lesions to the Secondary Somatosensory Area

- Tactile agnosia
  - *Tactile agnosia* is the umbrella term for the inability to attach meaning to sensory data.
  - Tactile agnosias include astereognosis, two-point discrimination disorder, agraphesthesia, and extinction of simultaneous stimulation (all described in the following sections).[4]

Gutman SA. *Quick Reference Neuroscience for Rehabilitation Professionals: The Essential Neurologic Principles Underlying Rehabilitation Practice, Third Edition* (pp 282-289). © 2017 Taylor & Francis Group.

Oliver Sacks Story

- Oliver Sacks describes a 60-year-old woman who was blind at birth, overprotected, and never encouraged to explore her environment with her hands.
- As an adult, she could not identify objects or sensations with her hands despite having intact sensory anatomy.
- Her sensory cortices had never been stimulated.
- At 60, she had to recreate the region in the cortical map for her hands by learning to use her hands to identify objects and sensations.
- This is an example of how the cortex is use-dependent.

Adapted from Sacks O. *The Man Who Mistook His Wife for a Hat.* New York, NY: Harper Perennial; 1987.

Impermanence of Cortically Based Sensory and Motor Functions

- The cortical representation for all sensory and motor functions is impermanent and use-dependent.
- This impermanence and use-dependence is true not only for the homunculi, but also for all areas of the cortex.
- For example, in people who become cortically deaf, regions of the auditory cortex may be reallocated for visual use.
- In people who become cortically blind, regions of the visual cortex may be reallocated for tactile and auditory use.[5]
- Primary sensation is mediated by the skin receptors, spinal nerves, spinal tracts (*dorsal columns* and spinothalamic tracts), and SS1.[1]

SOMATOSENSORY AND VISUAL CORTICES

Primary Somatosensory Cortex (SS1)
Secondary Somatosensory Area (SS2)
V3
V2
V1
Visual Cortices

Primary Somatosensory Area (SS1)
V3
V2
V1
V2
V3
Olfactory Cortex

Two Classifications of Sensation

Primary Sensation

- Primary sensation includes pain and temperature, light touch, pressure, vibration, and proprioception.[6]

Cortical Sensation

- Cortical sensations are mediated by SS2 and the posterior multimodal association cortex.
- Cortical sensations include the following tactile agnosias.
- **Astereognosis**
  - ○ The inability to identify objects by touch alone (sensory anatomy is intact; cortical interpretation is impaired).[7]
- **Two-point discrimination**
  - ○ Loss of the ability to determine whether one has been touched by 1 or 2 points (sensory anatomy is intact; the cortical interpretation of sensation is impaired).
  - ○ Two-point discrimination is evaluated by a standard instrument called an *aesthesiometer*.[8]
- **Agraphesthesia**
  - ○ Loss of the ability to interpret letters written on the contralateral hand of the affected side, despite intact sensory anatomy. Cortical interpretation of sensation is impaired.[9]
- **Extinction of simultaneous stimulation**
  - ○ Also called *double simultaneous extinction*.
  - ○ The patient is touched simultaneously on 2 different body regions: one on the involved side; one on the uninvolved side.
  - ○ Extinction occurs when the patient cannot feel the tactile sensation on the involved side (even though he or she could if the tactile sensation were applied only to the involved side).
  - ○ Extinction of simultaneous stimulation occurs because the neurons that carry tactile sensation from the involved side are cortically overridden by the neurons carrying sensation from the uninvolved side.[10]
- **Abarognosis**
  - ○ Loss of the ability to accurately estimate the weight of objects in relation to each other (sensory anatomy is intact; the cortical interpretation of sensation is impaired).[11]
- **Atopognosia**
  - ○ Loss of the ability to localize the exact origin of a sensation (sensory anatomy remains intact; cortical interpretation is impaired).[11]

VISUAL CORTEX

Primary Visual Cortex

- The primary visual cortex (V1) receives visual information from the optic tracts, lateral geniculate nuclei of the thalamus, and the superior colliculi of the midbrain.
- This neural region is responsible for the detection of visual input (not interpretation), such as the detection of shape, color, orientation, and direction.
- The primary visual cortex is located at the most posterior region of the occipital lobe.[12]

Lesions to the Primary Visual Cortex

- Lesions to the primary visual cortex result in loss of sight (despite intact visual anatomy).[13]

Lesions in the Primary Visual Cortex Produce Cortical Blindness

- When the primary visual cortex is lesioned, visual information travels through the retina, optic nerves, and optic tracts and to the lateral geniculate nucleus of the thalamus. Here, the visual information may be rerouted to the visual association areas rather than first proceeding to V1.

Sensory Signs and Symptoms	*Suspect*
• Astereognosis, agraphesthesia	• Contralateral parietal lobe impairment
• Decreased sensation to pin prick (hemihyperesthesia)	• Spinal cord tract damage
• Hyperesthesias only in the distal limbs	• Peripheral neuropathy

- Visual information may be processed unconsciously by the lateral geniculate nuclei. These nuclei form a primitive visual system that may have evolved to allow organisms the ability to respond immediately to visual data without the time needed for higher level cortical processing.
- The lateral geniculate nuclei are responsible for much of the visual processing of primitive organisms.
- In humans, this type of sight is known as *blind sight* or *unconscious sight*.
- When patients with V1 damage are asked to guess about observed objects in motion, or to distinguish colors, their ability to do so is better than chance.
- This suggests that visual information is in fact processed, but on a subcortical (or unconscious) level.
- Patients, however, are not consciously aware of having seen anything and are often surprised that their guesses are so accurate; their sight was not processed at a conscious level.[13]

Visual Association Areas (V2 and higher)

- The visual cortex has more than 30 specialized areas.
- V2 and higher are responsible for the interpretation of visual input.
- This is where meaning is attached to incoming visual data.
- V1 has a mature appearance at birth. The visual association areas do not. They appear to be dependent upon the acquisition of experience.[14]

Lesions to the Visual Association Areas

- Lesions to the visual association areas result in *visual agnosias*, an umbrella term that denotes the inability to attach meaning to visual data.[14]

V2

- V2 sends visual information from V1 to the appropriate visual association area for interpretation.
- V2 processes information for further refinement by the specialized visual association areas.
- This visual association area may be specialized to analyze spatial characteristics, color, figure-ground properties, and orientation.[14]

V3

- V3 is responsible for interpreting form discrimination, the ability to recognize identifiable shapes.[14]

Lesion to V3

- No one has ever reported a complete and exclusive loss of form vision.
- Area V3 forms a ring around V1 and V2. A lesion large enough to destroy all of V3 would almost certainly destroy V1, causing total blindness.
- V4 would also have to be knocked out because V4 plays a role in form discrimination (with regard to line orientation).[14]

V4

- V4 is responsible for the interpretation of color vision, line orientation, and geometric pattern.
- When people view an abstract color painting with no recognizable shapes, V4 has the highest cerebral blood flow on positron emission tomography (PET) scans.[15]

Lesion to V4

- A lesion to V4 produces achromatopsia, in which people only see shades of gray.
- This differs from color blindness due to damaged cone receptors in the retina.
- In achromatopsia, people cannot recall or bring up in memory what colors look like.
- If their retinas and V1 regions remain intact, their knowledge of form, depth, and motion are preserved.[15]

V5

- V5 is responsible for interpreting visual motion (identifying objects that are in motion).
- When people view a pattern of moving black and white squares on a computer screen, V5 has the highest cerebral blood flow on PET scans.[16]

Oliver Sacks Story

- Sacks described a man who was legally blind since early childhood. When the man's sight was surgically restored in his 40s, he could not integrate perception of color, form, and motion into a coherent visualization that had meaning, even though his visual anatomical structures were now intact.
- This suggests that the visual association areas only develop with direct experience and use.

Adapted from Sacks O. *An Anthropologist on Mars.* New York, NY: Vintage; 1995.

Depth Perception Develops Only From Experience

- Depth perception is the ability to interpret whether objects are closer or farther in relation to another object.
- Research has found that depth perception, like other cortical skills, develops only from experience.
- In cultures living in deep rain forests, where expansive views are prevented by the immense density of flora, people do not develop a sophisticated level of depth perception.

Sequence of Color Vision

- V1, the primary visual area, detects some type of visual information and sends it to V2 for further processing.
- V2 identifies that the visual information contains color and sends it to V4 for further processing.
- V4 interprets the color visual information. If V4 is damaged, people see the world in shades of gray.

Lesion to V5

- A lesion to V5 produces akinetopsia, in which people neither see nor understand the world in motion.
- While at rest, objects may be perfectly visible and understandable.
- Objects in motion appear to vanish.
- The other attributes of vision (color and form) remain intact.[16]

Two Visual Cortical Streams

- There appear to be 2 primary visual cortical streams[17]:
  1. *Dorsal stream*: this stream of visual information runs dorsally from V1 to the parietal lobe and is responsible for the analysis of visual motions and actions.
  2. *Ventral stream*: this stream of visual information stretches ventrally from V1 to the temporal lobe and is responsible for the perception of the visual world and object recognition.

Visual Regions Connect Together and Project to Surrounding Structures

- All visual areas connect directly and reciprocally with each other.
- The visual association areas project to the posterior multimodal association area, a cortical region where somatosensory, visual, and auditory information is integrated and interpreted in relation to each other. Here, visual information is integrated with other sensory data (eg, taste, sound, touch, smell).
- This information then travels to the hippocampus for the storage of visual memories. In the hippocampus, past visual memories are compared to new visual data for decision-making processes.
- Visual data also travel to other areas of the limbic system for emotional association. Here, visual information is compared to similar visual data that already have emotional associations. When a new visual stimulus is similar to stored visual memories having unhappy emotional associations, the novel visual stimulus can elicit the same sad feelings.[18]

AUDITORY CORTEX

Primary Auditory Cortex

- The primary auditory cortex (A1) is located within the *insula* in the temporal lobe and is responsible for detecting sounds from the environment.
- A1 sends auditory information to the auditory association areas for interpretation.[19]

Lesion to A1

- Unilateral deafness occurs if only one hemisphere is lesioned.
- Bilateral deafness occurs if both hemispheres are involved.
- Patients with cortical deafness resulting from a lesion to A1 may still have the ability to process auditory data on an unconscious level.
- This ability may be derived from the auditory pathway of the inferior colliculi (of the midbrain) and the medial geniculate nucleus (of the thalamus).
- Researchers have found that some patients with cortical deafness still retain the ability to startle in response to a loud noise. Such patients, however, are not consciously able to hear the noise.[19]

Auditory Association Areas

- There are several auditory association areas located throughout the cortex.
- These association areas are responsible for the interpretation of auditory data.
- The auditory association areas have not as yet been mapped as precisely as the visual association areas.
- Different auditory association areas interpret specific auditory information (eg, animal sounds, human language, the sounds of machinery).[20]

Lesion to the Auditory Association Areas

- A lesion to the auditory association areas results in *auditory agnosia*, an umbrella term that denotes the inability to attach meaning to specific sounds.[20]

Broca Area

- The Broca area is located only in the left hemisphere.
- This neural region mediates the motoric aspects of speech and is responsible for the verbal expression of language.
- Broca area is located just above the lateral fissure and sits within the inferior frontal gyrus of the premotor area.[21]

Lesion to Broca's Area

- Lesions to Broca's area produce expressive aphasia or nonfluent speech.
- Patients can understand what is spoken to them, but they cannot form meaningful sentences.[21]

Wernicke Area

- The Wernicke area is also located only in the left hemisphere and sits within the superior temporal gyrus in the temporal lobe.
- This language area is responsible for the comprehension of the spoken word.[22]

Lesion to Wernicke Area

- Lesions to the Wernicke area produce receptive aphasia.
- Patients cannot understand what is spoken to them.
- However, they can produce intact sentences (although the meaning of their words does not relate to anything that others have said to them).[22]

AUDITORY CORTICES

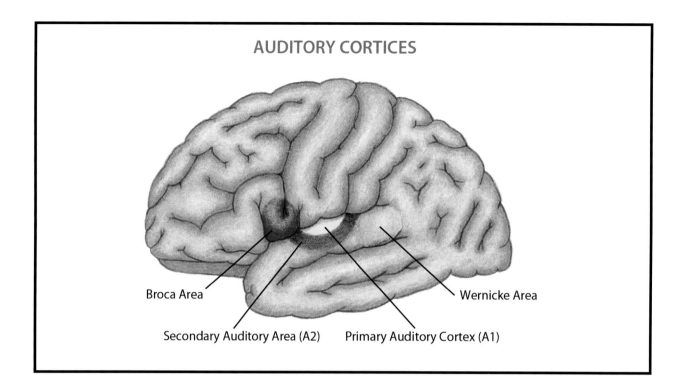

Broca Area

Wernicke Area

Secondary Auditory Area (A2)

Primary Auditory Cortex (A1)

REFERENCES

1. Feldman DE, Brecht M. Map plasticity in somatosensory cortex. *Science*. 2005;310(5749):810-815. doi:10.1126/science.1115807.

2. Wrigley PJ, Press SR, Gustin SM, et al. Neuropathic pain and primary somatosensory cortex reorganization following spinal cord injury. *Pain*. 2009;141(1):52-59. doi:10.1016/j.pain.2008.10.007.

3. Ruben J, Schwiemann J, Deuchert M, et al. Somatotopic organization of human secondary somatosensory cortex. *Cereb Cortex*. 2001;11(5):463-473. doi: 10.1093/cercor/11.5.463.

4. Binkofski F, Reetz K, Blangero A. Tactile agnosia and tactile apraxia: cross talk between the action and perception streams in the anterior intraparietal area. *Behav Brain Sci*. 2007;30(02):201-202. doi:10.1017/S0140525X07001409.

5. Kerr CE, Shaw JR, Wasserman RH, et al. Tactile acuity in experienced Tai Chi practitioners: evidence for use dependent plasticity as an effect of sensory-attentional training. *Exper Brain Res*. 2008;188(2):317-322. doi:10.1007/s00221-008-1409-6.

6. McGlone F, Reilly D. The cutaneous sensory system. *Neurosci Biobehav Rev*. 2010;34(2):148-159. doi:10.1016/j.neubiorev.2009.08.004.

7. Carlson MG, Brooks C. The effect of altered hand position and motor skills on stereognosis. *J Hand Surg*. 2009;34(5):896-899. doi:10.1016/j.jhsa.2009.01.029.

8. van Nes SI, Faber CG, Hamers RM, et al; PeriNomS Study Group. Revising two-point discrimination assessment in normal aging and in patients with polyneuropathies. *J Neurol Neurosurg Psychiatry*. 2008;79(7):832-834. doi:10.1136/jnnp.2007.139220.

9. Mørch CD, Andersen OK, Quevedo AS, Arendt-Nielsen L, Coghill RC. Exteroceptive aspects of nociception: insights from graphesthesia and two-point discrimination. *Pain*. 2010;151(1):45-52. doi:10.1016/j.pain.2010.05.016.

10. Birch HG, Belmont I, Karp E. The relation of single stimulus threshold to extinction in double simultaneous stimulation. *Cortex*. 1964;1(1):19-39. doi:10.1016/S0010-9452(64)80011-3.

11. Angel RW. Barognosis in a patient with hemiaraxia. *Ann Neurol*. 1980;7(1):73-77. doi: 10.1002/ana.410070113.

12. Li W, Piëch V, Gilbert CD. Perceptual learning and top-down influences in primary visual cortex. *Nat Neurosci*. 2004;7(6):651-657. doi:10.1038/nn1255.

13. Stoerig P. Functional rehabilitation of partial cortical blindness? *Restor Neurol Neurosci*. 2007;26(4-5):291-303.

14. Dougherty RF, Koch VM, Brewer AA, Fischer B, Modersitzki J, Wandell BA. Visual field representations and locations of visual areas V1/2/3 in human visual cortex. *J Vision*. 2003;3(10):586-98. doi:10.1167/3.10.1.

15. Bouvier SE, Engel SA. Behavioral deficits and cortical damage loci in cerebral achromatopsia. *Cereb Cortex*. 2006;16(2):183-191. doi:10.1093/cercor/bhi096.

16. Zeki S. Thirty years of a very special visual area, area V5. *J Physiol*. 2004;557(1):1-2. doi: 10.1113/jphysiol.2004.063040.

17. James TW, Humphrey GK, Gati JS, Menon RS, Goodale MA. Differential effects of viewpoint on object-driven activation in dorsal and ventral streams. *Neuron*. 2002;35(4):793-801. doi:10.1016/S0896-6273(02)00803-6.

18. Hasson U, Nir Y, Levy I, Fuhrmann G, Malach R. Intersubject synchronization of cortical activity during natural vision. *Science*. 2004;303(5664):1634-1640. doi:10.1126/science.1089506.

19. Weinberger NM. Specific long-term memory traces in primary auditory cortex. *Nat Rev Neurosci*. 2004;5(4):279-290. doi:10.1038/nrn1366.

20. Clarke S, Bellmann A, Meuli RA, Assal G, Steck AJ. Auditory agnosia and auditory spatial deficits following left hemispheric lesions: evidence for distinct processing pathways. *Neuropsychologia*. 2000;38(6):797-807. doi:10.1016/S0028-3932(99)00141-4.

21. Fadiga L, Craighero L, D'Ausilio A. Broca's area in language, action, and music. *Ann N Y Acad Sci*. 2009;1169(1):448-458. doi:10.1111/j.1749-6632.2009.04582.x.

22. Weiller C, Isensee C, Rijntjes M, et al. Recovery from Wernicke's aphasia: a positron emission tomographic study. *Ann Neurol*. 1995;37(6):723-732. doi:10.1002/ana.410370605.

Thalamus and Brainstem Sensory and Motor Roles
Function and Dysfunction

THALAMUS

- The thalamus is considered to be part of the diencephalon.
- This structure is a major relay and processing center for all types of sensory and motor information.
- There are 2 thalamic lobes, 1 in each hemisphere.
- The thalamus contains 26 pair of nuclei.
- Almost every major structure for sensory and motor data has connections with the thalamus. These include the cortex (all lobes), brainstem, reticular formation, hypothalamus, limbic system structures (eg, amygdala and hippocampus), basal ganglia, and cerebellum.
- Four of the most studied thalamic nuclei are as follows[1]:
    1. *Ventrolateral nucleus*: projects to the primary motor area (M1)
    2. *Lateral geniculate nucleus*: projects to the primary visual area (V1)
    3. *Medial geniculate nucleus*: projects to the primary auditory area (A1)
    4. *Ventral posterolateral nucleus*: projects to the primary somatosensory area (SS1)

Thalamic Pathways

Sensory Afferent Pathways

- Sensory receptors in the peripheral nervous system (PNS) project sensory messages to the spinal nerves. The spinal nerves carry sensory information to the spinal cord tracts. Sensory information is then projected to the brainstem, where it is processed by the reticular formation. Sensory information then travels to the thalamus and finally to the cortex (SS1).
- Sensory information may also be carried to the spinal cord (SC) from the spinal nerves in the PNS. Sensory information then travels from the SC to the brainstem, where it is projected through the middle cerebellar peduncle to the cerebellum. The cerebellum then sends the sensory information through the superior cerebellar peduncle to the thalamus. At the thalamic level, sensory information is either rerouted to the cortex or back down through the brainstem.[2,3]

Motor Efferent Pathways

- Motor messages are sent from the cortex (M1) to the thalamus. At the thalamic level, motor messages are sent down through the brainstem and SC to the muscles in the PNS.
- Motor messages may also project from the thalamus to the cerebellum, SC, and motor neurons in the ventral horn.[2,3]

Ansa Lenticularis Pathway

- The ansa lenticularis pathway carries motor messages from the basal ganglia to the ventrolateral nucleus of the thalamus. The information is then sent to M1.
- This pathway allows the basal ganglia, thalamus, and cortex to communicate with each other.[2,3]

Gutman SA. *Quick Reference Neuroscience for Rehabilitation Professionals:*
The Essential Neurologic Principles Underlying Rehabilitation Practice,
Third Edition (pp 290-295).
© 2017 Taylor & Francis Group.

Superior Colliculi Pathway

- The superior colliculi of the midbrain receive sensory messages from the optic pathways and the thalamic lateral geniculate nucleus.
- The superior colliculi then send this information to the thalamus via the medial longitudinal fasciculus.
- This pathway carries information that controls the position of the eyes and head in response to visual information.
- The pathway that carries visual information between the superior colliculi and the lateral geniculate nucleus forms a primitive visual system that is likely responsible for cortical sight or blind sight. This is the phenomenon in which patients with cortical blindness still retain the ability to process some visual information on an unconscious or subcortical level.[4]

Inferior Colliculi Pathway

- The inferior colliculi of the midbrain receive sensory information from the thalamic *medial* geniculate nucleus and the auditory cortex.
- The inferior colliculi then project this sensory information back to the thalamus and auditory cortex for the further processing of auditory information.
- This pathway is a primitive auditory pathway that allows sound to be processed on an unconscious or subcortical level. For example, patients with cortical deafness may still startle in response to the sound of a slammed door without consciously hearing the door slam shut.[5]

Thalamic Mediodorsal Nucleus Pathway

- The thalamic mediodorsal nucleus receives and projects sensory information to and from the amygdala, substantia nigra, and temporal cortex.
- When the mediodorsal nucleus is lesioned, memory loss occurs.[6]

Lesions to the Thalamus

Central Post-Stroke Pain

- Central post-stroke pain results from vascular insufficiency, or a cerebrovascular accident damaging the thalamus and/or adjacent areas of the CNS, and involves an alteration of sensory *perception*.
- Patients may become either hyper- or hyposensitive to sensation (particularly pain and noxious stimuli) on the contralateral side of the lesion.
- Initially, patients experience loss of sensation and tingling in the contralateral body. Several weeks after onset, patients develop burning, agonizing pain in the affected body parts.[7]

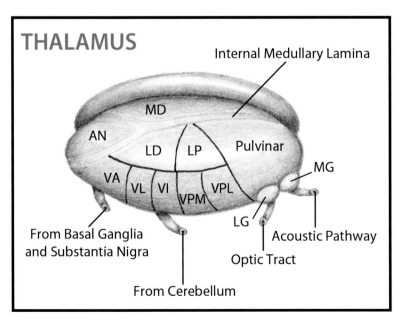

- AN = Anterior Nuclei
- LD = Lateral Dorsal Nucleus
- LG = Lateral Geniculate Nucleus
- LP = Lateral Posterior Nucleus
- MD = Mediodorsal Nucleus
- MG = Medial Geniculate Nucleus
- VA = Ventral Anterior Nucleus
- VI = Ventral Intermedial Nucleus
- VL = Ventrolateral Nucleus
- VPL = Ventral Posterolateral Nucleus
- VPM = Ventral Posteromedial Nucleus

Thalamic Tumors

- Sometimes patients present with specific symptoms, depending on which thalamic nuclei are involved:
  - A lesion to the ventrolateral nucleus destroys communication with M1. This results in paralysis of the involved body part.
  - A lesion to the lateral geniculate nucleus destroys communication with V1. This can result in cortical blindness.
  - A lesion to the medial geniculate nucleus destroys communication with A1. Cortical deafness or hyper-/hypo-sensitivity to sound can occur.
  - A lesion to the posterolateral nucleus destroys communication with SS1. Paresthesias, hypoesthesia, and/or causalgia can occur.
- Damage to the ventral posteromedial nucleus and the ventral posterolateral nucleus results in a loss of all forms of sensation, including light touch, tactile localization and discrimination, and proprioception from the contralateral side of the body.
- In other cases, a thalamic lesion results in dysfunction of neighboring structures, producing clinical symptoms that overshadow those produced by the thalamic disease. For example, a thalamic lesion may also involve the midbrain and, thus, result in coma.[7]

BRAINSTEM

- The brainstem is a phylogenetically old part of the brain that controls vegetative functions essential for survival: respiration and primitive stereotyped reflexes.
- The primitive stereotyped reflexes include the following:
  - Cough and gag reflex
  - Pupillary response
  - Spontaneous swallowing reflex
- The brainstem also controls the reticular formation.[8]

Reticular Formation

- The reticular formation is a poorly localized area of the brainstem.
- It resembles a net that is composed of nerve cells and fibers.
- The net extends up through the medulla, pons, and midbrain. Fibers connect it to the SC, hypothalamus, thalamus, and cortex.
- The reticular activating system is thought to be located diffusely in the rostral midbrain.
- The reticular inhibiting system is believed to be located diffusely from the caudal midbrain to the caudal medulla.
- Simplistically, the reticular formation acts as a screen for incoming sensory data to the cortex and outgoing motor information from the cortical and subcortical areas.[9]

Major Functions of the Reticular Formation

- Because the reticular formation has vast connections to all regions of the nervous system, it is believed to have many different types of function.
- Following are several of the most important and understood functions of the reticular formation.
- Regulation of consciousness
  - The reticular activating system is responsible for states of wakefulness.
  - Lesions to the reticular activating system result in a stuporous state. When the reticular activating system is lost, the reticular inhibitory system becomes dominant and causes heightened somnolence.
  - Conversely, the reticular inhibiting system is responsible for states of sleep and unconsciousness.
  - Lesions to the reticular inhibitory system result in constant wakefulness. When the reticular inhibitory system is lost, the reticular activating system becomes dominant and causes heightened arousal.[10]
- Control of muscle tone
  - The reticulospinal tracts can influence the activity of the alpha and gamma motor neurons.
  - This allows the reticular formation to influence muscle tone and reflex activity.
  - Along with the vestibulospinal and reticulospinal tracts, the reticular formation influences tone in antigravity muscles.[11]
- Control of pain
  - The reticular formation may have a key role in the gating mechanism for the control of pain.

- ○ The reticulospinal tracts are descending sensory tracts that receive pain information from the periphery through afferent spinal nerves that synapse in the reticular formation of the brainstem.
- ○ The reticulospinal tracts have their origin in the medullary reticular formation.
- ○ There, they travel to the raphe nuclei of the brainstem. The raphe nuclei are a group of nuclei located in the medulla. They are situated along the midline.
- ○ When the raphe nuclei become excited, they release endorphins through a descending pathway to the place of pain origin to decrease the pain sensation.[12]
- Regulation of circadian rhythms
  - ○ The reticular formation and the hypothalamus work conjointly in the regulation of circadian rhythms, or sleep and wake cycles.[13]

Reticular Activating System

- The reticular activating system is a subsystem of the reticular formation.
- The activating system alerts the cortex to attend to important incoming sensory information.
- This process is important for filtering unnecessary data so that people can focus on other activities more intently.
- When important sensory data is detected by the reticular activating system, it alerts the cortex, which then arouses the body and prepares it for activity.
- The cortex uses the thalamus, hypothalamus, limbic system, vestibular system, and autonomic nervous system (ANS) to arouse the body.[14]

Reticular Inhibiting System

- The reticular inhibiting system receives messages from the cortical and subcortical centers to calm the body in response to specific sensory data.
- The reticular inhibiting system works conjointly with the vestibular system to calm the body via such sensory stimulation as slow rocking, deep pressure, and vibration.[15]

Brainstem Damage and Disorders of Consciousness

- Severe brainstem damage can result in altered consciousness and coma.
- There are 2 basic types of disordered consciousness states involving the brainstem: persistent vegetative state and brain death.

Sensory Processing Disorders of the Reticular Formation

- In children with attention deficit hyperactivity disorder (ADHD), learning disability, autism, and tactile defensiveness, the reticular activating system may function in overdrive.
- These children cannot easily screen or filter extraneous sensory data. Thus, they react to almost all sensory stimulation in the environment in a random and disorganized fashion.
- Conversely, some children's reticular inhibiting system may function in overdrive. These children have difficulty registering the sensory information attempting to enter the central nervous system (CNS).
- Children with sensory processing disorders (or regulatory disorders) may seek specific types of stimulation in order to obtain the type of sensory data that their nervous systems require in order to develop and function optimally.
- Sensory integration treatment provides the child with sensory stimulation, which, over a period of time, may enhance the brain's ability to process sensory data more functionally.
- For children with hyper-reticular activating systems, slow rocking, deep pressure, and vibration may be the type of vestibular sensation needed to calm the body.
- For children with hyper-reticular inhibiting systems, sensory stimulation that arouses the brain may be needed.[16]

Pharmacologic Treatment for Sensory Processing Disorders

- Ritalin and other brands of methylphenidate are mild CNS stimulants used in the treatment of ADHD in children.
- Methylphenidate attempts to balance the divisions of the reticular formation. It can calm an overactive reticular activating system or stimulate the reticular activating system if it is sluggish.
- Methylphenidate targets impairment in the dopamine and norepinephrine neurotransmitter systems by increasing neurotransmission of both.[17]

Persistent Vegetative State

- Persistent vegetative state is considered to be a disorder of consciousness rather than coma.
- In a persistent vegetative state, the brainstem, including the reticular activating system, remains intact.
- The brunt of neurologic destruction is located in the cerebral hemispheres. Although PET and functional MRI studies have found some residual activation in some cortical regions in response to stimuli, such cortical activity is severed from reaching other regions required for awareness.
- In a vegetative state, patients are able to open their eyes and may display sleep-wake cycles but do not have cognitive function and awareness.
- A persistent vegetative state often results from cardiac or respiratory arrest causing a lack of blood flow (ischemia) and loss of oxygen (hypoxia) to the brain for several minutes.
- The brainstem is fairly resistant to ischemia and hypoxia. Four to 6 minutes of complete blood and oxygen loss to the brain can result in extensive cortical destruction while sparing the brainstem.
- After a period of days to a month, the patient will awaken into a condition of eyes-opened unconsciousness. This is called a *vegetative state*.
- Because the brainstem is spared, the cough, gag, and swallowing reflexes remain intact.
- This decreases the likelihood of respiratory infections and substantially lengthens life expectancy (particularly with life support technological systems).[18]

Brain Death

- Brain death occurs when all brainstem functions are lost.
- The heartbeat can continue because it is semi-autonomous from ANS regulation.
- This type of coma is a state of sleep-like (eyes-closed) unarousability due to extensive damage to the reticular activating system.
- The cough, gag, and swallowing reflexes are lost, leading to fatal respiratory infections within 6 months to 1 year.[19]

Cranial Nerve Nuclei Damage in the Brainstem

- The cranial nerve nuclei are located in the brainstem.
- They innervate ipsilateral body structures.
- Brainstem disorders depend upon which cranial nerve nuclei have been lost.
- See Section 8 for disorders of the cranial nerve nuclei.

Spinal Cord Tract Damage in the Brainstem

- Descending motor tracts and ascending sensory tracts travel through the brainstem and mediate motor and sensory functions of structures on the contralateral side of the body.
- When spinal cord tracts are lost due to brainstem damage, hemiplegia and hemiparesthesia on the contralateral side of the body result.
- See Sections 18 and 19 for spinal cord injuries and diseases.

Locked-In Syndrome

- Locked-in syndrome appears much like coma, but instead of losing consciousness, the patient remains aware yet has no means of communication other than eye movement.
- Such patients have lost the ability to speak and control muscles other than eyeball movement.
- Patients are able to move their eyes vertically and blink voluntarily. These movements can be used to respond to questions.
- Locked-in syndrome can result from infarction or hemorrhage in the ventral pons.
- The syndrome can be caused by traumatic brain injury, vascular diseases, demyelinating diseases, or drug overdose.
- The majority of patients with locked-in syndrome do not regain function; however, experimental research is attempting to help patients regain the ability to communicate.
- Researchers have successfully implanted electrodes into the motor cortex of several patients. The electrodes send messages to a computer that translates signals into cursor movements (on a computer screen). Patients can manipulate the cursor to spell or activate icons representing specific activities. While preliminary results have been successful, further research is needed before such techniques can become standard protocol.[20]

REFERENCES

1. Haber SN, Calzavara R. The cortico-basal ganglia integrative network: the role of the thalamus. *Brain Res Bull.* 2009;78(2):69-74. doi:10.1016/j.brainresbull.2008.09.013.

2. Sherman SM, Guillery RW. *Functional Connections of Cortical Areas: A New View from the Thalamus.* Cambridge, MA: MIT Press; 2013.

3. Jones EG. *The Thalamus.* 2nd ed. Cambridge, United Kingdom: Cambridge University Press; 2007.

4. May PJ. The mammalian superior colliculus: laminar structure and connections. *Prog Brain Res.* 2006;151:321-378. doi:10.1016/S0079-6123(05)51011-2.

5. Schreiner CE, Winer JA. *The Inferior Colliculus.* New York, NY: Springer; 2005.

6. Zikopoulos B, Barbas H. Prefrontal projections to the thalamic reticular nucleus form a unique circuit for attentional mechanisms. *J Neurosci.* 2006;26(28):7348-7361. doi:10.1016/S0165-0173(02)00181-9.

7. Montagna P, Provini F, Plazzi G, et al. Bilateral paramedian thalamic syndrome: abnormal circadian wake-sleep and autonomic functions. *J Neurol Neurosurg Psychiatry.* 2002;73(6):772-774. doi:10.1136/jnnp.73.6.772.

8. Joseph R. *Brain and Cerebellum: Medulla, Pons, Midbrain, Reticular Formation, Arousal, Vision, Hearing, Norepinephrine, Serotonin, Dopamine, Sleeping, Dreams, REM, Cranial Nerves, Motor Control.* Cambridge, MA: Cosmology Science; 2011.

9. Yeo SS, Chang PH, Jang SH. The ascending reticular activating system from pontine reticular formation to the thalamus in the human brain. *Front Hum Neurosci.* 2013;7:416. doi:10.3389/fnhum.2013.00416.

10. Vanini G, Wathen BL, Lydic R, Baghdoyan HA. Endogenous GABA levels in the pontine reticular formation are greater during wakefulness than during rapid eye movement sleep. *J Neurosci.* 2011;31(7):2649-2656. doi: 10.1523/JNEUROSCI.5674-10.2011.

11. Schepens B, Stapley P, Drew T. Neurons in the pontomedullary reticular formation signal posture and movement both as an integrated behavior and independently. *J Neurophysiol.* 2008;100(4):2235-2253. doi:10.1152/jn.01381.2007.

12. Lima D, Almeida A. The medullary dorsal reticular nucleus as a pronociceptive centre of the pain control system. *Prog Neurobiol.* 2002;66(2):81-108. doi:10.1016/S0301-0082(01)00025-9.

13. Malatesta M, Fattoretti P, Baldelli B, Battistelli S, Balietti M, Bertoni-Freddari C. Effects of ageing on the fine distribution of the circadian CLOCK protein in reticular formation neurons. *Histochem Cell Biol.* 2007;127(6):641-647. doi:10.1007/s00418-007-0284-8.

14. Nofzinger EA, Buysse DJ, Germain A, Price JC, Miewald JM, Kupfer DJ. Functional neuroimaging evidence for hyper-arousal in insomnia. *Am J Psychiatry.* 2004;161(11):2126-2128.

15. Steriade M. Sleep, epilepsy and thalamic reticular inhibitory neurons. *Trends Neurosci.* 2005;28(6):317-324. doi:10.1016/j.tins.2005.03.007.

16. Reynolds S, Lane SJ. Sensory overresponsivity and anxiety in children with ADHD. *Am J Occup Ther.* 2009;63(4):433-440. doi:10.5014/ajot.63.4.433.

17. Faraone SV, Buitelaar J. Comparing the efficacy of stimulants for ADHD in children and adolescents using meta-analysis. *Eur Child Adolesc Psychiatry.* 2010;19(4):353-364. doi:10.1007/s00787-009-0054-3.

18. Monti MM, Laureys S, Owen AM. The vegetative state. *BMJ.* 2010;341:292-296. doi:10.1136/bmj.c3765.

19. Bernat JL, Larriviere D. Areas of persisting controversy in brain death. *Neurology.* 2014;83(16):1394-1395. doi:10.1212/WNL.0000000000000883 1526-632X.

20. Stoll J, Chatelle C, Carter O, Koch C, Laureys S, Einhäuser W. Pupil responses allow communication in locked-in syndrome patients. *Curr Biol.* 2013;23(15):R647-R648. doi:10.1016/j.cub.2013.06.011.

Right vs Left Brain Functions and Disorders

HEMISPHERE DOMINANCE

- Generally, one side of the brain has dominant control.
- Specific individuals may be left or right brain dominant, although the left hemisphere is dominant in most people.
- Hemisphere dominance may be reversed in some people who are left-handed, or only certain brain functions may be dominant in the right hemisphere while other functions are within the domain of the left hemisphere.[1,2]

LEFT BRAIN FUNCTIONS

- The left hemisphere controls motor function on the right side of the body.
- This hemisphere also receives sensory information from the right side of the body.
- The left hemisphere has a role in language, specifically the interpretation and expression of aural and written words.
- The hemisphere is specialized for the interpretation of the concrete meanings of words (as opposed to the abstract or symbolic meaning).
- For example, the left hemisphere interprets the literal meaning of a story, but not the hidden or symbolic meaning.
- The left hemisphere controls concrete functions that can be easily observed and measured[3-5]:
  - Interpreting the concrete meaning of written or spoken words
  - Math calculations
  - Writing the letters of the alphabet
  - Reading a sentence
  - Categorizing shapes
  - Sequencing steps in a task

Gutman SA. *Quick Reference Neuroscience for Rehabilitation Professionals:*
The Essential Neurologic Principles Underlying Rehabilitation Practice,
Third Edition (pp 296-303).
© 2017 Taylor & Francis Group.

RIGHT BRAIN FUNCTIONS

- The right hemisphere controls motor function on the left side of the body.
- This hemisphere also receives sensory information from the left side of the body.
- It has a role in the interpretation of perception—how humans perceive their environment.
- The right hemisphere also has a role in the interpretation of information that is abstract and creative (as opposed to concrete and logical).
- This hemisphere controls abstract functions that cannot be easily observed—functions that relate to the perception of oneself in relation to the environment.
- It also has a role in language, but it is the interpretation of the abstract or symbolic meaning of a story or joke.
- This hemisphere is similarly responsible for interpreting someone's verbal tone and gestures; in other words, understanding the meaning behind the words.
- Perception includes visual and spatial perception, language perception, motor planning perception, body schema perception, tactile perception, and auditory perception.[6-8]

LEFT HEMISPHERE DISORDERS

- Damage to the left hemisphere can result in the following[9-11]:
  ○ Wernicke and Broca aphasia
  ○ Contralateral motor and sensory problems
  ○ Acalculia (the inability to calculate math problems)
  ○ Agraphia (the inability to write words that had been familiar preinjury/disease)
  ○ Alexia (the inability to read written words that had been familiar preinjury/disease)

RIGHT HEMISPHERE DISORDERS

- Right hemisphere disorders involve impairment in the recognition of physical reality.
- Such disorders distort physical reality—they distort the environment and/or one's own body perception[12-14]:
  ○ Visual-spatial disorders
  ○ Body schema perception disorders
  ○ Apraxias (motor planning perceptual problems)
  ○ Perceptual language disorders
  ○ Tactile perceptual disorders
  ○ Auditory perceptual disorders
  ○ Contralateral motor and sensory problems

THE CORRELATION BETWEEN ANATOMICAL DAMAGE AND SYMPTOMATOLOGY

- It is difficult to correlate precise anatomical damage with specific symptomatology.
- This is due to individual differences in human brains.
- Each human brain varies with regard to sulci and gyri patterns.
- It is also difficult to correlate damage and symptomatology because of neuroplasticity.

Savant Syndrome

- Savant syndrome generally occurs in people with IQs between 40 and 70 who have marked impairment in most daily living skills. Despite such impairment, people with savant syndrome possess highly sophisticated skills in areas such as music, art, mathematics, and memory.[15]
- For example, most people with musical savant syndrome have perfect pitch and can play musical instruments at an amazing skill level without any musical training.
- People with artistic savant syndrome are able to paint and sculpt perfect replicas of objects and people whose images are stored in their memory.
- People possessing mathematical savant syndrome can calculate with incredible speed and accuracy.
- Other people with savant syndrome can memorize many languages (but without understanding) or possess outstanding knowledge in areas such as history, statistics, and navigational abilities. Such people seem to have superior memory capabilities.
- One explanation for savant syndrome involves an overspecialization of the right hemisphere. Such overspecialization appears to occur concomitantly with damage to the left hemisphere.
- In the book *Cerebral Lateralization*,[16] the authors Geschwind and Galaburda suggest that, in utero, the left hemisphere completes its development later than the right hemisphere. Because of this lag in development, the left hemisphere is more vulnerable to prenatal influences for a longer period of time.
- Geschwind and Galaburda suggest that in male fetuses, circulating testosterone can slow brain growth and impair the development of neuronal connections in the left hemisphere. The right brain then becomes larger and more dominant in males in order to compensate for impairment in the left hemisphere.
- This theory seems to support the finding that savant syndrome occurs disproportionately in more male than female humans, at a 6:1 ratio. This greater male to female ratio is also seen in other forms of central nervous system (CNS) disorders such as dyslexia, delayed speech, delayed hand dominance, stuttering, attention deficit hyperactivity disorder (ADHD), learning disability, and autism.
- The skills that are associated with savant syndrome tend to be limited to right brain functions (ie, creativity, artistic skills, visuospatial abilities, and abstract functions), further supporting this theory.
- Researchers are beginning to use neurodiagnostic imaging scans to compare the left and right hemispheres in people with savant syndrome. Early studies have supported the idea that the left hemisphere has been impaired, thus giving rise to overdevelopment of the right hemisphere.
- Other researchers have found the emergence of savant-like skills in some patients with adult onset dementia. Such patients developed the ability to paint, draw, or play music with incredible precision. As in savant syndrome, single photon emission computed tomography (SPECT) scans showed that these patients had sustained damage to their left hemisphere as a result of the disease process.[17]
- Some researchers suggest that savant-like skills may lie dormant in the larger population. These researchers contend that the same neural circuitry that underlies savant skills is present in the larger population, but that the ability to access such skills becomes lost in a society that encourages left brain functions.[18]

NEUROPLASTICITY

- Neuroplasticity occurs when other areas of the brain assume the functions once mediated by regions that have been damaged.
- Human brains appear to possess a vast amount of brain matter that does not become active until damage occurs to other areas. At this time, those previously unused regions may become active and take over the function of damaged areas.
- It is possible that the same brain function may be shared by several, separate brain regions that lie dormant until injury/disease occurs. This may be the brain's evolutionary attempt at compensation.[19]
- Research has also shown that damage to regions of the homunculus can result in appropriation of cortical areas by adjacent regions.[20] For example, when the homunculi region representing the trunk is damaged, this region may be appropriated by the region representing the arm.
- Neuroplasticity is most viable in children because the CNS is not fully mature, but rather is still developing.
- The idea that the brain can change, or reorganize itself, in response to internal and external stimuli underlies all rehabilitation concepts.

Neuroplasticity Is Dependent Upon the Following

- Severity of neurologic damage
- Age (younger brains tend to have greater neuroplasticity)
- Premorbid health status
- Preinjury use of the damaged brain area: brain areas that were frequently used preinjury and then became damaged have a greater capacity to regain function. The more a brain region is used, the more it develops neuronal connections that can help in the recovery process.[21]

Constraint-Induced Movement Therapy

- Constraint-induced movement therapy (CIMT) is a rehabilitation technique in which a patient's unaffected limb is restricted in order to facilitate functional use of the affected limb.
- A patient's uninvolved extremity may be constrained for 30-minute practice sessions, 5 hours per day, over 10 days (dose and duration vary). During this time, patients participate in activity sessions that force them to use their affected limb.
- Repeated, task-specific practice with the affected extremity appears to enhance the growth and branching of dendrites and the remodeling of synaptic connections—or the mechanisms underlying neuroplasticity.
- Research regarding CIMT has demonstrated its effectiveness in patients who have sustained neurologic damage (eg, traumatic brain injury and stroke).
- Patient compliance can sometimes be difficult to obtain because patients with neurologic damage may fatigue easily or display anger in response to frustration caused by the restraint device. The high cost of CIMT may also be prohibitive.[22]

REFERENCES

1. Gazzaniga MS. Forty-five years of split-brain research and still going strong. *Nat Rev Neurosci*. 2005;6(8):653-659. doi:10.1038/nrn1723.

2. MacNeilage PF, Rogers LJ, Vallortigara G. Origins of the left and right brain. *Sci Am*. 2009;301(1):60-67. doi:10.1038/scientificamerican0709-60.

3. Janssen L, Meulenbroek RG, Steenbergen B. Behavioral evidence for left-hemisphere specialization of motor planning. *Exper Brain Res*. 2011;209(1):65-72. doi:10.1007/s00221-010-2519-5.

4. Vigneau M, Beaucousin V, Herve PY, et al. Meta-analyzing left hemisphere language areas: phonology, semantics, and sentence processing. *Neuroimage*. 2006;30(4):1414-1432. doi:10.1016/j.neuroimage.2005.11.002.

5. Rivera SM, Reiss AL, Eckert MA, Menon V. Developmental changes in mental arithmetic: evidence for increased functional specialization in the left inferior parietal cortex. *Cereb Cortex*. 2005;15(11):1779-1790. doi: 10.1093/cercor/bhi055.

6. Lindell AK. In your right mind: Right hemisphere contributions to language processing and production. *Neuropsychol Rev*. 2006;16(3):131-148. doi:10.1007/s11065-006-9011-9.

7. Gainotti G. Unconscious processing of emotions and the right hemisphere. *Neuropsychologia*. 2012;50(2):205-218. doi:10.1016/j.neuropsychologia.2011.12.005.

8. McGettigan C, Scott SK. Cortical asymmetries in speech perception: what's wrong, what's right and what's left? *Trends Cogn Sci*. 2012;16(5):269-276. doi:10.1016/j.tics.2012.04.006.

9. Ashkenazi S, Henik A, Ifergane G, Shelef I. Basic numerical processing in left intraparietal sulcus (IPS) acalculia. *Cortex*. 2008;44(4):439-448. doi:10.1016/j.cortex.2007.08.008.

10. Gorno-Tempini ML, Hillis AE, Weintraub S, et al. Classification of primary progressive aphasia and its variants. *Neurology*. 2011;76(11):1006-1014. doi:10.1212/ WNL. 0b013e31821103e6.

11. Cocchini G, Beschin N, Cameron A, Fotopoulou A, Della Sala S. Anosognosia for motor impairment following left brain damage. *Neuropsychology*. 2009;23(2):223. doi:10.1037/a0014266.

12. Farne A, Buxbaum LJ, Ferraro M, et al. Patterns of spontaneous recovery of neglect and associated disorders in acute right brain-damaged patients. *J Neurol Neurosurg Psychiatry*. 2004;75(10):1401-1410. doi:10.1136/jnnp.2002.003095.

13. Buxbaum LJ, Giovannetti T, Libon D. The role of the dynamic body schema in praxis: evidence from primary progressive apraxia. *Brain Cogn*. 2000;44(2):166-191. doi:10.1006/brcg.2000.1227.

14. Halligan PW, Fink GR, Marshall JC, Vallar G. Spatial cognition: evidence from visual neglect. *Trends Cogn Sci*. 2003;7(3):125-133. doi:10.1016/S1364-6613(03)00032-9.

15. Treffert DA. The savant syndrome: an extraordinary condition. A synopsis: past, present, future. *Philos Trans R Soc Lond B Biol Sci*. 2009;364(1522):1351-1357. doi:10.1098/rstb.2008.0326.

16. Geschwind N, Galaburda AM. *Cerebral Lateralization: Biological Mechanisms, Associations, and Pathology*. Cambridge, MA: MIT Press; 2003.

17. Mendez MF. Dementia as a window to the neurology of art. *Med Hypoth*. 2004;63(1):1-7. doi:10.1016/j.mehy.2004.03.002.

18. Snyder AW, Mulcahy E, Taylor JL, Mitchell DJ, Sachdev P, Gandevia SC. Savant-like skills exposed in normal people by suppressing the left fronto-temporal lobe. *J Integr Neurosci*. 2003;2(02):149-158. doi:10.1142/S0219635203000287.

19. Sagi Y, Tavor I, Hofstetter S, Tzur-Moryosef S, Blumenfeld-Katzir T, Assaf Y. Learning in the fast lane: new insights into neuroplasticity. *Neuron*. 2012;73(6):1195-1203. doi:10.1016/j.neuron.2012.01.025.

20. Dutta V. The phantom breast after mastectomy, the homunculus and the hole in the cortical map. *J Cancer Res Therapeut*. 2015;11(1):3-5. doi:10.4103/0973-1482.155090.

21. Wolf SL, Winstein CJ, Miller JP, et al; EXCITE Investigators. Effect of constraint-induced movement therapy on upper extremity function 3 to 9 months after stroke: the EXCITE randomized clinical trial. *JAMA*. 2006;296(17):2095-2104. doi:10.1001/jama.296.17.2095.

22. Cramer SC, Sur M, Dobkin BH, et al. Harnessing neuroplasticity for clinical applications. *Brain*. 2011;134(6):1591-1609. doi:10.1093/brain/awr039.

CLINICAL TEST QUESTIONS

Sections 23 to 25

1. Mr. Choi has been diagnosed with a tumor in his right secondary somatosensory area. As a result, he has difficulty identifying objects with his left hand (with vision occluded). The umbrella term for this disorder is called:
   a. tactile agnosia
   b. primary sensation

2. For example, when small objects are placed in Mr. Choi's left hand (with vision occluded), he cannot interpret them. This is called:
   a. two-point discrimination
   b. agraphesthesia
   c. astereognosis
   d. atopognosia

3. Mrs. Malinowski has a tumor located in V4. She is able to accurately see and interpret objects when they are still. However, she is unable to interpret objects in motion (such as moving cars on a street). This is referred to as:
   a. achromatopsia
   b. akinetopsia
   c. abarognosia
   d. topographical disorientation

4. Mrs. Novak had a left cerebral hemisphere stroke located in the inferior gyrus of the premotor area. She can understand language that is spoken to her, but when she tries to respond, she cannot form meaningful sentences. This type of aphasia is called _____.
   1. Broca aphasia
   2. Wernicke aphasia
   3. receptive aphasia
   4. expressive aphasia
   a. 1, 3
   b. 2, 3
   c. 1, 4
   d. 2, 4

5. Jose lost consciousness after a traumatic brain injury and has not regained it 2 months status post-injury. He is able to open his eyes and appears to display regular sleep-wake cycles, but does not have cognitive function or awareness. Jose's cough, gag, and swallowing reflexes all remain intact. This state of altered consciousness is called _____ and is caused by severe damage to the _____:
   1. brain death
   2. persistent vegetative state
   3. cortex
   4. brainstem
   a. 1, 3
   b. 2, 3
   c. 1, 4
   d. 2, 4

6. Jose's friend Alejandro, who was in the car accident with Jose, also sustained a traumatic brain injury. Alejandro is in a state of sleep-like (eyes closed) unarousability. All cognitive function has been lost as well as cough, gag, and swallowing reflexes. Alejandro's heartbeat continues from ANS regulation; however, Alejandro has been hooked up to life support because of a severe respiratory infection. This type of coma is called _____ and results from severe damage to the _____.
   1. brain death
   2. persistent vegetative state
   3. cortex
   4. brainstem
   a. 1, 3
   b. 2, 3
   c. 1, 4
   d. 2, 4

7. After a drug overdose that damaged her ventral pons, Lin lost all voluntary muscle control, including the ability to speak. The muscles controlling her eyeball movements are the only muscles over which she still retains control. Lin lies in a hospital bed and is conscious but cannot communicate. This state is called:
   a. brain death
   b. persistent vegetative state
   c. coma
   d. locked-in syndrome

8. After his stroke, Mr. Donatelli has difficulty expressing meaningful verbal communications to others and has hemiparesis and hemiparesthesia of his right side. His stroke likely occurred in which cerebral hemisphere?
   a. left
   b. right

9. After her stroke, Ms. Jenkins has developed hypersensitivity to sensation on the contralateral side of the lesion. The hypersensitivity progressed into burning, agonizing pain that causes Ms. Jenkins nausea and sleep disruption. This syndrome is called _____ and can result from _____.
   1. central post-stroke pain
   2. central hypersensitivity syndrome
   3. vascular insufficiency to the thalamus and nearby CNS structures
   4. vascular insufficiency to the sensory spinal cord tracts
   a. 1, 3
   b. 1, 4
   c. 2, 3
   d. 2, 4

10. Mr. Morrissey had a stroke to his brainstem, which damaged the structure responsible for states of wakefulness. As a result, he lies in a stuporous, unarousable state. The structure likely damaged was the:
    a. reticular inhibiting system
    b. reticular activating system

Answers

1. a
2. c
3. b
4. c
5. b
6. c
7. d
8. a
9. a
10. b

Perceptual Functions and Dysfunctions of the Central Nervous System

MULTIMODAL AREAS OF THE CENTRAL NERVOUS SYSTEM

- The multimodal areas of the central nervous system (CNS) are also called *convergence association areas.*[1,2]
- All sensory areas (as listed next) send information to the multimodal areas:
  - Somatosensory association area
  - Auditory association area
  - Visual association area
  - Motor association area (prefrontal cortex)
  - Olfactory cortex (piriform cortex in the temporal lobe)
  - Gustatory cortex (frontal insula)
- This information converges and becomes integrated together.
- There are 3 multimodal association areas in the brain:
  1. Posterior multimodal association area
  2. Anterior multimodal association area
  3. Limbic multimodal association area

Posterior Multimodal Association Area

- The posterior multimodal association area is located in the posterior of the brain in a region where the parietal, occipital, and temporal lobes meet.
- This posterior multimodal association area integrates sensory information processed by the somatosensory, visual, and auditory association areas, and the olfactory and gustatory cortices.
- This is where scent, vision, touch, taste, and sound are all connected to form a sensory experience.
- For example, the posterior multimodal association area combines the sound of the ocean, the color of the waves and crests, the feel of sand on one's feet, the taste of salt water in the air, and the smell of the sea all into one cohesive sensory experience.
- After integrating the 5 types of sensory data, the posterior multimodal association area then sends this data to the (1) anterior multimodal association area for the initiation of action in response to sensory data and to the (2) limbic multimodal association area to form memories associated with emotions generated by the sensory data.[3]

Anterior Multimodal Association Area

- The anterior multimodal association area is located in the prefrontal cortex, one storage area for motor plans.
- The anterior multimodal association area takes the integrated sensory data from the posterior multimodal association area and uses it to make decisions about which motor plan to implement.
- Once a decision is made, the anterior multimodal association area sends this information to the premotor area to access the appropriate motor plan.

Gutman SA. *Quick Reference Neuroscience for Rehabilitation Professionals: The Essential Neurologic Principles Underlying Rehabilitation Practice, Third Edition* (pp 304-315). © 2017 Taylor & Francis Group.

- Once the appropriate motor plan is accessed, the primary motor area (M1) implements the motor plan.
- For example, in response to the sensory data described previously, one may decide to implement the motor plans required for swimming in the ocean.[4-7]

Limbic Multimodal Association Area

- The limbic multimodal association area is located in the internal surfaces of the parietal, temporal, and frontal lobes and includes the hippocampal formation, cingulate gyrus, parahippocampal gyrus, and amygdala.
- The limbic multimodal association area takes the integrated sensory data from the anterior and posterior multimodal association areas and links it to emotions and motivations through memory. In other words, this association area is responsible for the generation of emotion in response to events, decides whether specific types of behaviors are rewarding and should be repeated, and forms memories of our emotions that guide future behaviors.
- For example, in response to the gustatory data evoked by eating an ice cream cone, the limbic association area generates positive emotions, decides that eating ice cream is internally rewarding and should be repeated, and forms a memory of the positive emotions associated with ice cream that guide our future ice cream–seeking behaviors.[4-7]

Impairment of the Multimodal Association Areas

- Because the multimodal association area in the right hemisphere plays an important role in perception (how one perceives the environment and one's relationship to the environment), damage to the right multimodal association area often results in perceptual disorders.[8]

Perceptual Impairment

- Perceptual impairment more often involves dysfunction of the right hemisphere (specifically the right posterior multimodal association area), rather than the left.
- Right hemisphere disorders of the posterior multimodal association area involve impairment in the recognition of physical reality.
- Physical reality becomes distorted.
- One's relationship to the environment becomes distorted. One's relationship to one's own body also becomes distorted.[8]

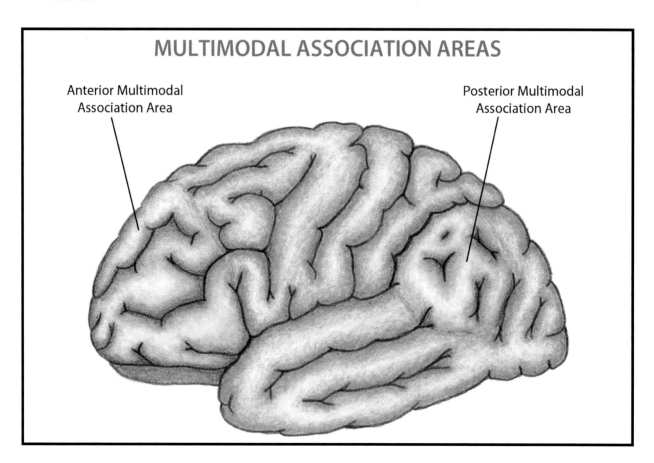

MULTIMODAL ASSOCIATION AREAS

Anterior Multimodal Association Area

Posterior Multimodal Association Area

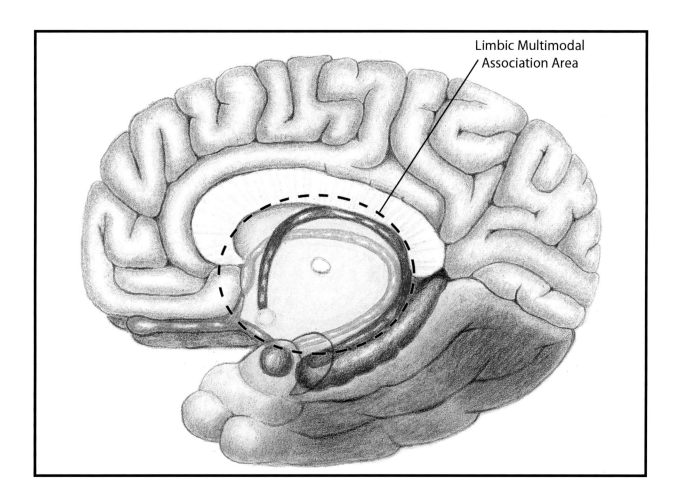

- There are several classifications of perception:
  - Visual perception (including spatial perception)
  - Body schema perception
  - Language perception (including expressive and receptive language perception)
  - Motor planning perception (or praxis)
  - Tactile perception
  - Auditory perception

VISUAL PERCEPTUAL DISORDERS

Visual Agnosia

- *Visual agnosia* is an umbrella term for the inability to identify and recognize familiar objects and people (although the visual anatomy remains intact).
- Lesions that cause visual agnosias are usually located in the right hemisphere in the posterior multimodal association area.[9]

Prosopagnosia

- Prosopagnosia is the inability to identify familiar faces because the individual cannot perceive the unique bone structure and facial muscle position that make each human face different from each other (a function of the right hemisphere).
- The left hemisphere specializes in identifying faces through facial details. A person with prosopagnosia may not be able to recognize friends and family, but he could recognize a particular face if it was characterized by a unique feature, such as a mole or scar. For example, a person may be able to identify his wife because she has a mole on her nose. This form of pattern recognition, however, causes the individual to think that everyone with a mole on her nose is his wife.[10]

Oliver Sacks Story

Prosopagnosia

- In *The Man Who Mistook His Wife For a Hat*, Oliver Sacks describes a 32-year-old patient who remained comatose for 3 weeks after a severe motor vehicle accident. As the patient regained consciousness and function, he began to complain of an inability to recognize familiar faces, even those of family members and close friends. There were 3 faces, however, which he could identify. All were work colleagues with unique distinguishing characteristics. One man had an eye-blinking tic; another had a large mole on his cheek; and the third was a tall, thin man whose skeletal structure made him stand out in crowds. The patient could recognize these men because of their single dominant feature. All other people could only be identified by their voices. In fact, the patient even had difficulty recognizing his own face in a mirror.

Simultanagnosia

- Sacks also describes a patient with simultanagnosia. When asked to view a *National Geographic* cover, the patient could only pick out isolated, small features: a bright color or shape; however, he was unable to integrate all pieces of the cover as a visual whole representing a specific scene, the Sahara dunes. Instead, the patient began compensating for his inability by inventing nonexistent images. He began describing a landscape of tiny guest houses with parasols lining the beach, all the while looking past the magazine cover into midair.

Adapted from Sacks O. *The Man Who Mistook His Wife for a Hat.* New York, NY: Harper Perennial; 1987.

Simultanagnosia

- Simultanagnosia involves difficulty interpreting a visual stimulus as a whole.
- Patients often confabulate to compensate for what they cannot interpret visually.[11]
- For example, when asked to look out a window and describe the view, a person may be able to visually interpret isolated objects in her visual field (such as a person walking by or flowers in a window box), but would be unable to integrate all visual data in order to understand that she was viewing a city street with moving cars, shops, and people.

Metamorphopsia

- Metamorphopsia involves a visual distortion of the physical properties of objects so that objects appear bigger, smaller, or heavier than they really are.[12]
- For example, a person with metamorphopsia may cut his food into tiny pieces because he perceives them as larger. He may open his mouth wide to receive each piece, perceiving that the food is larger on his fork.

Color Agnosia

- In color agnosia patients display an inability to attach appropriate colors to specific objects.
- In other words, they do not appear to know the color of common objects.[13]
- For example, a patient might think that bananas are blue.

Color Anomia

- Patients have lost the names for colors.[13,14]
- However, they would continue to recognize that a blue banana was strange.

Cerebral Achromatopsia

- Cerebral achromatopsia is a condition that occurs when V4 is lost and the world appears in shades of gray.
- The memory of color is erased.
- Color agnosia and color anomia differ from cerebral achromatopsia. In color agnosia, patients remember colors but can no longer associate color and objects correctly. Similarly, in color anomia, patients remember colors but can no longer remember the names for specific colors.[15]

VISUAL-SPATIAL PERCEPTUAL DYSFUNCTION

Right-Left Discrimination Dysfunction

- Involves difficulty understanding and using the concepts of right and left[16]
- Quick screen:
  - Ask the patient to point to left and right body parts.
  - Give the patient left/right directions around the halls of the treatment facility. Assess how well patients are able to use left/right commands as they negotiate changes in direction.

Figure-Ground Discrimination Dysfunction

- Involves difficulty distinguishing the foreground from the background[17]
- Quick screen:
  - Ask the patient to pick out forks from a drawer of disorganized utensils.
  - Using a plate of food, observe whether a patient can distinguish the potatoes from the background of the white dish.

Form-Constancy Dysfunction

- Involves difficulty attending to subtle variations in form or changes in form, such as a size variation of the same object. The ability to correctly observe that an object has constant physical attributes—when viewed from different distances, vantage points, or under different light sources—is impaired.[17]
- Quick screen:
  - Can the patient still identify an object when it is turned on its side or placed upside down?
  - Can a patient identify a group of shapes as triangles when they are placed at different distances from the viewer?
  - Can the patient identify the same object when it is placed under different light sources?

Position in Space Dysfunction

- Involves difficulty with concepts relating to positions such as up/down, in/out, behind/in front of, or before/after[17]
- Quick screen:
  - Give the patient directions using the terms listed previously.
  - Place the pencil on top of the box and place the box inside the drawer.
  - Take the pot from underneath the sink and place it on the counter. Put the rice inside the pot.

Topographical Disorientation

- Involves difficulty comprehending the relationship of one location to another[18]
- Quick screen:
  - Can the patient find his or her way around the hospital using written directions or a pictorial map?

Depth Perception Dysfunction (Stereopsis)

- Involves difficulty determining whether one object is closer to the patient than another object[19]
- Quick screen:
  - Can the patient determine whether objects in the natural environment are near or far in relation to each other and in relation to the patient?

BODY SCHEMA PERCEPTUAL DYSFUNCTION

- Body schema is the awareness of spatial characteristics of one's own body, an awareness formed by current and previous sensory input.
- It is the neural perception of one's body in space.
- This neural perception is derived from a synthesis of tactile, proprioceptive, and pressure sensory associations about the body and its parts.
- This perceptual disorder is also referred to as *somatagnosia*.
- Body schema perceptual dysfunction is more likely to occur as a result of right hemisphere lesions in the posterior multimodal association area.
- However, as with all of the perceptual disorders, body schema perceptual dysfunction can also result from left hemisphere lesions.[20]

Body Schema Differs From Body Image

- Body image is the emotional and cognitive assessment one holds about one's body.
- For example, patients with an amputated hand may have a body image of impairment; they may emotionally feel that their body is now damaged. Their body schema, however, may involve phantom pain in which they can feel their amputated hand. The pain of the phantom sensation may be experienced as cramping and burning.
- Patients with anosognosia (a severe neglect syndrome) often have positive thoughts about their body image, believing that all of their limbs are intact and functional, despite having a hemiplegic left side. Their body schema tells them that they have no left side. Because they are not processing the neural input from their left limbs, they have no awareness that the left side of their body exists and is hemiplegic.[20]

Finger Agnosia

- Finger agnosia involves an impaired perception concerning the relationship of the fingers to each other.
- It also involves an impaired identification and localization of one's own fingers.[21]
- Quick screen:
  - Ask the patient to tap his or her index finger or to touch his or her ring finger with the thumb.

Unilateral Neglect

- Involves the inability to integrate and use perceptions from the left side of the body or the left side of the environment.
- The awareness of the left side of the environment is lost temporarily.
- Patients more often have a left neglect rather than a right neglect, although right neglect syndromes occur as well.
- Right neglect syndromes tend to resolve more quickly than left neglect syndromes.
- A left neglect often results from a lesion to the right hemisphere's posterior multimodal association area.
- Patients with unilateral neglect can be trained to heighten their awareness of the left (or right) side of their bodies and environments.[22]
- Quick screen:
  - Ask the patient to (a) draw a clock and a human figure, (b) read a paragraph, or (c) perform a "cross-out the Hs" worksheet.
  - Observe the patient while eating a meal. Check whether the patient attends to both sides of the plate or ignores one half.

Anosognosia

- Anosognosia is extensive neglect and failure to recognize one's own body paralysis on one side.
- While patients with unilateral neglect can usually be taught to enhance their awareness of the left side of the body and environment, patients with anosognosia cannot be taught in the same way.
- Anosognosia is accompanied by a strange affective dissociation. Patients show extraordinary indifference to their affected limb.
- They have no concept that they have a paralyzed limb.
- Patients may ask the hospital staff to "take the arm away with the lunch tray."
- Anosognosia is usually a transient state of the acute cerebrovascular accident patient. Anosognosia will usually resolve as the patient recovers.
- Right hemisphere lesions cause more severe neglect syndromes than do left hemisphere lesions.
- Left neglect syndromes resolve less readily than right neglect.
- Patients who are several months post–neurologic damage are more likely to display left neglect. Right neglect syndromes more commonly clear by several months post neurologic insult.
- Sometimes patients with severe left neglect must live with their neglect syndrome for the remainder of their lives, particularly if the patient is elderly or the neurologic damage is severe.[23]

Double Simultaneous Extinction (Extinction of Simultaneous Stimulation)

- Double simultaneous extinction is categorized as a cortical somatosensory association disorder.
- However, it is also considered to be a form of attentional neglect.
- The therapist touches the patient on 2 body regions: first, on the involved limb, and second, on the uninvolved limb. The patient's eyes are closed.
- The patient is able to feel the tactile stimulus on both the involved and uninvolved limbs.
- Then, the therapist touches the patient on the same body regions simultaneously.

- Extinction occurs when the patient cannot feel the tactile sensation on the involved side (even though he or she could when the tactile sensation was only applied to the involved side).
- As the neurons mediating tactile sensation recover on the involved side, they can be overridden by tactile stimulation on the uninvolved side.
- This is called a *limited attention recovery phase*.
- As the neurologic damage resolves, the phenomenon of double simultaneous extinction disappears.[24]

LANGUAGE PERCEPTION DYSFUNCTION

Aphasia

- *Aphasia* means impairment in the expression and/or comprehension of language.
- There are 2 primary classifications of aphasia: receptive and expressive.[25]

Receptive Aphasia

- Receptive aphasia is impairment in the comprehension of language.
  - Wernicke aphasia involves difficulty comprehending the literal interpretation of language. Wernicke aphasia always results from a left hemisphere lesion in the brain region referred to as the *Wernicke area*.[26]
  - Alexia is the inability to comprehend the written word; also the inability to read. Alexia can occur as a result of lesions to either hemisphere; more often the left hemisphere is lesioned.[27]
  - Dyslexia is the impaired ability to read. It is a language problem in which the ability to break down words into their most basic units—phonemes—is impaired.[28]
  - Asymbolia is difficulty comprehending gestures and symbols. Usually the left hemisphere is lesioned.[29]
  - Aprosodia is impaired comprehension of tonal inflections used in conversation. Patients have difficulty perceiving the emotional tone of someone's conversation. Aprosodia usually results from a right hemisphere lesion.[30]

Receptive Aphasia in the Right vs Left Hemisphere

- Patients with receptive aphasia from a left hemisphere lesion can still perceive and accurately interpret the emotional tones of a conversation, even though they cannot understand the concrete meaning of the words.
- Patients with receptive aphasia from a right hemisphere lesion can understand the concrete meaning of the words but not the emotional tone of conversations.[30]

Expressive Aphasia

- Expressive aphasia involves difficulty expressing clear, meaningful language.
  - Broca aphasia is an expressive language disorder in which patients can understand what is spoken to them, but they cannot express their ideas in an understandable way. Often, they speak gibberish or sentences that do not make sense. Patients with Broca aphasia commonly display word finding difficulties in which they either (a) cannot complete sentences because they cannot retrieve the correct words, or (b) they mistakenly use the wrong word. Broca aphasia always results from a left hemisphere lesion in the brain region referred to as *Broca area*.[31]
  - Anomia is the inability to remember and express the names of people and objects. The individual may know the person but cannot remember his or her name. Anomia differs from prosopagnosia; in prosopagnosia, individuals do not recognize familiar faces. Lesions resulting in anomia can occur in either hemisphere.[32]
  - Agrammation is the inability to arrange words sequentially so that they form intelligible sentences. It occurs as a result of left hemisphere lesions.[33]
  - Agraphia is the inability to write intelligible words and sentences. It occurs as a result of left hemisphere lesions.[34]
  - Acalculia is the inability to calculate mathematical problems and results from an acquired neurological lesion. Dyscalculia is difficulty calculating math and results from a developmental disability. Lesions that result in acalculia occur in the left hemisphere.[35]
  - Alexithymia is the inability to express one's emotions through words. Dyslexithymia involves difficulty attaching words to feelings. These can occur as a result of either left or right hemisphere damage.[36]

Differences in Male and Female Language Processing

- Research has shown that women tend to use both hemispheres in the processing of language. They use the left hemisphere to interpret the concrete meaning of words and sentences and the right hemisphere to interpret the emotions attached to those words and sentences.
- Women are also more able to attach words to their emotions. This requires the ability to use the left hemisphere to attach words to emotions generated in the right hemisphere.
- Men predominantly use the left hemisphere to process language. Because they do not as readily integrate both hemispheres in language processing, they may have more difficulty attaching words to their emotions. This is referred to as *dyslexithymia*.[37]

PERCEPTUAL MOTOR DYSFUNCTION

- Perceptual motor dysfunction involves the *apraxias* or motor planning impairments.
- Apraxia can result from either right or left hemisphere lesions, but it usually results from right hemisphere lesions of the anterior multimodal cortex, the premotor area, and/or the primary motor cortex.
- Patients with apraxia have a distorted perception of the motor strategies required to negotiate their environment.[38]
- There are several classifications of apraxia:
  - Ideational apraxia
  - Ideomotor apraxia I and II
  - Dressing apraxia
  - Two- and 3-dimensional constructional apraxia

Ideational Apraxia

- Ideational apraxia involves an inability to cognitively understand the motor demands of the task.
- For example, a patient may not understand that a shirt is an article of clothing to be worn on the torso and upper extremities.[39]

Ideomotor Apraxia I

- Ideomotor apraxia involves the loss of the kinesthetic memory of motor patterns; essentially, the motor plan for a specific task is lost.
- In ideomotor apraxia I, the patient cannot access the appropriate motor plan. She can cognitively understand the motor demands of the task but cannot translate that understanding into appropriate motor movements. For example, a patient can understand that a shirt is an article of clothing to be worn on the torso and upper extremities, but she cannot access these motor plans.[40]

Ideomotor Apraxia II

- In ideomotor apraxia II, the patient cannot implement the appropriate motor plan. She understands the motor demands of the task, but when she attempts to implement the appropriate motor plan, an inappropriate one is activated. For example, when the patient is shown a toothbrush, she understands that this is a self care item used for cleaning teeth. When she attempts to activate the motor plan for teeth brushing, however, another motor plan becomes activated instead and she attempts to brush her hair with the toothbrush.[40]

Dressing Apraxia

- Dressing apraxia is a form of ideomotor apraxia involving an inability to dress oneself due to impairment in either (a) body schema perception or (b) perceptual motor functions.
- Example: Patients may attempt to put their arms through pant legs or dress only one-half of their body.[41]

Two- and Three-Dimensional Constructional Apraxia

- This type of apraxia involves an inability to copy 2- and 3-dimensional designs or models.
- A patient who is an architect may be unable to draw 2-dimensional blueprints.
- A patient who is a building contractor may be unable to put together a wooden birdhouse kit.
- Patients with constructional apraxia due to a right hemisphere lesion draw objects or put pieces of a kit together in a spatially disorganized way.
- Patients with constructional apraxia due to a left hemisphere lesion draw objects that lack detail. Three-dimensional objects are correctly spatially organized, but pieces are often left out.[42]

TACTILE PERCEPTUAL DYSFUNCTION

Tactile Agnosia

- *Tactile agnosia* is the umbrella term for the inability to attach meaning to somatosensory data.
- Tactile agnosia commonly results from lesions to the secondary somatosensory area (SS2).
- The anatomy for touch and pain/temperature receptors remains intact.
- The ability to attach meaning to somatosensory data is referred to as *cortical sensation* (as opposed to *primary sensation*).[43]

Cortical Sensation

- Cortical sensation includes the following forms of tactile agnosia:
  - Astereognosis is the inability to identify objects by touch alone. Astereognosis can be further broken down into ahylognosia and amorphognosia.[44]
    - Ahylognosia is the inability to discriminate between different types of materials by touch alone.[45]
    - Amorphognosia is the inability to discriminate between different forms/shapes by touch alone.[46]
  - Two-point discrimination is the loss of the ability to determine whether one has been touched by 1 or 2 points. An esthesiometer is the instrument used to assess 2-point discrimination.[47]
  - Agraphesthesia is the loss of the ability to interpret letters written on the contralateral hand.[48]
  - Double simultaneous extinction is the inability to determine that one has been touched on both the involved side and the uninvolved side; the neural sensation of the uninvolved side overrides the ability to perceive touch on the involved side.[24]
  - Abarognosis is the inability to accurately estimate the weight of objects, particularly in comparison to each other.[49]
  - Atopognosia is the inability to accurately perceive the exact location of a sensation.[49]

AUDITORY PERCEPTUAL DYSFUNCTION

Auditory Agnosia

- *Auditory agnosia* is the umbrella term for the inability to attach meaning to sound.
- This condition commonly occurs concomitantly with other communication disorders.
- The external anatomy responsible for hearing remains intact. Instead, lesions involve the posterior multimodal association area, particularly the association areas of the temporal lobe.
- Lesions to the left auditory association areas result in an inability to attach meaning to language. Language can be heard, but not interpreted.
- Lesions to the right auditory association areas produce an inability to attach meaning to non-language sounds. For example, a patient may be unable to interpret the sound of a train whistle.
- Sometimes patients cannot distinguish between sounds. For example, a patient with auditory agnosia may be unable to distinguish the sound of a train from the sound of thunder and wind.[50]

Other Perceptual Phenomena

Synesthesia

- Synesthesia is a perceptual phenomenon involving the ability to combine senses in response to specific stimuli.
- For example, some people have the ability to see colors when they hear music. These people report that specific musical notes are associated with specific colors. Such colors are always elicited whenever certain musical notes are heard.
- Others have the ability to see colors when reading the alphabet. These people report that specific letters are always associated with specific colors.[51]

Migraine-Induced Auras

- Fifteen percent of people who experience migraines also experience auras that precede migraine headaches.
- Auras are cortically generated perceptions or hallucinations; they occur as a precursor to migraine headaches.
- Auras can involve all types of sensory phenomena (eg, odors, colors, sounds, tastes) but most often occur in the form of visual symptoms, such as flashing lights, blotting out of vision, and sparkling, colored moving lines.
- Auras involve a sequence of neurologic events leading from cortical excitation of nerve cells to activation of pain-sensitive structures. While the actual aura is a cortically generated hallucination, the pain of the headache likely involves dysfunction in the nerves to major blood vessels in the head.
- Auras tend to develop gradually over 5 to 20 minutes and last for approximately 60 minutes. They often serve as a warning to patients that a migraine headache will occur shortly. The headache itself can last up to 72 hours.
- Many people with creative talents who experience migraine-induced auras report that the aura can be inspirational to their work. The author of *Alice in Wonderland*, Lewis Carroll, was reported to have experienced migraine-induced auras. Such auras purportedly served as inspiration for many of the unique phenomena written about in the book.[52]

REFERENCES

1. Kayser C, Logothetis NK. Do early sensory cortices integrate cross-modal information? *Brain Struct Funct.* 2007;212(2): 121-132. doi:10.1007/s00429-007-0154-0.

2. Eckert MA, Kamdar NV, Chang CE, Beckmann CF, Greicius MD, Menon V. A cross-modal system linking primary auditory and visual cortices: evidence from intrinsic fMRI connectivity analysis. *Hum Brain Mapp.* 2008;29(7):848-857. doi: 10.1002/hbm.20560.

3. Downar J, Crawley AP, Mikulis DJ, Davis KD. A multimodal cortical network for the detection of changes in the sensory environment. *Nat Neurosci.* 2000;3(3):277-283. doi:10.1038/72991.

4. Damasio AR. The brain binds entities and events by multiregional activation from convergence zones. *Neural Comput.* 1989;1(1):123-132. doi:10.1162/neco.1989.1.1.123.

5. Driver J, Noesselt T. Multisensory interplay reveals crossmodal influences on 'sensory-specific' brain regions, neural responses, and judgments. *Neuron.* 2008;57(1):11-23. doi:10.1016/j.neuron.2007.12.013.

6. Nolte J, Sundsten J. *The Human Brain: An Introduction to Its Functional Anatomy.* Vol. 5. St. Louis, MS: Mosby; 2002.

7. Schmahmann JD, Pandya DN, Wang R, et al. Association fibre pathways of the brain: parallel observations from diffusion spectrum imaging and autoradiography. *Brain.* 2007;130(3):630-653. doi.org/10.1093/brain/awl359.

8. Kucharska-Pietura K, Phillips ML, Gernand W, David AS. Perception of emotions from faces and voices following unilateral brain damage. *Neuropsychologia.* 2003;41(8):1082-1090. doi:10.1016/S0028-3932(02)00294-4.

9. Aviezer H, Hassin RR, Bentin S. Impaired integration of emotional faces and affective body context in a rare case of developmental visual agnosia. *Cortex.* 2012;48(6):689-700. doi:10.1016/j.cortex.2011.03.005.

10. Ramon M, Busigny T, Rossion B. Impaired holistic processing of unfamiliar individual faces in acquired prosopagnosia. *Neuropsychologia.* 2010;48(4):933-944. doi:10.1016/j.neuropsychologia.2009.11.014.

11. Chechlacz M, Rotshtein P, Hansen PC, Riddoch JM, Deb S, Humphreys GW. The neural underpinings of simultanagnosia: Disconnecting the visuospatial attention network. *J Cogn Neurosci.* 2012;24(3):718-735. doi:10.1162/jocn_a_00159.

12. Miwa H, Kondo T. Metamorphopsia restricted to the right side of the face associated with a right temporal lobe lesion. *J Neurol.* 2007;254(12):1765-1767. doi:10.1007/s00415-007-0671-z.

13. Cavina-Pratesi C, Kentridge RW, Heywood CA, Milner AD. Separate channels for processing form, texture, and color: Evidence from fMRI adaptation and visual object agnosia. *Cereb Cortex.* 2010;20(10):2319-2332. doi:10.1093/cercor/bhp298.

14. Roux FE, Lubrano V, Lauwers-Cances V, Mascott CR, Démonet JF. Category-specific cortical mapping: color-naming areas. *J Neurosurg.* 2006;104(1):27-37.

15. Celesia GG. Visual perception and awareness. *J Psychophysiol.* 2015;24(2):62-67. doi:10.1027/0269-8803/a000014.

16. Auer T, Schwarcz A, Aradi M, et al. Right–left discrimination is related to the right hemisphere. *Laterality.* 2008;13(5): 427-438. doi:10.1080/13576500802114120.

17. Tsai CL, Wilson PH, Wu SK. Role of visual–perceptual skills (non-motor) in children with developmental coordination disorder. *Hum Mov Sci.* 2008;27(4):649-664. doi:10.1016/j.humov.2007.10.002.

18. Iaria G, Bogod N, Fox CJ, Barton JJ. Developmental topographical disorientation: case one. *Neuropsychologia.* 2009;47(1):30-40. doi:10.1016/j.neuropsychologia.2008.08.021.

19. Parker AJ. Binocular depth perception and the cerebral cortex. *Nat Rev Neurosci.* 2007;8(5):379-391. doi:10.1038/nrn2131.

20. De Vignemont F. Body schema and body image—pros and cons. *Neuropsychologia.* 2010;48(3):669-680. doi:10.1016/j.neuropsychologia.2009.09.022.

21. Ardila A, Concha M, Rosselli M. Angular gyrus syndrome revisited: acalculia, finger agnosia, right-left disorientation and semantic aphasia. *Aphasiology.* 2000;14(7):743-754. doi:10.1080/026870300410964.

22. Danckert J, Ferber S. Revisiting unilateral neglect. *Neuropsychologia.* 2006;44(6):987-1006. doi:10.1016/j.neuropsychologia.2005.09.004.

23. Orfei MD, Robinson RG, Prigatano GP, et al. Anosognosia for hemiplegia after stroke is a multifaceted phenomenon: a systematic review of the literature. *Brain.* 2007;130(12):3075-3090. doi:10.1093/brain/awm106.

24. Baylis GC, Simon SL, Baylis LL, Rorden C. Visual extinction with double simultaneous stimulation: what is simultaneous?. *Neuropsychologia.* 2002;40(7):1027-1034. doi:10.1016/S0028-3932(01)00144-0.

25. Gorno-Tempini ML, Hillis AE, Weintraub S, et al. Classification of primary progressive aphasia and its variants. *Neurology.* 2011;76(11):1006-1014. doi:10. 1212/ WNL. 0b013e31821103e6.

26. Kurland J, Baldwin K, Tauer C. Treatment-induced neuroplasticity following intensive naming therapy in a case of chronic Wernicke's aphasia. *Aphasiology.* 2010;24(6-8):737-751. doi:10.1080/02687030903524711.

27. Kleinschmidt A, Cohen L. The neural bases of prosopagnosia and pure alexia: recent insights from functional neuroimaging. *Curr Opin Neurol.* 2006;19(4):386-391. doi:10.1097/01.wco.0000236619.89710.ee.

28. Vidyasagar TR, Pammer K. Dyslexia: a deficit in visuo-spatial attention, not in phonological processing. *Trends Cogn Sci.* 2010;14(2):57-63. doi:10.1016/j.tics.2009.12.003.

29. Goldenberg G, Hartmann K, Schlott I. Defective pantomime of object use in left brain damage: apraxia or asymbolia? *Neuropsychologia.* 2003;41(12):1565-1573. doi:10.1016/S0028-3932(03)00120-9.

30. Leon SA, Rodriguez AD. Aprosodia and its treatment. *Perspect Neurophysiol Neurogenic Speech Lang Disord.* 2008;18(2): 66-72. doi:10.1044/nnsld18.2.66.

31. Boo M, Rose ML. The efficacy of repetition, semantic, and gesture treatments for verb retrieval and use in Broca's aphasia. *Aphasiology.* 2011;25(2):154-175. doi:10.1080/02687031003743789.

32. Fridriksson J. Preservation and modulation of specific left hemisphere regions is vital for treated recovery from anomia in stroke. *J Neurosci.* 2010;30(35):11558-11564. doi: 10.1523/JNEUROSCI.2227-10.2010.

33. Kim M, Thompson CK. Patterns of comprehension and production of nouns and verbs in agrammatism: implications for lexical organization. *Brain Lang.* 2000;74(1):1-25. doi:10.1006/brln.2000.2315.

34. Sheldon CA, Malcolm GL, Barton JJ. Alexia with and without agraphia: an assessment of two classical syndromes. *Can J Neurol Sci.* 2008;35(05):616-624. doi:10.1017/S0317167100009410.

35. Ashkenazi S, Henik A, Ifergane G, Shelef I. Basic numerical processing in left intraparietal sulcus (IPS) acalculia. *Cortex.* 2008;44(4):439-448. doi:10.1016/j.cortex.2007.08.008.

36. Berthoz S, Artiges E, Van de Moortele PF, et al. Effect of impaired recognition and expression of emotions on frontocingulate cortices: an fMRI study of men with alexithymia. *Am J Psychiatry.* 2002;159(6):961-967. doi.org/10.1176/appi.ajp.159.6.961.

37. Ingalhalikar M, Smith A, Parker D, et al. Sex differences in the structural connectome of the human brain. *Proc Natl Acad Sci.* 2014;111(2):823-828. doi: 10.1073/pnas.1316909110.

38. Goldenberg G. Apraxia: The cognitive side of motor control. *Cortex.* 2014;57:270-274. doi:10.1016/j.cortex.2013.07.016.

39. Chainay H, Humphreys GW. Ideomotor and ideational apraxia in corticobasal degeneration: a case study. *Neurocase.* 2003;9(2):177-186. doi:10.1076/neur.9.2.177.15073.

40. Sunderland A, Shinner C. Ideomotor apraxia and functional ability. *Cortex.* 2007;43(3):359-367. doi:10.1016/S0010-9452(08)70461-1.

41. Fitzgerald LK, McKelvey JR, Szeligo F. Mechanisms of dressing apraxia: a case study. *Cogn Behav Neurol.* 2002;15(2):148-155.

42. Laeng B. Constructional apraxia after left or right unilateral stroke. *Neuropsychologia.* 2006;44(9):1595-1606. doi:10.1016/j.neuropsychologia.2006.01.023.

43. Hömke L, Amunts K, Bönig L, et al. Analysis of lesions in patients with unilateral tactile agnosia using cytoarchitectonic probabilistic maps. *Hum Brain Mapp.* 2009;30(5):1444-1456. doi:10.1002/hbm.20617.

44. Mulcahey MJ, Kozin S, Merenda L, et al. Evaluation of the box and blocks test, stereognosis and item banks of activity and upper extremity function in youths with brachial plexus birth palsy. *J Pediatr Orthop.* 2012;32:S114-S122. doi:10.1097/BPO.0b013e3182595423.

45. Carello C, Kinsella-Shaw J, Amazeen EL, Turvey MT. Peripheral neuropathy and object length perception by effortful (dynamic) touch: A case study. *Neurosci Lett.* 2006;405(3):159-163. doi:10.1016/j.neulet.2006.06.047.

46. Kubota S, Yamada M, Satoh H, Tsujihata M. A pure form of amorphognosia: a case report. *J Neurol Sci.* 2013;333:e181-e182. doi:10.1016/j.jns.2013.07.741.

47. van Nes SI, Faber CG, Hamers RM, et al; PeriNomS Study Group. Revising two-point discrimination assessment in normal aging and in patients with polyneuropathies. *J Neurol Neurosurg Psychiatry.* 2008;79(7):832-834. doi:10.1136/jnnp.2007.139220.

48. Drago V, Foster PS, Edward D, Wargovich B, Heilman KM. Graphesthesia: a test of graphemic movement representations or tactile imagery?. *J Int Neuropsychol Soc.* 2010;16(01):190-193. doi.org/10.1017/S1355617709990762.

49. Hsu HY, Kuo LC, Jou IM, Chen SM, Chiu HY, Su FC. Establishment of a proper manual tactile test for hands with sensory deficits. *Arch Phys Med Rehabil.* 2013;94(3):451-458. doi:10.1016/j.apmr.2012.07.024.

50. Saygin AP, Leech R, Dick F. Nonverbal auditory agnosia with lesion to Wernicke's area. *Neuropsychologia.* 2010;48(1):107-113. doi:10.1016/j.neuropsychologia.2009.08.015.

51. Brang D, Hubbard EM, Coulson S, Huang M, Ramachandran VS. Magnetoencephalography reveals early activation of V4 in grapheme-color synesthesia. *Neuroimage.* 2010;53(1):268-274. doi:10.1016/j.neuroimage.2010.06.008.

52. Dalkara T, Nozari A, Moskowitz MA. Migraine aura pathophysiology: the role of blood vessels and microembolisation. *Lancet Neurol.* 2010;9(3):309-317. doi:10.1016/S1474-4422(09)70358-8.

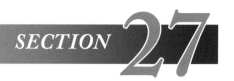
Blood Supply of the Brain
Cerebrovascular Disorders

MAJOR ARTERIES

Internal Carotids (2)

Route

- The internal carotids rise from the common carotid artery and enter the brain at the level of the optic chiasm.

Supply

- These are the major arteries that supply the brain.[1]

Vertebral Arteries (2)

Route

- The vertebral arteries run along the lateral aspect of the medulla.
- They connect to form the basilar artery at the base of the pons-medulla junction.
- They give rise to the anterior spinal artery.

Supply

- These arteries supply the lateral medulla areas.[2]

Anterior Spinal Artery (1)

Route

- The anterior spinal arteries begin as 2 small branches that become 1 main artery.
- The 2 anterior spinal branches rise off of the vertebral arteries and become 1 main artery that travels along the anterior surface of the medulla and spinal cord.

Supply

- The spinal artery supplies the anterior portion of the medulla and spinal cord.[3]

THREE ARTERIES THAT SUPPLY THE CEREBELLUM

Posterior Inferior Cerebellar Arteries (2)

Route

- The posterior inferior cerebellar arteries rise from the vertebral arteries at the medulla level.

Supply

- They supply part of the dorsolateral medulla (including the cerebellar peduncles), the inferior surface of the cerebellum, and the deep cerebellar nuclei.[4]

Gutman SA. *Quick Reference Neuroscience for Rehabilitation Professionals:*
The Essential Neurologic Principles Underlying Rehabilitation Practice,
Third Edition (pp 316-328).
© 2017 Taylor & Francis Group.

Anterior Inferior Cerebellar Arteries (2)

Route

- The anterior inferior cerebellar arteries rise from the vertebral arteries at the pons-medulla junction.

Supply

- They supply the inferior surface of the cerebellum and the deep cerebellar nuclei.[5]

Superior Cerebellar Arteries (2)

Route

- The superior cerebellar arteries rise from the basilar artery at the pons-midbrain junction.

Supply

- They supply the superior aspect of the cerebellum and parts of the deep cerebellar nuclei.[6]

Basilar Artery (1)

- The basilar artery does not supply the cerebellum. But it does give rise to the superior cerebellar arteries.

Route

- Travels along the anterior aspect of the pons.
- Gives rise to the superior cerebellar arteries.

Supply

- Supplies the anterior and lateral aspects of the pons.[7]

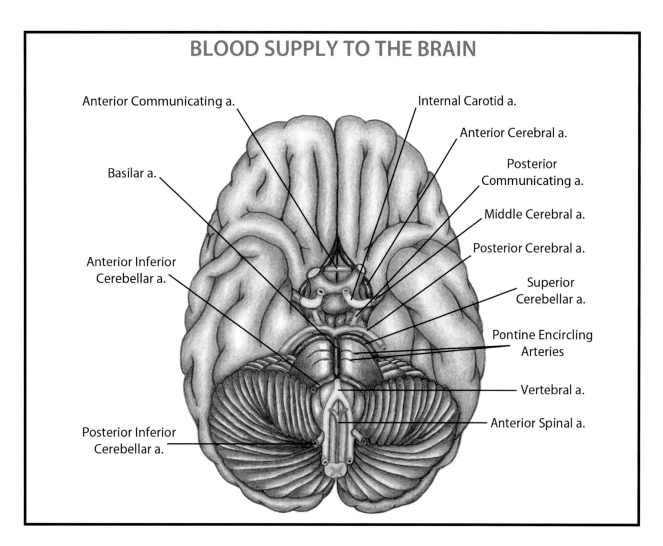

BLOOD SUPPLY TO THE BRAIN

Anterior Communicating a.
Internal Carotid a.
Anterior Cerebral a.
Posterior Communicating a.
Basilar a.
Middle Cerebral a.
Posterior Cerebral a.
Anterior Inferior Cerebellar a.
Superior Cerebellar a.
Pontine Encircling Arteries
Vertebral a.
Anterior Spinal a.
Posterior Inferior Cerebellar a.

Three Main Cerebral Arteries

Posterior Cerebral Arteries (2)

Route

- The posterior cerebral arteries rise from the basilar artery.

Supply

- They supply the medial and inferior surfaces of the temporal and occipital lobes, the thalamus, and the hypothalamus.[8]

Middle Cerebral Arteries (2)

Route

- The middle cerebral arteries rise from the internal carotids and travel through the lateral fissure to the brain's surface.

Supply

- These arteries supply the lateral surfaces of the frontal, temporal, and parietal lobes.
- They also supply the inferior surface of part of the frontal and temporal lobes.[9]

Anterior Cerebral Arteries (2)

Route

- The anterior cerebral arteries rise from the internal carotids.

Supply

- These arteries supply the superior, lateral, and medial aspects of the frontal and parietal lobes.
- They also supply part of the basal ganglia and the corpus callosum.[10]

Communicating Arteries and Multiple Encircling Arteries

- The communicating arteries provide blood supply pathways to the major cerebral arteries.
- The multiple pontine encircling arteries provide a blood supply pathway to the pons.

Posterior Communicating Arteries (2)

Route

- The posterior communicating arteries connect the internal carotids and the posterior cerebral arteries.

Supply

- They supply the diencephalon, internal capsule, and optic chiasm.[11]

Anterior Communicating Artery (1)

- The anterior communicating artery connects the 2 anterior cerebral arteries.[12]

Pontine Encircling Arteries (Multiple)

Route

- These arteries rise from the basilar artery and wrap around the pons.

Supply

- They supply the lateral and posterior portions of the pons.[13]

Circle of Willis

- The circle of Willis is a circuit of interconnecting arteries that function to prevent lack of blood flow to the brain due to occlusion.
- Components of the circle of Willis include the following[14]:
  - Posterior cerebral arteries
  - Posterior communicating arteries
  - Internal carotid arteries
  - Anterior cerebral arteries
  - Anterior communicating artery

CIRCLE OF WILLIS

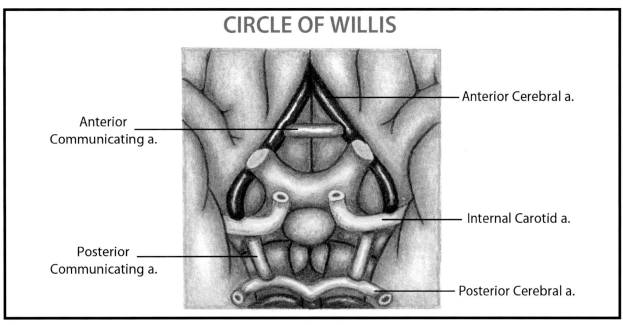

Anterior Communicating a.

Anterior Cerebral a.

Internal Carotid a.

Posterior Communicating a.

Posterior Cerebral a.

BLOOD SUPPLY OF SPECIFIC BRAIN REGIONS

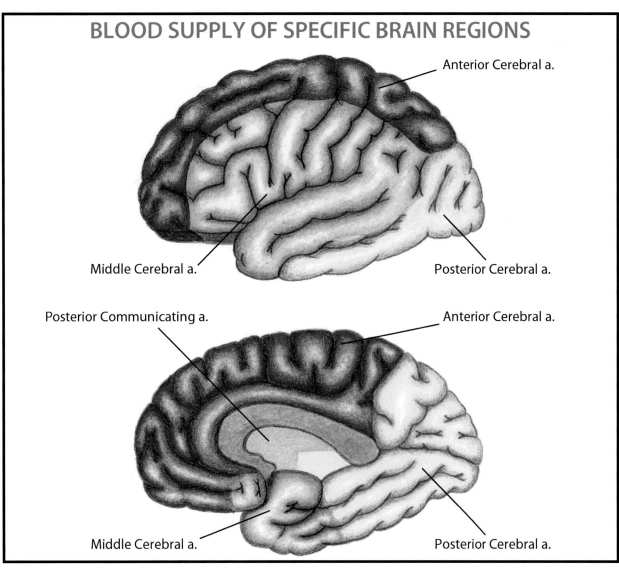

Anterior Cerebral a.

Middle Cerebral a.

Posterior Cerebral a.

Posterior Communicating a.

Anterior Cerebral a.

Middle Cerebral a.

Posterior Cerebral a.

COMMON AREAS OF ARTERIAL OCCLUSION IN THE CORTEX

Middle Cerebral Arterial Occlusion

- The middle cerebral arteries are the most common site of occlusion resulting in cerebrovascular accident (CVA).
- The middle cerebral arteries supply the lateral surfaces of the frontal, temporal, and parietal lobes, and the inferior surface of portions of the frontal and temporal lobes.[9]

Middle Cerebral Arterial Occlusion in the Left Hemisphere

- An occlusion in the middle cerebral artery in the left hemisphere may result in the following:
  - *Contralateral hemiplegia* (on the right side of the body): the primary motor area is lesioned.
  - *Contralateral hemiparesthesia* (on the right side of the body): the primary somatosensory area is lesioned.
  - *Aphasia*: Broca or Wernicke area may be lesioned. Other language areas may also be damaged, resulting in different types of aphasia.
  - *Cognitive involvement*: impairment in cognitive function results from a frontal lobe lesion.
  - *Affective involvement*: often when the left hemisphere is lesioned, the patient may display emotional lability and depression. This is sometimes referred to as a *catastrophic response*.[15]

Middle Cerebral Arterial Occlusion in the Right Hemisphere

- An occlusion in the middle cerebral artery in the right hemisphere may result in the following:
  - *Contralateral hemiplegia* (on the left side of the body): the primary motor area is lesioned.
  - *Contralateral hemiparesthesia* (on the left side of the body): the primary somatosensory area is lesioned.
  - *Perceptual deficits*: left neglect syndromes are common with damage to the right hemisphere, particularly to the posterior multimodal association area.
  - *Apraxia*: the anterior multimodal association area, premotor area, and/or primary motor cortex may be lesioned.
  - *Cognitive involvement*: impairment in cognitive function results from a frontal lobe lesion.
  - *Affective involvement*: often when the right hemisphere is lesioned, the patient may display euphoria or report a sense of well-being. If a neglect syndrome is present, the patient is often unaware of his or her deficits.[15]

Posterior Cerebral Arterial Occlusion

- The posterior cerebral arteries supply the medial and inferior surfaces of the temporal and occipital lobes.
- These arteries also help to supply the thalamus and the hypothalamus; however, a lesion to a posterior cerebral artery will likely not affect the thalamic and hypothalamic functions.
- A lesion to one of the posterior cerebral arteries may result in the following:
  - Memory loss due to temporal lobe involvement
  - Visual perceptual deficits result from damage of the occipital lobe and the posterior multimodal association area.
  - Visual field cuts result from occlusion to the optic chiasm. The optic chiasm is supplied by the posterior communicating arteries, which connect to the posterior cerebral arteries.[8,16]

Anterior Cerebral Arterial Occlusion

- The anterior cerebral arteries supply the superior, lateral, and medial aspects of the frontal and parietal lobes.
- These arteries also help to supply portions of the basal ganglia and corpus callosum.
- A lesion to one of the anterior cerebral arteries may result in the following:
  - *Contralateral hemiplegia*: often of the lower extremities; the primary motor area is lesioned.
  - *Contralateral hemiparesthesia*: often of the lower extremities; the primary somatosensory area is lesioned.
  - *Cognitive involvement*: due to frontal lobe involvement
  - *Apraxia*: the anterior multimodal association area, premotor area, and/or primary motor area may be lesioned.
  - *Affective involvement*: if the left hemisphere is lesioned, emotional lability and depression may occur. If the right hemisphere is lesioned, euphoria or emotional dissociation may occur.[10,17]

CEREBELLAR ARTERIAL OCCLUSION

- The 3 major symptoms of cerebellar disorders include the following:
  1. Incoordination
  2. Ataxia
  3. Intention tremors

Posterior Inferior Cerebellar Arterial Occlusion

- The posterior inferior cerebellar arteries supply the cerebellar peduncles.
- Cerebellar arterial occlusion often involves the brainstem structures that are supplied by the cerebellar arteries.[4]
  - *Ipsilateral hypertonicity and hyperactive reflexes*: because the posterior and anterior spinocerebellar tracts travel through the superior cerebellar peduncle, damage to the superior cerebellar peduncles may result in ipsilateral hypertonicity and hyperactive reflexes.
  - *Vertigo, nausea, nystagmus, diplopia*: because the posterior inferior cerebellar arteries also supply blood to the medulla, an occlusion to this artery may also result in vertigo, nausea, nystagmus, and diplopia as a result of vestibular nerve nuclei loss.
  - Ipsilateral loss of pain and temperature on the face (due to loss of the spinothalamic tract).
  - Contralateral loss of pain and temperature on the trunk and extremities (due to loss of the spinothalamic tract).
  - Dysphagia and dysarthria due to involvement of the nucleus ambiguous.
  - Ipsilateral Horner syndrome (miosis, ptosis) due to vestibular nuclei involvement.

Anterior Inferior Cerebellar and Superior Cerebellar Arterial Occlusion

- Occlusion to either of these 2 arteries may result in the following[5,6]:
  - Ipsilateral ataxia
  - Ipsilateral hypotonicity and hyporeflexia
  - Dysmetria
  - Adiadochokinesia (and dysdiadochokinesia)
  - Movement decomposition
  - Asthenia
  - Rebound phenomenon
  - Staccato voice
  - Ataxic gait
  - Intention tremors
  - Incoordination
  - Nystagmus
- Occlusion to these arteries may also result in the following, due to the arteries' connection to the blood supply of the medulla:
  - Vestibular signs (nystagmus, vertigo, nausea)
  - Ipsilateral loss of pain and temperature on the face (due to loss of the spinothalamic tract)
  - Contralateral loss of pain and temperature on the trunk and extremities (due to loss of the spinothalamic tract)
  - Dysphagia
  - Dysarthria
  - Bell palsy

OCCLUSION OF ARTERIES THAT SUPPLY THE BRAINSTEM

Anterior Spinal Artery Occlusion

- The anterior spinal arteries supply the anterior spinal cord and medulla.[3]
  - Bilateral motor function loss at and below the lesion level if bilateral corticospinal tract involvement occurs.
  - Bilateral loss of pain and temperature at and below the lesion level if bilateral spinothalamic tract involvement occurs.

Vertebral Arterial Occlusion
- The vertebral arteries supply the lateral aspect of the low medulla, including the accessory nuclei.[18]
- Dysphagia may occur if the *accessory nerve* nuclei are lost.

Basilar Arterial Occlusion
- The basilar artery supplies the pons, including the corticospinal tracts and the abducens, trigeminal, and facial nerve nuclei.[7,19]
  - Contralateral hemiplegia can occur if the opposite corticospinal tract is lost.
  - Contralateral sensory loss of the body can occur if the opposite dorsal column tract is lost.
  - Ipsilateral sensory loss of the face can occur if the same side trigeminal nerve nuclei are lost.
  - Medial or internal strabismus can occur if the abducens nerve nuclei are lost.
  - Ipsilateral loss of the masseter reflex and the corneal reflex can also occur if the same side trigeminal nerve nuclei are lost.
  - Bell palsy and hyperacusis can occur if the facial nerve nuclei are lost.
  - Deviation of the tongue to the affected side results if the hypoglossal nerve nuclei are involved.
  - Nystagmus and balance disturbances can result if the vestibular nuclei are involved.

Cerebrovascular Accident

- *CVA*, or *stroke*, is an umbrella term applied to conditions in which blood flow to cerebral vessels becomes disrupted, either from clotting or rupture.
- There are 2 primary types of CVA: ischemic and hemorrhagic.
- Ischemic strokes are the most common type of CVA and result from thrombosis (static clot) or emboli (traveling clot).[20]
- Hemorrhagic strokes involve bleeding into brain tissue and can result from hypertension, aneurysms, or head injury. Hemorrhagic strokes are the most fatal type.[21]
- Risk factors include the following:
  - Age
  - Sex (men have a 19% greater risk of stroke than women)
  - Race (Blacks have a 60% greater risk than the general population)
  - Hypertension
  - High cholesterol levels
  - Cigarette smoking
  - Diabetes mellitus
  - Prior stroke
  - Obesity
  - Heart disease

Thrombotic Strokes
- Thrombi are clots formed by plaque development in a vessel wall.
- These are the most common type of ischemic strokes and occur in atherosclerotic blood vessels.
- Common sites of plaque formation include larger vessels of the brain, including the origin of the internal carotid arteries, the vertebral arteries, and the junction of the basilar and vertebral arteries.
- Thrombotic strokes usually occur gradually over several days.
- They are frequently seen in older persons with arteriosclerotic heart disease.
- This type of stroke is not associated with exertion or activity and can occur when the person is at rest.[22]

(continued)

Cerebrovascular Accident

(continued)

Lacunar Infarcts

- Lacunar infarcts are small clots located in the deep regions of the brainstem and subcortical structures.
- They are often found in single deeply penetrating arteries that supply the internal capsule, basal ganglia, and brainstem.
- They commonly result from occlusion of the smaller branches of the large cerebral arteries, most notably the middle and posterior cerebral arteries. Sometimes lacunar infarcts can also occur in the anterior cerebral, vertebral, and basilar arteries.
- Because they are small, lacunar infarcts usually do not cause severe impairment.[23]

Embolic Strokes

- Emboli are clots that dislodge from their site of origin and travel to a cerebral blood vessel, where they become trapped and interrupt blood flow.
- Embolic strokes often affect the smaller cerebral vessels. The most frequent site is the middle cerebral artery.
- This type of stroke commonly has a sudden onset and is associated with the presence of cardiac disease (eg, rheumatic heart disease, ventricular aneurysm, and bacterial endocarditis). Cardiac embolism can also occur after a recent myocardial infarction.[24]

Hemorrhagic Stroke

- Hemorrhagic strokes are frequently fatal.
- However, if patients can survive the initial hemorrhagic damage, prognosis is generally good.
- Hemorrhagic strokes involve bleeding into brain tissue after the rupture of a blood vessel wall.
- This type of stroke results in edema and compression of brain tissue that, if not medically treated immediately, can be fatal.
- Hemorrhagic strokes commonly occur suddenly and are associated with exertion and activity.[21]
- Aneurysmal subarachnoid hemorrhage
  - An aneurysm is a bulge occurring in a blood vessel wall as a result of clot formation.
  - Most aneurysms are small saccular structures called *berry aneurysms*.
  - Berry aneurysms commonly occur in the circle of Willis or the junction of 2 vessels.
  - Aneurysms tend to enlarge with time and weaken vessel walls until rupture occurs.[25]

Transient Ischemic Attack

- Transient ischemic attacks (TIAs) are sometimes referred to as *mini strokes*.
- They are characterized by focal ischemic cerebral incidents that last less than 24 hours; most TIAs usually last less than 1 to 2 hours.
- The causes of TIAs include atherosclerotic disease and emboli.
- TIAs may provide a warning of an impending larger stroke.
- Signs include the following[26]:
  - Numbness and mild weakness on one side of the body
  - Transient visual disturbances (eg, blurred vision, fading vision)
  - Dizziness
  - Falls
  - Confusion and possible blackout

References

1. Silvestrini M, Cagnetti C, Pasqualetti P, et al. Carotid wall thickness and stroke risk in patients with asymptomatic internal carotid stenosis. *Atherosclerosis.* 2010;210(2):452-457. doi:10.1016/j.atherosclerosis.2009.12.033.

2. Sato K, Ogoh S, Hirasawa A, Oue A, Sadamoto T. The distribution of blood flow in the carotid and vertebral arteries during dynamic exercise in humans. *J Physiol.* 2011;589(11):2847-2856. doi:10.1113/jphysiol.2010.204461.

3. Tsai YD, Liliang PC, Chen HJ, Lu K, Liang CL, Wang KW. Anterior spinal artery syndrome following vertebroplasty: a case report. *Spine.* 2010;35(4):E134-E136. doi: 10.1097/BRS.0b013e3181b52221.

4. Peluso JP, Van Rooij WJ, Sluzewski M, Beute GN, Majoie CB. Posterior inferior cerebellar artery aneurysms: incidence, clinical presentation, and outcome of endovascular treatment. *Am J Neuroradiol.* 2008;29(1):86-90. doi: 10.3174/ajnr. A0758.

5. Lee H, Sohn SI, Cho YW, et al. Cerebellar infarction presenting isolated vertigo frequency and vascular topographical patterns. *Neurology.* 2006;67(7):1178-1183. doi:10. 1212/ 01. wnl. 0000238500. 02302. b4.

6. Kumral E, Kısabay A, Ataç C. Lesion patterns and etiology of ischemia in superior cerebellar artery territory infarcts. *Cerebrovasc Dis.* 2005;19(5):283-290. doi:10.1159/000084496.

7. Schonewille WJ, Wijman CA, Michel P, et al; BASICS Study Group. Treatment and outcomes of acute basilar artery occlusion in the Basilar Artery International Cooperation Study (BASICS): a prospective registry study. *Lancet Neurol.* 2009;8(8):724-730. doi:10.1016/S1474-4422(09)70173-5.

8. Hendrikse J, van der Grond J, Lu H, van Zijl PC, Golay, X. Flow territory mapping of the cerebral arteries with regional perfusion MRI. *Stroke.* 2004;35(4):882-887. doi:10.1161/01.STR.0000120312.26163.EC.

9. Arnold M, Schroth G, Nedeltchev K, et al. Intra-arterial thrombolysis in 100 patients with acute stroke due to middle cerebral artery occlusion. *Stroke.* 2002;33(7):1828-1833. doi:10.1161/01.STR.0000020713.89227.B7.

10. Kang SY, Kim JS. Anterior cerebral artery infarction stroke mechanism and clinical-imaging study in 100 patients. *Neurology.* 2008;70(24 Part 2):2386-2393. doi:10. 1212/ 01. wnl. 0000314686. 94007.d0.

11. Golshani K, Ferrell A, Zomorodi A, Smith TP, Britz GW. A review of the management of posterior communicating artery aneurysms in the modern era. *Surg Neurol Int.* 2010;1:88. doi:10.4103/2152-7806.74147.

12. Castro MA, Putman CM, Sheridan MJ, Cebral JR. Hemodynamic patterns of anterior communicating artery aneurysms: a possible association with rupture. *Am J Neuroradiol.* 2009;30(2):297-302. doi:10.3174/ajnr.A1323.

13. Kumral E, Bayülkem G, Evyapan D. Clinical spectrum of pontine infarction. *J Neurol.* 2002;24(12):1659-1670. doi:10.1007/ s00415-002-0879-x.

14. Hendrikse J, van Raamt AF, van der Graaf Y, Mali WP, van der Grond J. Distribution of cerebral blood flow in the circle of Willis. *Radiology.* 2005;235(1):184-189. doi:10.1148/radiol.2351031799.

15. Walz B, Zimmermann C, Böttger S, Haberl RL. Prognosis of patients after hemicraniectomy in malignant middle cerebral artery infarction. *J Neurol.* 2002;249(9):1183-1190. doi:10.1007/s00415-002-0798-x.

16. Hallacq P, Piotin M, Moret J. Endovascular occlusion of the posterior cerebral artery for the treatment of p2 segment aneurysms: retrospective review of a 10-year series. *Am J Neuroradiol.* 2002;23(7):1128-1136.

17. Kumral E, Bayulkem G, Evyapan D, Yunten N. Spectrum of anterior cerebral artery territory infarction: clinical and MRI findings. *Eur J Neurol.* 2002;9(6):615-624. doi: 10.1046/j.1468-1331.2002.00452.x.

18. Cloud GC, Markus HS. Diagnosis and management of vertebral artery stenosis. *Q J Med.* 2003;96(1):27-54. doi:10.1093/ qjmed/hcg003.

19. Mattle HP, Arnold M, Lindsberg PJ, Schonewille WJ, Schroth G. Basilar artery occlusion. *Lancet Neurol.* 2011;10(11): 1002-1014. doi:10.1016/S1474-4422(11)70229-0.

20. Jauch EC, Saver JL, Adams HP, et al. Guidelines for the early management of patients with acute ischemic stroke a guideline for healthcare professionals from the American Heart Association/American Stroke Association. *Stroke.* 2013;44(3): 870-947. doi: 10.1161/STR.0b013e318284056a.

21. González-Pérez A, Gaist D, Wallander MA, McFeat G, García-Rodríguez LA. Mortality after hemorrhagic stroke. Data from general practice (The Health Improvement Network). *Neurology.* 2013;81(6):559-565. doi:10. 1212/ WNL. 0b013e31829e6eff.

22. Stam J. Thrombosis of the cerebral veins and sinuses. *N Engl J Med.* 2005;352(17):1791-1798. doi:10.1056/NEJMra042354.

23. Chen X, Wen W, Anstey KJ, Sachdev PS. Prevalence, incidence, and risk factors of lacunar infarcts in a community sample. *Neurology.* 2009;73(4):266-272. doi:10. 1212/ WNL. 0b013e3181aa52ea.

24. Goldhaber SZ, Bounameaux H. Pulmonary embolism and deep vein thrombosis. *Lancet*. 2012;379(9828):1835-1846. doi:10.1016/S0140-6736(11)61904-1.

25. Connolly ES, Rabinstein AA, Carhuapoma JR, et al. Guidelines for the management of aneurysmal subarachnoid hemorrhage a guideline for healthcare professionals from the American Heart Association/American Stroke Association. *Stroke*. 2012;43(6):1711-1737. doi:10.1161/STR.0b013e3182587839.

26. Furie KL, Kasner SE, Adams RJ, et al. Guidelines for the prevention of stroke in patients with stroke or transient ischemic attack a guideline for healthcare professionals from the American Heart Association/American Stroke Association. *Stroke*. 2011;42(1):227-276. doi10.1161/STR.0b013e3181f7d043.

CLINICAL TEST QUESTIONS

Sections 26 to 27

1. Mrs. Elliot has had a benign brain tumor removed from area V4 of the occipital lobe. After recovery from surgery, she reports that she sees the world in shades of gray and cannot remember what objects looked like in color. She believes that she always saw objects as gray and does not recognize any change in her visual perception. Ophthalmological tests confirm that all visual anatomical structures are intact (all rods and cones are functional). Seeing everything as shades of gray as a result of cortical loss of area V4 is called:
   a. color anomia
   b. achromatopsia
   c. metamorphopsia
   d. simultanagnosia

2. After Mr. Li's stroke, his therapist has observed visual-spatial problems. The therapist gives a pencil, eraser, and small box to Mr. Li and asks him to follow her directions: "Put the box on top of the table. Place the eraser inside of the box. Place the pencil next to the box." Mr. Li has difficulty following these directions. This visual-spatial problem is known as:
   a. figure-ground discrimination disorder
   b. topographical disorientation
   c. position in space dysfunction
   d. right-left discrimination disorder

3. Andrew, who sustained a traumatic brain injury 5 years ago, now lives in a supervised apartment in the community, which he shares with a roommate. Although Andrew only lives 1 mile from the bank, he continuously gets lost each time he attempts to walk to the bank from his house. This visual-spatial disorder is called:
   a. position in space dysfunction
   b. right-left discrimination disorder
   c. figure-ground discrimination disorder
   d. topographical disorientation

4. Mr. Tarantino had a right hemisphere stroke and as a result has hemiplegia and hemiparesthesia in both left upper and lower extremities. Despite this severe impairment, Mr. Tarantino is cheerful and has no awareness of his deficits. This morning, he asked his nurse to remove the leg that was in his bed all night. This severe neglect syndrome is called:
   a. anosognosia
   b. unilateral neglect
   c. body image dysphoria
   d. aggramation

5. Along with Wernicke aphasia, Ms. Walsh has difficulty understanding gestures and symbols commonly used in social communication. This form of receptive aphasia is called:
   a. aprosodia
   b. dyslexia
   c. asymbolia
   d. dyslexithymia

6. When given a toothbrush, Mr. Samuelson verbally indicates that a toothbrush is used to clean teeth; but when he attempts to use it, he instead brushes his hair with it. This motor planning problem is called:
   a. ideational apraxia
   b. ideomotor apraxia

7. When Samantha hears music, she also sees the music as colors. The ability to generate multiple sensations in response to a single sensory experience is called _____ and is a perceptual phenomenon.
   a. synesthesia
   b. chromathesia

8. Mr. Owusu sustained a left hemisphere middle cerebral arterial stroke. He may experience all of the following except for which one?
   a. right side hemiplegia and hemiparesthesia
   b. cognitive impairment
   c. affective (emotional) involvement
   d. ataxic gait

9. Ms. Brayden had a cerebrovascular accident caused by an occlusion to the superior cerebellar arteries. She may experience all of the following except for which one?
   a. ataxic gait
   b. hypotonicity and hyporeflexia
   c. dysmetria and nystagmus
   d. loss of pain and temperature on the contralateral side

10. Mr. Kagan is experiencing numbness and weakness in his left arm and leg, blurred vision, dizziness, and confusion. His daughter calls 911, because she recognizes these signs as indicative of a:
    a. visual-perceptual disorder
    b. migraine-induced aura
    c. transient ischemic attack
    d. tactile agnosia

Answers

1. b
2. c
3. d
4. a
5. c
6. b
7. a
8. d
9. d
10. c

Commonly Used Neurodiagnostic Tests

LUMBAR PUNCTURE (SPINAL TAP)

- A lumbar puncture is an invasive procedure used to remove a sample of cerebrospinal fluid (CSF) from the sub-arachnoid space for diagnostic evaluation.
- As a result of the technological advancement of other diagnostic evaluations, lumbar punctures are no longer commonly used in the assessment of central nervous system (CNS) disorders.
- Lumbar punctures are used to do the following:
  - Collect CSF to detect pathological conditions
  - Measure CSF pressure in the diagnosis of hydrocephalus
  - Administer contrast dye to the spinal canal during imaging scans
  - Administer anesthesia to the spinal cord for surgical procedures
  - Relieve hydrocephalus
- Disorders in which lumbar punctures are indicated include the following:
  - CNS infection (eg, meningitis, encephalitis)
  - Space-occupying lesions of the subarachnoid space
  - Multiple sclerosis
  - Acute inflammatory demyelinating polyneuropathy (Guillain-Barré syndrome)
  - Neuroimmunologic disorders
- The procedure involves the insertion of a hollow needle between the third and fourth lumbar vertebrae into the spinal canal; however, the needle does not contact spinal nerves.
- Most often, 5 to 20 mL of CSF is collected and measured with a manometer attached to the needle.
- The CSF is then evaluated for cell counts, biochemical and immunologic studies, and microbiologic analysis.
- While the procedure is safe, some patients experience a spinal headache afterward, caused by minimal CSF leakage.[1]

MYELOGRAM

- A myelogram is an invasive procedure that uses x-ray technology or computed tomography (CT) and contrast agents to evaluate the condition of the spine, spinal canal, spinal cord, spinal nerve roots, and vertebral discs.
- A lumbar puncture is used to draw CSF for testing. A contrast agent is then injected into the spinal canal, and an x-ray fluoroscope then records images produced by the contrast material.
- While regular x-rays of the spine only allow observation of the bones, the contrast agent used in a myelogram appears white on x-rays, allowing detailed observation of the spinal cord, nerves, and spinal canal.
- Myelograms can be used to evaluate and diagnose the following:
  - Spinal cord tumors
  - Spinal abscesses
  - Herniated discs causing nerve root impingement
- Myelography has been largely replaced by CT and magnetic resonance imaging (MRI).[2]

Gutman SA. *Quick Reference Neuroscience for Rehabilitation Professionals: The Essential Neurologic Principles Underlying Rehabilitation Practice, Third Edition* (pp 330-337).
© 2017 Taylor & Francis Group.

ELECTROENCEPHALOGRAPHY

- An electroencephalogram (EEG) is a noninvasive test that is able to record neural electrical patterns or brain waves.
- Most neurologic imaging scans have replaced the EEG in the determination of the exact location of anatomic pathology.
- The EEG is currently used as a pathophysiological tool able to identify abnormal cerebral function that cannot be visualized through radiographic or magnetic imaging scans.
- The EEG is most commonly used in the evaluation of the following:
  - Seizures (transient state): while the EEG is useful for the evaluation of seizures, it is not useful for the evaluation of headache or dizziness.
  - Epilepsy
  - Herpes simplex encephalitis (evolving condition)
  - Dementia (global disorder)
  - Sleep disorders
- The EEG is able to measure the changing electrical potentials on the scalp in response to a controlled stimulus.
- Electrodes are placed on the scalp over specific brain regions (and attached with an adhesive substance). Electrodes are able to detect the small electrical signals that form brain waves and transmit these signals to the EEG machine.[3]
- Limitations of the EEG include the following:
  - The test cannot detect brainstem activity well.
  - An EEG is not useful in the diagnosis of brain death.

EVOKED POTENTIALS

- Evoked potential tests measure neural electrical activity in response to stimulation of specific nerve pathways.
- Evoked potentials can identify slowed electrical conduction caused by demyelination even when such damage is too subtle to be detected on neurological exam.
- Wires are placed on the scalp over stimulated brain regions. Sensory input is then administered and neural responses recorded.
- Evoked potentials are used in the assessment of several sensory organs, including those related to vision, audition, and tactile sensation.[4]

Visual System

- Visual evoked potentials are recorded over the occipital region in response to a controlled stimulus.
- This assessment can detect pre- and postchiasmal lesions and asymptomatic optic neuritis. Because pathology of the optic nerves is poorly detected by MRI, visual evoked potentials have become an important adjunctive tool in the diagnosis of optic nerve lesions.[5]

Auditory System

- Auditory evoked potentials are used in the evaluation of brainstem structures and auditory functions.
- Five specific waves are recorded from the vestibulocochlear nerve, the cochlear nucleus, the superior olivary complex, the lateral lemniscus, and the inferior colliculus.
- Auditory evoked potentials can detect physiologic lesions that are below the resolution limit of neurologic imaging techniques.[6]

Somatosensory System

- Upper extremity somatosensory evoked potentials are recorded following stimulation of the median nerve.
- Lower extremity somatosensory evoked potentials are recorded following stimulation of the posterior tibial nerve.
- Somatosensory evoked potentials can aid in the diagnosis of multiple sclerosis because multiple sclerosis plaques in the spinal cord are difficult to detect using MRI.[7]

Electromyography and Nerve Conduction Studies

- Electromyography (EMG) and nerve conduction studies are valuable in the assessment and diagnosis of peripheral nerve and muscular disorders.
- EMG involves the recording of spontaneous, voluntary, and electrically stimulated muscle activity through small intramuscular needle electrodes.
- An EMG involves the insertion of very thin needles into specific muscles under evaluation. Each needle contains an electrode that is attached to a wire; the wire transmits signals to an oscilloscope, which records electrical signals in the form of wave patterns.
- Nerve conduction velocity (NCV) involves electrical stimulation of a peripheral nerve. The peripheral nerve's rate of transmission (or speed of conduction) and amplitude of response are then measured.
- NCV procedures involve the taping of small pads to the skin surface along the path of a nerve. These pads electrically stimulate the nerve under evaluation. Nerve signal conduction pathology is detected as the electrical current travels along the nerve and is picked up by the surface pads.
- EMG and NCV yield data that can determine the distinction among the following:
  - Primary motor neuron disease vs muscular disease
  - Demyelinating vs axonal neuropathy
  - Nerve root vs plexus disorders
- For example, these evaluations can determine the difference between motor neuron diseases (such as amyotrophic lateral sclerosis) and muscle disorders (such as myotonic dystrophy).
- EMG and NCV can also determine the presence and location of mononeuropathy. The most common entrapment syndrome best detected by an EMG is carpal tunnel syndrome.[8]

ANGIOGRAPHY

- Angiography is a neurological imaging method used to see the internal structure of blood vessels and organs.
- Radiopaque contrast agents are injected into structures and then viewed using x-ray fluoroscopy.

Cerebral Angiography

- Cerebral angiography is used to observe the blood vessels of the brain for narrowing or blockage.
- Angiography is an invasive procedure that involves entering a catheter into the body to inject contrast material through the carotid arteries (which supply the brain).
- Insertion of the catheter is usually made in the femoral artery. After insertion, the catheter is guided through the arterial system to the exact cerebral position under evaluation.
- X-ray fluoroscopy is then used to image the contrast material as it flows through the blood vessels.
- Cerebral angiography is most commonly performed after other tests (such as a CT scan) have detected pathology.
- The procedure provides a good visualization of the neurologic vascular system and is commonly used prior to neurosurgical procedures.[9]
- Cerebral angiography is particularly useful in the detection of the following:
  - Acute cerebrovascular accident (CVA)
  - Cerebral anastomoses and occlusions
  - Aneurysm
  - Arteriovenous malformation
  - Tumor
  - Arterial stenosis

Magnetic Resonance Angiography

- Magnetic resonance angiography (MRA) uses MRI technology to detect and diagnose cerebrovascular disease and cardiac disease.
- MRA is a noninvasive method of evaluating cerebrovascular structures without the use of contrast material. Sometimes, however, contrast material is administered to enhance resolution.
- This technique is widely used to detect diseased intracranial arteries.
- For example, MRA can detect aneurysms that cannot be observed by conventional angiography.[10]

Computerized Tomography Angiography

- Computerized tomographic angiography (CTA) is a noninvasive imaging method that uses CT to observe blood flow throughout the brain and body.
- CT combines the use of x-rays with computer analysis of images.
- X-rays are passed through the patient's body from different angles to produce cross-sectional images. These images are then assembled by computer into three-dimensional photos.
- CTA is able to detect transient ischemic attacks (TIA) in order to prevent a full CVA.
- Examining cerebral arteries using CTA may also help in the correct diagnosis of patients who report headache, dizziness, tinnitus, and/or syncope.[11]

MAGNETIC RESONANCE IMAGING

- MRI uses magnets and radio waves to detect subtle electromagnetic fields in the brain.
- Radiofrequency waves are directed at protons (the nuclei of hydrogen atoms). Protons emit radio signals that can be computer-processed to form an image.
- Images can be viewed in cross-sectional slices of the coronal, sagittal, and horizontal planes. Such cross-sectional slices can be as thin as one-quarter of an inch.
- MRI is a noninvasive procedure that does not require the injection of contrast material and does not expose the patient to ionizing radiation.
- It is valuable for providing images of the heart, large blood vessels, soft tissues, and brain.
- MRI is more sensitive than CT.
- Because MRI offers high-resolution images in multiple planes, it has become the preferred clinical and research tool for anatomic imaging.[12]
- Diagnoses in which MRI is most useful include the following:
  - Arteriosclerosis
  - Arteriovenous malformations
  - Vertebral disc disease
  - Spinal stenosis
  - Spinal metastases
  - Chiari malformation
  - Spina bifida
  - Spinal cord tumors
  - Demyelinating and degenerative brain disorders
  - Brain hemorrhages, infarcts, and space-occupying lesions

FUNCTIONAL MAGNETIC RESONANCE IMAGING

- Functional magnetic resonance (fMRI) is a noninvasive tool that combines the high resolution of conventional MRI with the opportunity to measure brain function and metabolic processes during neurologic activity.
- fMRI is able to detect small changes in the magnetic resonance signal resulting from an increase or decrease in blood oxygen level. Changes in blood oxygen level occur in response to the cellular activity of brain structures.
- This imaging technique allows researchers to examine how brain structures function in various neurologic pathologies, particularly neurobehavioral disorders (eg, schizophrenia, depression, autism).
- Researchers can use fMRI to determine which brain regions are responsible for functions such as cognition, language and speech, movement, and sensation.
- fMRI allows researchers to better understand how a normal, diseased, or injured brain is working.
- Additionally, neurosurgeons frequently use fMRI to map the brain for surgical procedures.[13]

DIFFUSION TENSOR IMAGING

- Diffusion tensor imaging (DTI) is a form of MRI.
- While MRIs allow precise examination of the nerve cell bodies that make up the gray matter, DTI provides the opportunity for researchers and clinicians to image the axons that make up the white matter with great specificity. DTI captures neural fiber connectivity and networks both in living beings and in post-mortem organisms.
- In DTI, radiofrequency and magnetic field gradient pulses are used to track water molecule movement in the brain.
- Researchers commonly use DTI to study neuronal network dysfunction in neurodegenerative diseases such as Parkinson, Huntingdon, multiple sclerosis, epilepsy, Alzheimer, schizophrenia, cognitive impairment, and developmental disorders (eg, dyslexia, autism spectrum disorders, and attention deficit hyperactivity disorder).
- DTI can also be used to localize lesions in traumatic brain injury, tumors, and stroke.
- It is hoped that the vast body of knowledge emerging from DTI studies can, in the future, be used clinically for treatment planning, detection of preclinical markers, and detection of microstructural abnormalities before disease progression.[14]

COMPUTED TOMOGRAPHY

- CT involves the absorption of photons by tissues to generate data that, after computerized processing, are presented in a familiar grayscale format.
- In CT scans of the brain, numerous x-rays are passed through the skull and brain at various angles and then joined together to produce cross-sectional images of structures.
- CT is a noninvasive procedure; however, contrast dye may be injected intravenously to enhance resolution.
- While MRIs are more sensitive than CT scans, CTs are better than MRIs in the detection of fresh blood within cranial spaces. For this reason, it is the preferred method of imaging a CVA.[15]
  - Emergency CT scans are used to rule out hemorrhage in the case of CVA. This knowledge is important when considering whether to administer anticoagulant (blood thinning) drugs, which are contraindicated in hemorrhagic stroke.
  - In the subacute phase of CVA, CT scans are used to detect edema and infarction.
- CT scans are particularly effective in the detection of the following:
  - Subarachnoid hemorrhages
  - Subdural collections of blood
  - Neoplasms
  - Vascular anomalies (eg, aneurysms and arteriovenous malformations)

NUCLEAR MAGNETIC RESONANCE SPECTROSCOPY

- Nuclear magnetic resonance spectroscopy, also called *NMR spectroscopy*, is an imaging technique that applies computer software programming to the traditional MRI hardware.
- NMR spectroscopy is used to determine the molecular structure of a compound or to determine the compound's presence.
- It is based on the idea that nuclei of certain atoms have characteristic properties. As a result, signals can be received and displayed as an image.
- NMR spectroscopy is noninvasive and does not expose the patient to ionizing radiation.
- It is an important tool in the diagnosis and monitoring of the following[16]:
  - Progression of CVA
  - Ischemic injury
  - Intracranial tumors
  - Multiple sclerosis
  - Dementia
  - Encephalopathies
- NMR spectroscopy is most commonly used as an adjunct to MRI when differential diagnoses cannot be otherwise made. For example, it is used to do the following:
  - Differentiate CVAs from neoplasms
  - Make clearer diagnoses when recurrent tumor, neoplasia, and necrosis cannot be otherwise diagnosed

POSITRON EMISSION TOMOGRAPHY

- Positron emission tomography (PET) involves the measurement of positron emission from an injected radionuclide.
- A PET scan is an integration of 2 technologies: CT and radioactive tracers.
- The tracer is a radioactively labeled substance that is injected into the body and emits gamma rays. Gamma rays can be detected by PET in order to observe various metabolic processes in the brain and body. The tracers are similar to the contrast agents used in CT and MRI technologies.
- When the tracer is absorbed into the body, the patient is then scanned. PET is able to collect information emitted by the tracer and transforms it into 2-dimensional cross-sectional images.
- The radioisotopes used in PET to label tracers can be detected by the scanner but pass through the body safely.
- Like fMRI, PET is able to measure cellular changes resulting from increases or decreases in blood oxygen and glucose levels. In other words, PET measures changes in regional cerebral blood flow when people perform specific activities (within the confines of the PET scanner).
- In addition to blood oxygen and glucose levels, PET can measure the following:
  - Blood flow
  - Blood volume
  - Tissue acidity
  - Drug activity
- PET is also the preferred tool to measure the growth rate of malignant tumors.
- Both PET and fMRI have enabled researchers to examine how neuroanatomical structures function in neurobehavioral disorders.
- Because PET requires a cyclotron to produce isotopes, its use is limited to major research and medical centers.
- Like fMRI, PET requires intravenous injection of radioactive material.[17]

SINGLE PHOTON EMISSION COMPUTED TOMOGRAPHY

- Single photon emission computed tomography (SPECT) employs radiation detectors to determine the location of a tracer drug in the brain.
- Simplistically, SPECT is a form of nuclear imaging that is primarily used to view how blood flows through arteries and veins in the brain.
- Like PET, SPECT is based on the 2 technologies of CT and radioactive tracers.
- Just prior to the scan, patients are injected with a tracer chemical that is radioactively labeled and emits gamma rays. Gamma rays can be detected by the SPECT scanner.
- The computer then collects the information emitted by the gamma rays and transforms them into two-dimensional cross-sectional images.
- SPECT differs from PET in that the SPECT tracer remains in the bloodstream rather than being absorbed by surrounding tissues. This limits detection of images to regions of blood flow.
- SPECT uses a tracer with a long half-life, making possible studies that involve a prolonged series of scans over a 4-hour period.
- Like PET and fMRI, SPECT can be used to determine which brain regions are active during functional task performance. SPECT, however, has a poorer resolution than fMRI, making it less efficient in the examination of neurobehavioral disorders.
- While SPECT has less sensitivity than PET, it is less expensive and more available than PET.[18]

Neurologic Indications for Computed Tomography
- Acute cerebrovascular disease
- Acute head trauma
- Extracerebral tumors (particularly meningiomas)
- Intracranial calcification or osseous lesions
- Lumbar spine presurgical planning
- Subarachnoid hemorrhage

Neurologic Indications for Magnetic Resonance Imaging
- Cervical spine damage
- Demyelinating disorders
- Head trauma (after acute phase)
- Inflammatory disorders
- Intracranial tumors
- Osseous vertebral column metastases
- Posterior fossa and craniovertebral junction lesions
- Seizures
- Spinal cord lesions

REFERENCES

1. Peterson MA, Pisupati D, Heyming TW, Abele JA, Lewis RJ. Ultrasound for routine lumbar puncture. *Acad Emerg Med.* 2014;21(2):130-136. doi: 10.1111/acem.12305.

2. Song KJ, Choi BW, Kim GH, Kim JR. Clinical usefulness of CT-myelogram comparing with the MRI in degenerative cervical spinal disorders: is CTM still useful for primary diagnostic tool? *J Spinal Disord Tech.* 2009;22(5):353-357. doi:10.1097/BSD.0b013e31817df78e.

3. Schomer DL, Da Silva FL. *Niedermeyer's Electroencephalography: Basic Principles, Clinical Applications, and Related Fields.* 5th ed. Philadelpia, PA: Lippincott Williams & Wilkins; 2012.

4. Colon E, Visser SL, de Weerd JPC, Zonneveldt A. *Evoked Potential Manual: A Practical Guide to Clinical Applications.* New York, NY: Springer; 2013.

5. Tobimatsu S, Celesia GG. Studies of human visual pathophysiology with visual evoked potentials. *Clin Neurophysiol.* 2006;117(7):1414-1433. doi:10.1016/j.clinph.2006.01.004.

6. Picton T. *Human Auditory Evoked Potentials.* San Diego, CA: Plural; 2010.

7. Cruccu G, Aminoff MJ, Curio G, et al. Recommendations for the clinical use of somatosensory-evoked potentials. *Clin Neurophysiol.* 2008;119(8):1705-1719. doi:10.1016/j.clinph.2008.03.016.

8. Weiss LD, Weiss JM, Silver JK. *Easy EMG: A Guide to Performing Nerve Conduction Studies and Electromyography.* 2nd ed. Elsevier Health Sciences; 2015.

9. Bradac GB. *Cerebral Angiography: Normal Anatomy and Vascular Pathology.* 2nd ed. New York, NY: Springer; 2014.

10. Carr JC, Carroll TJ, eds. *Magnetic Resonance Angiography: Principles and Applications.* New York, NY: Springer; 2011.

11. Rubin GD, Rofsky NM, eds. *CT and MR Angiography: Comprehensive Vascular Assessment.* Philadelphia, PA: Lippincott, Williams, & Wilkins; 2008.

12. Bushong SC, Clarke G. *Magnetic Resonance Imaging: Physical and Biological Principles.* 4th ed. St. Louis, MS: Mosby; 2014.

13. Huettel SA, Song AW, McCarthy G. *Functional Magnetic Resonance Imaging.* 3rd ed. Saunderland, MA: Sinauer; 2014.

14. Soares JM, Marques P, Alves V, Sousa N. A hitchhiker's guide to diffusion tensor imaging. *Front Neurosci.* 2013;7:31. doi:10.3389/fnins.2013.00031.

15. Romans L. *Computed Tomography for Technologists: A Comprehensive Text.* Philadelphia, PA: Lippincott, Williams, & Wilkins; 2010.

16. Keeler J. *Understanding NMR Spectroscopy.* 2nd ed. New York, NY: Wiley; 2010.

17. Saha GB. *Basics of PET Imaging: Physics, Chemistry, and Regulations.* 2nd ed. New York, NY: Springer; 2010.

18. Wernick MN, Aarsvold JN, eds. *Emission Tomography: The Fundamentals of PET and SPECT.* San Diego, CA: Elsevier; 2004.

Neurotransmitters
The Neurochemical Basis of Human Behavior

- Neurotransmitters are chemicals that relay and modulate messages between neurons.
- Much of human behavior is mediated by the action of neurotransmitters in the brain. Researchers are also demonstrating that behavioral pathology is largely due to imbalances in one or more neurotransmitter systems. Physical diseases may also be due to specific neurotransmitter pathway disturbances (eg, Parkinson disease).
- Neurotransmitters are chemicals that are stored in and released from the terminal boutons of neurons; they are released into the synaptic cleft.
- Once in the synaptic cleft, neurotransmitters can be destroyed by enzymatic degraders, chemical substances that break down a neurotransmitter so that the postsynaptic neuron can repolarize in order to fire again.
- Neurotransmitters can also be reabsorbed by the presynaptic terminal boutons in a process called *reuptake*.
- Sometimes there is a decrease in the number of receptors for a neurotransmitter on the postsynaptic neuron due to long-term exposure to the neurotransmitter. This is called *downregulation*.
- Neurotransmitters can be classified into 4 major groups:
  1. Amino acids (eg, glutamate, gamma-aminobutyric acid [GABA], aspartic acid, glycine)
  2. Peptides (eg, vasopressin, somatostatin)
  3. Monoamines (norepinephrine, dopamine, serotonin)
  4. Acetylcholine (ACh)
- There are multiple neurotransmitter systems in the brain (and in the enteric nervous system).
- In the peripheral nervous system (PNS), only 2 neurotransmitters are used: ACh and norepinephrine.
- Neurotransmitters can be excitatory or inhibitory, depending on which receptor sites they bind to. They work like the brain's brake and accelerator systems.[1-3]

MAJOR NEUROTRANSMITTERS ABOUT WHICH INFORMATION IS KNOWN

- ACh
- Gamma-aminobutyric acid (GABA)
- Glutamate (GLU)
- Dopamine (DA)
- Serotonin (5-HT)
- Norepinephrine (NE)
- Substance P
- Endorphins
- Histamine

Gutman SA. *Quick Reference Neuroscience for Rehabilitation Professionals: The Essential Neurologic Principles Underlying Rehabilitation Practice, Third Edition* (pp 338-352).
© 2017 Taylor & Francis Group.

ACETYLCHOLINE

- ACh was the first neurotransmitter to be discovered.
- In the PNS, ACh is the major neurotransmitter that controls muscle action. There are comparatively few ACh receptors in the brain.
- In the PNS, this neurotransmitter most often has excitatory effects and facilitates action at the neuromuscular junction.
- In the central nervous system (CNS), ACh is part of the cholinergic system and has an inhibitory effect.
- Excessive levels of ACh at the motor end plates of the neuromuscular junction can result in dyskinesia. Dyskinesia is a hyperkinetic motor disorder characterized by involuntary muscle contractions.
- Deficient levels of ACh at the neuromuscular junction can result in paralysis.
- In the CNS, ACh plays a role in regulating the autonomic nervous system (ANS), such as in the regulation of heart rate.
- There are 2 main classes of ACh:
  1. A fast-acting receptor called *nicotinic*, which is activated by the toxin in tobacco
  2. A slow-acting receptor named *muscarinic*, which is activated by the toxin muscarine (found in poisonous mushrooms)
- Acetylcholinesterase (AChE) is the enzymatic degrader that will stop the action of ACh at the neuromuscular junction. The effects of nerve agents (used as chemical weapons) such as sarin gas work because they inhibit AChE. This results in a painful continuous stimulation of muscles and glands.[4]
- Certain insecticides, similarly, work because they inhibit AChE in insects.
- Some snake venoms contain toxins that can block nicotinic receptors and cause paralysis. In addition, curare is a nicotinic blocking agent extracted from plants. Curare has been used as a poison (placed on arrowheads) by certain South American indigenous groups.
- Botulin is also a poison that works as an ACh blocking agent causing paralysis. Botox, which is a botulin derivative, has become a popular cosmetic treatment to diminish facial wrinkles by temporarily paralyzing the responsible muscles.[5]

Alzheimer Disease

- A shortage of ACh in the brain has been implicated as a contributing factor in Alzheimer disease. Certain drugs that inhibit AChE have been found to have some effectiveness in treatment of the disease.[6]

Myasthenia Gravis

- Myasthenia gravis is a disease characterized by muscle weakness and fatigue. The disease occurs when the body inappropriately produces antibodies against ACh receptors. This causes ACh transmission to become impaired. Drugs that inhibit AChE have been found to be effective in the treatment of myasthenia gravis.[7]

GAMMA-AMINOBUTYRIC ACID

- GABA is the major inhibitory neurotransmitter of the brain.
- It essentially turns off the function of cells and acts like a brake on excitatory neurotransmitters that can cause anxiety.
- Without inhibitory neurotransmitters like GABA, brain cells would fire uncontrollably (as in epileptic seizures).
- GABA is most highly concentrated in the substantia nigra and globus pallidus. Other neural areas of high GABA concentration include the hypothalamus, periaqueductal gray matter (of the midbrain), and hippocampus.
- There are 2 known GABA receptors: GABA-A and GABA-B.
  1. GABA deficiency is implicated in anxiety disorders, insomnia, and epilepsy.
  2. GABA excess is implicated in memory loss and the inability for new learning.
- Preliminary research suggests that agents that can block GABA-B may improve learning and memory.[8]

GABA and Anxiety Disorders

- People who experience anxiety and panic attacks may have an imbalance in the GABA system involving a depletion of this neurotransmitter.
- Benzodiazepines are a class of drugs (eg, Xanax [alprazolam], Valium [diazepam], Ativan [lorazepam]) used in the treatment of anxiety disorders.
- These drugs work by enhancing the effect of GABA on GABA-A receptors.
- Prolonged use of benzodiazepines results in adaptation; in other words, GABA receptors increase in number or sensitivity to the drug, making it less effective over time (referred to as *downregulation*).
- Larger doses of benzodiazepines are then needed to provide relief from anxiety. This is called *tolerance*.
- Stopping the use of benzodiazepines can result in diminished sensitivity of GABA receptors, causing heightened anxiety.
- Many dietary supplement companies sell GABA as a sleep aid and antianxiety treatment; however, research demonstrating the effectiveness of such aids has not been extensively conducted.[8,9]

GLUTAMATE

- Glutamate, also known as glutamic acid or GLU, is the most common neurotransmitter in the CNS and may account for as much as half of all neurotransmitters in the brain.
- It is one of the major excitatory neurotransmitters of the CNS and is believed to have a significant role in learning and memory.
- Some researchers believe that glutamate can be used to enhance memory and new learning in Alzheimer disease.[10]
- Disordered glutamate mechanisms have been identified in several neurological disorders, including Huntington disease, ischemia, autism, multiple sclerosis, Parkinson disease, schizophrenia, seizures, Alzheimer disease, and amyotrophic lateral sclerosis.[11-13]
- Glutamate also serves as a precursor for the synthesis of the inhibitory neurotransmitter GABA.
- It is present in a wide variety of foods and is responsible for the taste sense of umami (ie, meaty or hearty). The sodium salt of glutamic acid (monosodium glutamate) is a common food additive used to enhance flavor.

Epileptic Seizures

- Overactivity of glutamate may produce epileptic seizures.
- There is a delicate balance between excitation and inhibition in the brain.
- In epilepsy, the brain's chemistry may have tilted too far toward excitation.[14]
- Some researchers suggest that any disorder, such as Alzheimer disease, schizophrenia, Parkinson disease, epilepsy, or cerebrovascular accident (CVA), may essentially involve an imbalance in one or more neurotransmitter systems.

Excitotoxicity

- An excess of glutamate can produce neuronal damage and cell death, or excitotoxicity. Frequently, trauma to the brain (eg, CVA, head injury) will trigger an excess release of glutamate, resulting in the cell death of many more neurons than had occurred in the original trauma.
- For example, in CVA, researchers believe that it is not just oxygen deprivation that kills brain cells but also the release of too much glutamate.
- When the brain experiences a series of crises, glutamate is released 1000 times more than its normal level.
- This may serve as the organism's way of facilitating a painless death process when severe CNS trauma occurs.
- Physicians, in their attempt to save an individual's life, inadvertently stop the release of glutamate after it has already killed off an extensive amount of brain cells.
- Often, glutamate release is responsible for the greatest damage in traumatic brain injuries and CVAs, rather than the initial injury.
- Researchers are attempting to develop drugs that can immediately prevent the release of glutamate after a severe brain injury.
- However, such drugs would have to be administered in the first hours after injury, and often patients are not transported to hospital emergency departments in time.
- Another suggested strategy involves the development of drugs that could cause glutamate to bind with neighboring neurons without killing them. Essentially, researchers would be changing the way that glutamate works in the brain.[15]

DOPAMINE

- The dopamine system has major effects on the motor system, cognition, and motivation and reward.
- Researchers have identified several sources of dopamine in the CNS, including the substantia nigra of the midbrain, the tegmentum of the midbrain, and the arcuate nucleus of the hypothalamus.[16]

Dopaminergic Tracts in the Brain

- The nigrostriatal tract travels from the substantia nigra to the striatum and accounts for most of the brain's dopamine.
- The tuberoinfundibular tract travels from the arcuate nucleus of the hypothalamus to the pituitary stalk. This pathway controls the release of the hormone *prolactin* through D2 receptors.[17]
- The mesolimbic tract travels from the ventral tegmental area to parts of the limbic system.
- The mesocortical tract travels from the ventral tegmental area to the neocortex, particularly the prefrontal area.[16,17]

Parkinson Disease

- Dopamine affects the basal ganglia and thus influences movement.
- Loss of dopamine from the substantia nigra and the nigrostriatal pathway is believed to be the primary cause of Parkinson disease, causing paucity of movement, festinating gait, and masked face.
- Precursors to dopamine, such as L-dopa, can alleviate some of the symptoms of Parkinson disease.[18]

Schizophrenia

- Too much dopamine has been implicated in schizophrenia, causing hallucinations, delusions, disorganized thinking, and paucity of thought.
- Dopamine neurons in the mesolimbic pathway are associated with psychosis and schizophrenia.
- Phenothiazines are a class of antipsychotic drugs that block D2 dopamine receptors. These drugs can effectively reduce psychotic symptoms.
- Drugs such as amphetamines and cocaine greatly increase dopamine levels and can cause psychosis.
- Most modern antipsychotic medications are designed to block function of dopamine receptors to some degree.
- Conversely, blockage of D2 dopamine receptors has been associated with depression relapse. Such blockage can reduce the effectiveness of the class of antidepressant medications known as selective serotonin reuptake inhibitors (SSRIs).
- Older classifications of drugs used to treat schizophrenia would often cause Parkinsonian-like symptoms called *tardive dyskinesia*. Tardive dyskinesia is a hyperkinetic motor disorder characterized by involuntary muscle contractions: lip smacking, repetitive tongue protrusion, and blepharospasm. Clozapine is a newer class of antipsychotic drug that reduces the effects of schizophrenia without inducing Parkinsonism.[19,20]

The Reward System and Addiction

- Dopamine has a significant role in the brain's reward system and is commonly released in response to highly pleasurable experiences, such as eating and sexual activity.
- Dopamine is also strongly involved in the process of addiction.
- When drugs such as heroin, amphetamines, and cocaine are ingested, dopamine levels rise to unnaturally high levels in the brain. This accounts for the high experienced in response to addictive substances.
- This unnatural boost of dopamine acts like an assault on the brain. To counteract the assault, the brain begins to decrease its natural production of dopamine, causing severe craving for the addictive substance.[21]

Cognitive Function

- Dopamine disorders in the frontal lobes are believed to be responsible for a decline in cognitive functions such as memory, attention, and problem solving.
- Some researchers suggest that diminished dopamine concentrations in the prefrontal cortex are a contributing factor in attention deficit hyperactivity disorder (ADHD) and the negative symptoms of depression and schizophrenia (eg, social withdrawal, apathy, anhedonia).[19,22,23]

SEROTONIN

- Serotonin is synthesized in serotonergic neurons in the CNS and gastrointestinal (GI) tract. It is synthesized from the amino acid tryptophan.
- In the CNS, the neurons of the raphe nuclei of the medulla are the principle source of serotonin release.
- There are at least 15 serotonin systems in the CNS.
- Serotonin has been implicated in sleep, emotional control and equanimity, pain regulation, emesis (vomiting), and carbohydrate feeding behaviors (or the binging behaviors that occur in certain eating disorders).[24]

Regulation of Circadian Rhythms and Sleep-Wake Cycles

- The richest concentration of serotonin in the body is found in the pineal gland, although this gland does not use serotonin as a neurotransmitter. Rather, the pineal gland uses serotonin to synthesize melatonin, a substance that is important in the regulation of circadian rhythms, diurnal patterns, and sleep-wake cycles.
- The suprachiasmatic nucleus (SCN) of the hypothalamus is extensively innervated by serotonergic input from the raphe nucleus and is responsible for regulating circadian rhythms.
- Low serotonin levels may disrupt SCN regulation of circadian rhythms, as seen in seasonal affective disorder.
- Depletion of serotonin may also be related to the disruption of sleep-wake cycles seen in aging.[25]

Depression, Anger, Obsessive-Compulsive Disorder

- Low levels of serotonin are associated with depression and suicidal behavior.[24]
- SSRIs are a classification of antidepressants that increase the brain's levels of serotonin by blocking the reuptake of serotonin in the presynaptic neuron.[26]
- Kramer's Kindling Theory of Depression is an attempt to describe the physiologic process of chronic, recurrent depression. The first 3 or 4 depressive episodes (which may be minor) can cause a permanent change in the serotonin system. With each successive depressive episode, the synaptic vessels produce and release less serotonin. Once the serotonin system becomes less responsive, it may never return to its normal activity level without intervention.[27]
- Low levels of serotonin have also been associated with aggression, anger, and violence. Some researchers have suggested that impulsivity and aggression may be inversely correlated with the responsiveness of one's serotonin system. The less active or responsive a serotonin system is, the more impulsively and aggressively a person may behave. SSRIs have been used effectively to reduce levels of anger, irritability, and depression.[28]
- In addition to depression and anger, too little serotonin has also been associated with obsessive-compulsive disorder (OCD). The SSRIs have shown some effectiveness in the treatment of OCD.[29]

Appetite and Eating Disorders

- Serotonin levels also play a role in appetite and carbohydrate feeding behaviors.
- Low serotonin levels have been shown to be related to increased appetite and carbohydrate craving. Studies of patients with bulimia have demonstrated that low serotonin levels are present in patients demonstrating binging behaviors.
- The antidepressant Prozac (fluoxetine) has been used effectively to treat patients with binging and compulsive eating disorders.[30]

NOREPINEPHRINE

- Also called *noradrenalin*
- Most norepinephrine pathways in the brain have their origin in the locus ceruleus (a nucleus in the pons).
- Norepinephrine and ACh are the only 2 neurotransmitters used in the PNS.
- In the CNS, norepinephrine is released from the medulla (of the adrenal glands) as a hormone into the blood.
- Norepinephrine is also a neurotransmitter released from noradrenergic neurons during synaptic transmission.[31]

Alertness and Attention

- Noradrenergic neurons that project from the locus ceruleus of the reticular activating system play a major role in wakefulness/arousal.
- Because of this connection to the reticular activating system, norepinephrine is important in the active surveillance of one's surroundings by increasing attendance to sensory information from the environment. It has thus become an important agent in pharmaceutical intervention for people with ADHD because it appears to enhance concentration and cognitive organization.[32]

- Psychostimulant medications (such as Ritalin [methylphenidate], Concerta [methylphenidate], Dexedrine [dextro-amphetamine], and Adderall [dextroamphetamine, amphetamine]) are commonly prescribed to increase norepinephrine and dopamine levels in people with ADHD.[33]
- Strattera (atomoxetine) is a selective norepinephrine reuptake inhibitor sometimes used in the treatment of ADHD that only affects norepinephrine, rather than dopamine.
- As a result, Strattera has a lower potential for abuse and can remain active in the body for longer periods of time. Strattera has been shown to be effective for some patients with ADHD.

Stress Hormone

- As a stress hormone, norepinephrine is essential in activating the sympathetic nervous system to produce the fight/flight response, increase heart rate, release energy from fat storage, and increase muscle preparedness.
- Overactivity of the norepinephrine system produces fear, anxiety, and panic (through the action of cortical and limbic regions).
- Beta-blocking agents such as propranolol prevent norepinephrine from binding to beta receptors. This prevents sweating, rapid heart beat (tachycardia), and other sympathetic nervous system signs that may occur in stressful situations.[34]
- Musicians, actors, and public speakers commonly use beta blockers before performances to reduce sympathetic nervous system signs and to enhance calmness.

Depression

- Low levels of norepinephrine have been implicated in depression.
- Serotonin-norepinephrine reuptake inhibitors (SNRIs) are a class of antidepressants that increase the amount of serotonin and norepinephrine available in the brain.
- There is recent evidence that SNRIs may increase dopamine levels as well.
- Like the SSRIs, the SNRIs have shown effectiveness in the treatment of depression.[35]

SUBSTANCE P

- Substance P is classified as a neuropeptide that functions as a neurotransmitter and neuromodulator.
- In the CNS, substance P is associated with mood regulation, anxiety, stress, neurogenesis, respiratory rhythm, neurotoxicity, vasodilation, nausea and emesis, and pain perception.
- Substance P acts as a neurotransmitter in the nociceptive pathway and is involved in the transmission of pain signals from peripheral receptors to the CNS. The nociceptive pathway mediates the sensation of pain.
- Substance P is found in the dorsal horn of the spinal cord, substantia nigra, amygdala, hypothalamus, and cerebral cortex.[36]
- Some researchers have suggested that substance P may play a role in fibromyalgia. The pain reliever capsaicin (the active ingredient in peppers) has been shown to reduce substance P levels by reducing the number of C fiber nerves or causing these nerves to be less sensitive.[37]
- The vomiting center in the medulla consists of high levels of substance P along with other neurotransmitters (eg, dopamine, histamine, serotonin). The activation of substance P in the vomiting center activates the vomiting reflex. A substance P antagonist, Emend (aprepitant), is used as an antiemetic to treat chemotherapy-related nausea.

OPIOID PEPTIDES

- Opioid peptides include endorphins, enkephalins, and dynorphins.
- These peptides are neurotransmitters produced in the pituitary gland and hypothalamus. The highest concentration of opioid receptors is found in the sensory, limbic, and hypothalamic regions of the CNS. The amygdala and periaqueductal gray (of the midbrain) have particularly high concentrations of opioid receptors.
- The opioids resemble opiates (opium, morphine, heroin) in their ability to produce analgesia and feelings of well-being. They are sometimes referred to as the *body's natural painkillers* or *natural morphine.*
- The opioids have a major role in the perception of pleasure produced by the mesocorticolimbic system, the brain's reward system. Along with dopamine, the opioids may contribute to the mechanisms underlying addiction.
- The primary action of the opioids is the inhibition of nociceptive or pain information. Endorphins work conjointly with substance P as a pain modulator.[38] The analgesic capsaicin (the active ingredient in peppers) has been shown to stimulate the release of endorphins. Capsaicin in the form of a topical cream has been used effectively in the treatment of certain types of chronic pain.

- Some researchers have found that endorphin release may underlie the placebo effect in the treatment of pain.
- Other studies have found that acupuncture may trigger the production of endorphins and thus produce pain relief.[39]
- In addition to modulating pain, opioid peptides have a role in cardiac, gastric, and vascular functions.
- Low levels of opioid peptides have also been associated with anxiety and panic.
- There is evidence, too, that some opioid peptides play a role in satiety and appetite control.[40]

HISTAMINE

- Histamine is a chemical that acts as a neurotransmitter and functions in inflammatory responses, GI processes, and sleep regulation.
- Much of the histamine in the body is produced in mast and white blood cells. Histamine is also stored and released in the cells of the GI tract and in the tuberomammillary nucleus of the hypothalamus.
- Histamine is released in response to allergic reaction and causes (1) vasodilation and increased blood flow and (2) increased fluid secretion at the infection site. Vasodilation allows white blood cells to act at the infection site, and fluid helps wash the infection site of allergens and poisons. At the molecular level, histamine stimulates macrophage responses and T cell function, both necessary in the antibody response.
- In GI tract function, histamine acts to generate stomach acid and increase gastric motility.
- Histamine also functions in wakefulness and alertness. Older antihistamines that can cross the blood-brain barrier produce drowsiness; newer antihistamines that do not cross the blood-brain barrier do not induce sleep.[41]

NEUROTRANSMITTERS CAN OVERLAP IN FUNCTION

- Several different neurotransmitters can regulate the same behaviors.
- This redundancy in the regulation of functions is seen throughout the CNS and the PNS.
- This redundancy is likely the nervous system's way of creating a foolproof system, akin to having back-up systems if something goes wrong. This mechanism may have developed as an evolutionary safeguard for the survival of human beings.
- Dopamine, serotonin, and opioid peptides appear to regulate functions and disorders involving the experience of anger, depression, anxiety, and addictive behaviors.[17,24,38]
- Norepinephrine also appears to regulate well-being, anxiety, and arousal.[35]
- GABA and glutamate have shared roles in memory and learning.[8,10]
- ACh and dopamine have shared roles in the regulation of motor activity.[4,16]
- Neurotransmitters involved in wakefulness and consciousness include norepinephrine, dopamine, ACh, histamine, and glutamate.[10,19,32]
- Neuropeptides involved in wakefulness and consciousness include corticotropin-releasing hormone, thyrotropin-releasing hormone, and vasoactive intestinal peptide. Deficiency in one or more of these substances can produce somnolence (sleep).[40]

Role of Neurotransmitters in the Treatment of Depression

- Depression is a serious clinical disorder that affects approximately 16% of the population at least once in their lives.
- The average age of onset is the mid to late 20s; it affects women more than men at a 2 to 1 ratio.
- Depression is often characterized by the following: anhedonia (loss of interest in once enjoyable activities); sadness; fear; hopelessness; helplessness; guilt; difficulty concentrating; decreased memory functions; loss of energy; psychomotor agitation; and changes in sleep patterns, appetite, and weight.
- The etiology of depression may have multiple contributing factors including heredity, physiology, medical conditions, and diet.
- Several neurotransmitters have been implicated in the cause of depression including serotonin, norepinephrine, and dopamine.[42]

(continued)

Role of Neurotransmitters in the Treatment of Depression

(continued)

Selective Serotonin Reuptake Inhibitors

- The SSRIs are a class of antidepressants currently considered as standard first-line agents.
- Researchers have suggested that low levels of serotonin play a major role in the etiology of depression.
- The SSRIs may work, in part, by preventing the reabsorption of serotonin into nerve cells, thus increasing the amount available for use by the brain.
- SSRIs include fluoxetine (Prozac), paroxetine (Paxil), escitalopram (Lexapro), citalopram (Celexa), and sertraline (Zoloft).
- While these antidepressants work as effectively as older classes, they have fewer side effects and thus may be easier to tolerate.[43]

Norepinephrine Reuptake Inhibitors

- Researchers have found that in some patients, low levels of norepinephrine may be a factor in the etiology of depression.
- Norepinephrine reuptake inhibitors (NRIs) are a newer class of antidepressants that block the reabsorption of norepinephrine into the presynaptic neuron, thus increasing the amount available for use by the brain.
- Because norepinephrine is one of the neurochemicals believed to regulate concentration and motivation, the NRIs are thought to have a positive effect on alertness and attention as well as mood.
- NRIs include such drugs as reboxetine (Edronax) and atomoxetine (Strattera).[44]

Serotonin-Norepinephrine Reuptake Inhibitors

- SNRIs are a newer class of antidepressant drug that works on both norepinephrine and serotonin. Recent research suggests that the SNRIs may also affect dopamine levels.
- They are typically used as second-line agents when patients do not respond to SSRI treatment.
- Like the SSRIs, they have fewer side effects than the older classes of antidepressants but are about as effective.
- Examples include venlafaxine (Effexor) and duloxetine (Cymbalta).[45]

Norepinephrine-Dopamine Reuptake Inhibitors

- Bupropion (Wellbutrin) is a norepinephrine-dopamine reuptake inhibitor (NDRI) that is believed to inhibit the reuptake of dopamine.
- It also blocks the reuptake of serotonin and norepinephrine, but to a much lesser extent when compared with the tricyclic drugs.
- Bupropion has been shown to be effective in some patients.
- Common side effects include increased restlessness, agitation, and insomnia, which may be intolerable to some patients.
- When administered in higher doses, bupropion may cause seizures and is thus contraindicated in patients with seizure disorders.
- Bupropion is also contraindicated in patients with anorexia nervosa, as this antidepressant may stimulate appetite loss.[46]

Tricyclic Antidepressants

- The tricyclics are the oldest class of antidepressants and include drugs such as amitriptyline and desipramine.
- The tricyclics block the reuptake of norepinephrine and serotonin.
- While their effectiveness is equal or greater to the SSRIs, they are no longer commonly used because of their side effects, which are more severe than those of the SSRIs. An overdose of tricyclic drugs also has the potential to be lethal.
- Generally, tricyclic drugs are used when patients do not respond to the SSRIs, NRIs, SNRIs, and NDRIs.[47]

Monoamine Oxidase Inhibitors

- Monoamine oxidase inhibitors (MAOIs) block the enzyme monoamine oxidase, which breaks down serotonin and norepinephrine.
- The MAOIs are as or more effective than the tricyclics but are rarely used because of their potentially fatal interactions with certain foods and drugs.
- MAOIs such as Nardil (phenelzine) may be used when patients are not responsive to the SSRIs, NRIs, SNRIs, NDRIs, or tricyclic drugs. Patients using an MAOI must remain on a restricted diet to avoid drug and food interactions.
- A new MAOI has recently been developed called *moclobemide* (Manerix). This drug is referred to as a *reversible inhibitor* of monoamine oxidase A. Because it uses a very specific chemical pathway in the brain, it does not pose the threat of fatal drug/food interactions, and patients taking moclobemide do not have to remain on a restricted diet.[48]

Role of Neurotransmitters in the Treatment of Obsessive-Compulsive Disorder

- OCD is a type of anxiety disorder involving obsessive thoughts and worries. To alleviate the obsessive worries, people engage in compulsive behaviors that become ritualistic (ie, performed repeatedly in the same way).
- Examples of OCD include a fear of dirt and germs (eg, compulsive hand washing rituals), checking disorders (eg, checking repeatedly to see if the door is locked), counting disorders (ie, compulsions to ritualistically count such things as floor tiles), and hoarding disorders (ie, fear of throwing anything away in case it may one day be needed).
- Approximately 2.5% of the population will experience some form of OCD at some point in their lives.
- The disorder occurs equally among men and women and all age groups.
- Researchers believe that the etiology of OCD involves genetics and an imbalance in certain neurotransmitter systems.[42]
- Some researchers have suggested that OCD can sometimes be caused by a streptococcal infection occurring in childhood. Researchers found that a high rate of strep infections occurred in the 3-month period prior to the onset of OCD symptoms. A child who experienced several strep infections had nearly 14 times the average risk of developing OCD in the following year. It is suggested that antibodies recruited to defeat the infection attacked other body systems, including the basal ganglia, a neural region implicated in OCD.[49]
- PET scans of people diagnosed with OCD have shown malfunction in a neural circuit connecting the frontal lobes and the basal ganglia. The basal ganglia normally filter messages to and from the frontal lobes regarding body movements. In OCD, dysfunction of this circuit may lead to the obsessional thoughts and ritualistic compulsive behaviors seen in the disorder.
- Neurotransmitters that are found in the pathway between the frontal lobes and the basal ganglia include serotonin and dopamine.[50]
- The role of these neurotransmitters, however, is unclear. The SSRIs have some effectiveness in the treatment of OCD, while drugs that increase the activity of dopamine worsen symptoms of the disorder.[51]

Antidepressant Drug Treatment

- The primary choice for drug treatment of OCD is currently the SSRIs: fluoxetine (Prozac), fluvoxamine (Luvox), sertraline (Zoloft), paroxetine (Paxil), escitalopram (Lexapro), or citalopram (Celexa).
- Venlafaxine (Effexor), an SNRI, has become a recent alternative.[51]
- Some researchers believe that clomipramine (Anafranil), a tricyclic antidepressant, may be the most effective treatment currently available. Clomipramine blocks the reuptake of norepinephrine and serotonin from the presynaptic neuron.
- Generally, OCD requires higher doses of the antidepressant drugs listed previously than are normally administered in the treatment of depression. The antidepressants also take longer to work when treating OCD than when treating depression: usually as long as 3 months (compared with 2 to 4 weeks in the treatment of depression).
- Approximately half of all treated patients experience some relief from symptoms but frequently relapse when drug treatment is stopped. If treatment is continued, approximately 80% experience a reduction of symptoms but not a complete cessation. In most cases, the disorder remains throughout life and worsens if left untreated.[52]

Role of Neurotransmitters in the Treatment of Anxiety Disorders

- Anxiety disorders involve excessive fear, worries, and physiological distress that interfere with one's daily function.
- Physical symptoms of anxiety disorders can include shortness of breath, palpitations, chest pain, psychomotor agitation, restlessness, sweating, and choking sensations.
- Anxiety disorders include panic attack, agoraphobia, OCD, post-traumatic stress disorder (PTSD), generalized anxiety disorder, acute stress disorder, social phobia, and specific phobia.
- Recent research suggests that anxiety disorders may be caused by abnormalities in the function of several neurotransmitter systems.[42]

(continued)

Role of Neurotransmitters in the Treatment of Anxiety Disorders

(continued)

- Primary neurotransmitters that have been shown to play a role in the etiology of anxiety disorders include serotonin, norepinephrine, GABA, and dopamine.[53]
- Currently, the most effective pharmaceutical agents in the treatment of anxiety disorders affect the GABA and serotonin systems.
- Drugs that are primarily used to treat anxiety are called *anxiolytics.*

Benzodiazepines

- The benzodiazepines are a class of drugs that were developed in the 1950s and 1960s.
- Common benzodiazepines include alprazolam (Xanax), diazepam (Valium), lorazepam (Ativan), clonazepam (Klonopin), and triazolam (Halcion).
- Benzodiazepines are highly effective anxiolytics that work quickly and are well tolerated.
- The disadvantages of using benzodiazepines include drowsiness, impaired memory, and incoordination. In addition, physical dependence can develop after long-term use, along with the occurrence of withdrawal symptoms upon discontinuation.[54]

Selective Serotonin Reuptake Inhibitors

- While the SSRIs were developed as antidepressants, they have been shown to have some efficacy in the treatment of anxiety disorders.
- Because they are well tolerated, have fewer side effects than older classes of antidepressants, and lack the potential for physical dependence (as seen with benzodiazepines), the SSRIs have become first-line agents in the treatment of anxiety.
- The benzodiazepines are primarily recommended as adjunctive treatment for anxiety disorders; however, they are still used when patients are unresponsive to or cannot tolerate the SSRIs.[55]

Serotonin and Norepinephrine Reuptake Inhibitors

- Venlafaxine (Effexor) is an SNRI that has recently been approved for the treatment of generalized anxiety disorder.
- There is evidence, too, that venlafaxine's effectiveness may extend to other forms of anxiety disorders.
- As with the SSRIs, side effects may be poorly tolerated by some patients. Common side effects include weight gain, sexual dysfunction, and agitation.[55]

GABA-Enhancing Pharmaceuticals

- Researchers have begun to generate evidence that the neurotransmitter GABA has a significant role in the etiology of anxiety and other mood disorders.
- A large amount of research data now suggests that drugs affecting the GABA system are highly effective in the treatment of anxiety.
- Such drugs include the benzodiazepines and certain anticonvulsant drugs including tiagabine, valproate, vigabatrin, and gabapentin. In the past several years, anticonvulsant drugs have been commonly used as mood stabilizers in the treatment of bipolar and unipolar depression.[56]
- These GABA-enhancing drugs have demonstrated effectiveness in the treatment of anxiety.[57] Tiagabine, topiramate, valproate, and carbamazepine (all anticonvulsant drugs with GABA-enhancing properties) have shown effectiveness in the treatment of PTSD. One characteristic of PTSD is nighttime awakening from vivid and frightening dreams. Tiagabine in particular has been found to normalize sleep disturbances and reduce the frequency of flashbacks in PTSD.[58]
- Tiagabine enhances CNS GABA transport through its unique ability to inhibit GABA reuptake. Currently, tiagabine is the only available selective GABA reuptake inhibitor. Tiagabine increases available extracellular GABA by up to 200%.
- Gabapentin increases GABA primarily by enhancing release of the neurotransmitter from glia cells. Gabapentin has been shown to have anxiolytic effects similar to those of the benzodiazepines and diazepam, but without the memory impairment often seen in long-term benzodiazepine use. Gabapentin has also been shown to be effective in panic disorder, social phobia, OCD, and PTSD.[57]
- Both tiagabine and gabapentin appear to have the same high effectiveness as the benzodiazepines but do not produce the physical dependence or withdrawal symptoms upon discontinuation that are characteristic of the benzodiazepines.[56,57]

Role of Neurotransmitters in the Treatment of Eating Disorders

- Today, most researchers believe that the etiology of eating disorders is multifactorial and includes genetic, neurotransmitter, and hormonal abnormalities in addition to cultural ones.
- Anorexia nervosa is characterized by severe reduction in food intake (to the point of starvation), extreme weight loss, distorted body image, and obsession with weight and food.
- Bulimia nervosa is characterized by repeated episodes of uncontrollable binge eating followed by self-induced purging (eg, vomiting, laxative abuse, excessive exercise).
- More than 90% of patients diagnosed with an eating disorder are adolescent or young adult women. For many years, this finding was interpreted as evidence that social and cultural expectations of thinness lay at the center of the disorders' etiology.
- In recent years, however, an increasing amount of research has pointed to genetic, neurochemical, and hormonal abnormalities as primary factors underlying eating disorder etiology.[42,59]

Serotonin

- Abnormalities in the serotonergic pathways have been connected to the onset and persistence of eating disorders. A growing body of research indicates that increased serotonin levels in the brain may be responsible for anorexic behavior, while decreased serotonin levels may account for bulimic behaviors.
- A large amount of evidence has been generated showing that increased serotonin activity is associated with appetite suppression. Drugs that suppress appetite and are used in the treatment of obesity work by increasing serotonin levels in the brain. Researchers have suggested that increased serotonin levels may account for the food restriction that is a common characteristic of anorexia.[60,61]
- Conversely, decreased levels of serotonin are related to increased appetite. High serotonin levels may account for the gnawing hunger and inability to feel satiated that is characteristic of bulimia.[60,61]
- People with bulimia may have disturbances in their satiation response center. The brain's satiety center lies in the ventromedial hypothalamus. When this part of the brain is stimulated, feelings of satiety occur and eating stops. In contrast, the lateral hypothalamus governs hunger. When it is stimulated, feelings of hunger ensue and eating behaviors are triggered. Normally, these 2 hypothalamic systems work cooperatively to maintain normal weight and eating patterns. When pathology occurs in the system, eating disorders can emerge.[60,61]
- Serotonin has been linked to feelings of well-being and satiation. After eating a carbohydrate-rich diet, the body converts these sugars to *tryptophan*, the precursor of serotonin. People with bulimia may engage in binge-eating behaviors in an attempt to raise their own serotonin levels.[60,61]
- Conversely, people with anorexia may have an overactive serotonergic system, leading to abnormally high levels of brain serotonin. The food restriction that is commonly seen in anorexia may be a self-imposed attempt to lower serotonin levels. Very high levels of serotonin have been correlated with nervousness, irritation, and jitteriness. People with anorexia may be using food restriction as a way to control these uncomfortable feelings.[60,61]
- Some researchers have also suggested that people with eating disorders may become addicted to fasting or binge eating. Fasting and binge eating both trigger opioid and dopamine release in the brain, just as other addictive substances and behaviors do. People with eating disorders may become addicted to the chemicals released in the brain's reward center during fasting and binge eating.[60,61]

Comorbid Disorders: Depression, Eating Disorders, and Obsessive-Compulsive Disorder

- There is a high comorbidity between depression and eating disorders. Because many people with eating disorders also have depression, researchers have proposed a physiological link between these 2 pathologies. Low levels of serotonin and norepinephrine have been found in both people with depression and people with eating disorders.[62]
- SSRIs and SNRIs are 2 classes of antidepressant drug that have been found to be effective in the treatment of both depression and anorexia.[63]
- Researchers have also found a high comorbidity between bulimia and OCD. A disproportionately high number of people with bulimia also have OCD. Similarly, people with OCD frequently possess some form of abnormal eating behaviors. Again, biochemical similarities between the 2 groups have been found to exist largely within the serotonin system.
- The hormone vasopressin has also been found to be abnormal in both people with eating disorders and people with OCD. Researchers have found that vasopressin levels are abnormally elevated in patients with OCD, anorexia, and bulimia. Vasopressin is normally released in response to either physical or emotional stress. Abnormally elevated levels of vasopressin may contribute to the obsessive behavior seen in some patients with eating disorders.[64]

Role of Neurotransmitters in the Treatment of Schizophrenia

- Schizophrenia is a serious psychiatric disorder characterized by disorganized thinking and perception.
- Positive symptoms of schizophrenia (the presence of abnormal behaviors) include hallucinations, delusions, disorganized speech and cognition, severely disorganized behavior, and catatonic behavior.
- Negative symptoms of schizophrenia (the absence of normal behaviors) include social withdrawal, isolation, poor self-care, blunted mood and affect, and lack of spontaneous thinking.
- Schizophrenia affects 1 in 100 people and occurs in all cultures and socioeconomic groups. Men and women are affected equally, but the typical age of onset differs by gender (male average age of onset occurs in the early 20s; female average age of onset occurs in the late 20s).[42]

Neural Regions Involved in Schizophrenia

- Brain abnormalities have been found in several consistent areas including the frontal lobe, temporal lobe, limbic system (specifically the cingulate gyrus, amygdala, and hippocampus), thalamus, and cerebellum. All of these areas have been found to have decreased volumes in people with schizophrenia.
- Additionally, many studies have found a general decrease in cortical mass, as demonstrated by abnormally widened sulci, enlarged ventricular spaces, and decreased volumes of gray and white matter.
- Imaging scans have also demonstrated decreased cerebral blood flow and glucose metabolism in the frontal lobe.[65]

Neurotransmitters Involved in Schizophrenia

- The dopamine hypothesis of schizophrenia suggests that the disease is caused by an overactive dopamine system. Excessive dopamine can be responsible for disruptions in motor, cognitive, and emotional function.
- Studies have shown that excessive amounts of dopamine can induce psychosis. Recent studies have demonstrated that reduced numbers of D1 dopamine receptors may increase dopamine levels in the brain.[66]
- While dopamine abnormalities have been considered to be the primary factor in the etiology of schizophrenia, researchers have also begun to compile evidence that other neurotransmitters may also play significant roles. These include serotonin, glutamate, GABA, and acetylcholine. [67]
- For example, because irregularly low levels of glutamate receptors have been found in the postmortem brains of adults diagnosed with schizophrenia, it has been suggested that glutamate system deficits may contribute to schizophrenia. Dysfunction of the glutamate system has been linked to poorer cognitive function and can influence dopamine levels.
- Researchers have proposed that the etiology of schizophrenia either involves an imbalance in a single neurotransmitter, such as dopamine, that pathologically affects other neurotransmitters or that the cause of schizophrenia involves an imbalance of multiple neurotransmitter systems.[67]

Pharmaceutical Intervention

- Drug treatment for schizophrenia involves 2 main categories: first-generation antipsychotic drugs and second-generation antipsychotic drugs.
- First-generation antipsychotic drugs include chlorpromazine, fluphenazine, and haloperidol. These drugs are dopamine antagonists, which work by stopping dopamine from binding to its receptor. First-generation antipsychotics have a high risk of dangerous side effects including tardive dyskinesia (uncontrolled motor movements).
- Second-generation antipsychotic drugs include clozapine, olanzapine, risperidone, quetiapine, amisulpride, and ziprasidone. Second-generation antipsychotics are dopamine and serotonin antagonists. These drugs work by preventing dopamine and serotonin from binding to their receptor sites. They have considerably fewer side effects than first-generation drugs and are thus more widely prescribed.[68]

REFERENCES

1. Andreassi JL. *Psychophysiology: Human Behavior & Physiological Response.* 4th ed. New York, NY: Psychology Press; 2013.

2. Kruk ZL. *Neurotransmitters and Drugs.* New York, NY: Springer; 2014.

3. Del Arco A, Mora F. Neurotransmitters and prefrontal cortex–limbic system interactions: implications for plasticity and psychiatric disorders. *J Neural Transm.* 2009;116(8):941-952. doi:10.1007/s00702-009-0243-8.

4. Hurst R, Rollema H, Bertrand D. Nicotinic acetylcholine receptors: from basic science to therapeutics. *Pharmacol Therapeut.* 2013;137(1):22-54. doi:10.1016/j.pharmthera.2012.08.012.

5. Lund BM, Peck MW. *Clostridium Botulinum. Guide to Foodborne Pathogens.* 2nd ed. Wiley; 2013.

6. Hernandez CM, Dineley KT. α7 nicotinic acetylcholine receptors in Alzheimer's disease: neuroprotective, neurotrophic or both? *Curr Drug Targets.* 2012;13(5):613-622. doi:10.2174/138945012800398973.

7. Verschuuren JJ, Huijbers MG, Plomp JJ, et al. Pathophysiology of myasthenia gravis with antibodies to the acetylcholine receptor, muscle-specific kinase and low-density lipoprotein receptor-related protein 4. *Autoimmun Rev.* 2013;12(9): 918-923. doi:10.1016/j.autrev.2013.03.001.

8. Gao Y, Heldt SA. *Gamma-Aminobutyric Acid. Phobias: The Psychology of Irrational Fear.* Santa Barbara, CA: ABC-CLIO; 2015.

9. Möhler H. The GABA system in anxiety and depression and its therapeutic potential. *Neuropharmacology.* 2012;62(1): 42-53. doi:10.1016/j.neuropharm.2011.08.040.

10. Boulware MI, Heisler JD, Frick KM. The memory-enhancing effects of hippocampal estrogen receptor activation involve metabotropic glutamate receptor signaling. *J Neurosci.* 2013;33(38):15184-15194. doi: 10.1523/JNEUROSCI.1716-13.2013.

11. Ahmed I, Bose SK, Pavese N, et al. Glutamate NMDA receptor dysregulation in Parkinson's disease with dyskinesias. *Brain.* 2011;134(Pt 4):979-86. doi:10.1093/brain/awr028.

12. Ramoz N, Reichert JG, Smith CJ, et al. Linkage and association of the mitochondrial aspartate/glutamate carrier SLC25A12 gene with autism. *Am J Psychiatry.* 2014;161(4):662-669. doi:10.1176/appi.ajp.161.4.662.

13. Goff DC, Coyle JT. The emerging role of glutamate in the pathophysiology and treatment of schizophrenia. *Am J Psychiatry.* 2014;158(9):1367-1377. doi.org/10.1176/appi.ajp.158.9.1367.

14. Naylor DE. Glutamate and GABA in the balance: convergent pathways sustain seizures during status epilepticus. *Epilepsia.* 2010;51(s3):106-109. doi: 10.1111/j.1528-1167.2010.02622.x.

15. Nguyen D, Alavi MV, Kim KY, et al. A new vicious cycle involving glutamate excitotoxity, oxidative stress and mitochondrial dynamics. *Cell Death Disease.* 2011;2(12):e240. doi:10.1038/cddis.2011.117.

16. Gantz SC, Ford CP, Neve KA, Williams JT. Loss of Mecp2 in substantia nigra dopamine neurons compromises the nigrostriatal pathway. *J Neurosci.* 2011;31(35):12629-12637. doi: 10.1523/JNEUROSCI.0684-11.2011.

17. Beaulieu JM, Gainetdinov RR. The physiology, signaling, and pharmacology of dopamine receptors. *Pharmacol Rev.* 2011;63(1):182-217. doi:10.1124/pr.110.002642.

18. Sánchez-Danés A, Richaud-Patin Y, Carballo-Carbajal I, et al. Disease-specific phenotypes in dopamine neurons from human iPS-based models of genetic and sporadic Parkinson's disease. *EMBO Mol Med.* 2012;4(5):380-395. doi:10.1002/emmm.201200215.

19. Howes OD, Kambeitz J, Kim E, et al. The nature of dopamine dysfunction in schizophrenia and what this means for treatment: meta-analysis of imaging studies. *Arch Gen Psychiatry.* 2012;69(8):776-786. doi:10.1001/archgenpsychiatry.2012.

20. Seeman P. All roads to schizophrenia lead to dopamine supersensitivity and elevated dopamine D2High receptors. *CNS Neurosci Therapeut.* 2011;17(2):118-132. doi: 10.1111/j.1755-5949.2010.00162.x.

21. Volkow ND, Wang GJ, Fowler JS, Tomasi D, Telang F. Addiction: beyond dopamine reward circuitry. *Proc Natl Acad Sci U S A.* 2011;108(37):15037-15042. doi: 10.1073/pnas.1010654108.

22. Tye KM, Mirzabekov JJ, Warden MR, et al. Dopamine neurons modulate neural encoding and expression of depression-related behaviour. *Nature.* 2013;493(7433):537-541. doi:10.1038/nature11740.

23. Volkow ND, Wang GJ, Newcorn JH, et al. Motivation deficit in ADHD is associated with dysfunction of the dopamine reward pathway. *Mol Psychiatry.* 2011;16(11):1147-1154. doi:10.1038/mp.2010.97.

24. Risch N, Herrell R, Lehner T, et al. Interaction between the serotonin transporter gene (5-HTTLPR), stressful life events, and risk of depression: a meta-analysis. *JAMA.* 2009;301(23):2462-2471. doi:10.1001/jama.2009.878.

25. Ciarleglio CM, Resuehr HES, McMahon DG. Interactions of the serotonin and circadian systems: nature and nurture in rhythms and blues. *Neuroscience.* 2011;197:8-16. doi:10.1016/j.neuroscience.2011.09.036.

26. Thase ME, Haight BR, Richard N, et al. Remission rates following antidepressant therapy with bupropion or selective serotonin reuptake inhibitors: a meta-analysis of original data from 7 randomized controlled trials. *J Clin Psychiatry.* 2005;66(8):974-981.

27. Kramer PD. *Listening to Prozac.* Revised ed. New York, NY: Penguin Books; 2007.

28. Hakulinen C, Jokela M, Hintsanen M, et al. Serotonin receptor 1B genotype and hostility, anger and aggressive behavior through the lifespan: the Young Finns study. *J Behav Med.* 2013;36(6):583-590. doi:10.1007/s10865-012-9452-y.

29. Matsumoto R, Ichise M, Ito H, et al. Reduced serotonin transporter binding in the insular cortex in patients with obsessive-compulsive disorder: a [11 C] DASB PET study. *Neuroimage.* 2010;49(1):121-126. doi:10.1016/j.neuroimage.2009.07.069.

30. Lee. Y, Lin PY. Association between serotonin transporter gene polymorphism and eating disorders: a meta-analytic study. *Int J Eat Disord.* 2010;43(6):498-504. doi: 10.1002/eat.20732.

31. Aston-Jones G, Cohen JD. An integrative theory of locus coeruleus-norepinephrine function: adaptive gain and optimal performance. *Annu Rev Neurosci.* 2005;28:403-450. doi:10.1146/annurev.neuro.28.061604.135709.

32. Howells FM, Stein DJ, Russell VA. Synergistic tonic and phasic activity of the locus coeruleus norepinephrine (LC-NE) arousal system is required for optimal attentional performance. *Metabol Brain Dis.* 2012;27(3):267-274. doi:10.1007/s11011-012-9287-9.

33. Arnsten AF. Stimulants: therapeutic actions in ADHD. *Neuropsychopharmacology.* 2006;31(11):2376-2383. doi:10.1038/sj.npp.1301164.

34. Flannery G, Gehrig-Mills R, Billah B, Krum H. Analysis of randomized controlled trials on the effect of magnitude of heart rate reduction on clinical outcomes in patients with systolic chronic heart failure receiving beta-blockers. *Am J Cardiol.* 2008;101(6):865-869. doi:10.1016/j.amjcard.2007.11.023.

35. Machado M, Einarson TR. Comparison of SSRIs and SNRIs in major depressive disorder: a meta-analysis of head-to-head randomized clinical trials. *J Clin Pharm Therapeut.* 2010;35(2):177-188. doi:10.1111/j.1365-2710.2009.01050.x.

36. Abrahamsen B, Zhao J, Asante CO, et al. The cell and molecular basis of mechanical, cold, and inflammatory pain. *Science.* 2008;321(5889):702-705. doi:10.1126/science.1156916.

37. Finan PH, Zautra AJ. Fibromyalgia and fatigue: central processing, widespread dysfunction. *Phys Med Rehabil.* 2010;2(5):431-437. doi:10.1016/j.pmrj.2010.03.021.

38. Udenfriend S, Meienhofer J, eds. *Opioid Peptides: Biology, Chemistry, and Genetics: The Peptides: Analysis, Synthesis, Biology.* Vol. 6; reprint of original edition. New York, NY: Academic Press; 2014.

39. Sun Y, Gan TJ, Dubose JW, Habib AS. Acupuncture and related techniques for postoperative pain: a systematic review of randomized controlled trials. *Br J Anaesth.* 2008;101(2):151-160.doi: 10.1093/bja/aen146.

40. Gosnell BA, Levine AS. Reward systems and food intake: role of opioids. *Int J Obesity.* 2009;33:S54-S58. doi:10.1038/ijo.2009.73.

41. Haas HL, Sergeeva OA, Selbach O. Histamine in the nervous system. *Physiol Rev.* 2008;88(3):1183-1241. doi:10.1152/physrev.00043.2007.

42. American Psychiatric Association. *Diagnostic and Statistical Manual of Mental Disorders.* 5th ed. Arlington, VA: American Psychiatric Association; 2013.

43. Hedges DW, Brown BL, Shwalb DA, Godfrey K, Larcher AM. The efficacy of selective serotonin reuptake inhibitors in adult social anxiety disorder: a meta-analysis of double-blind, placebo-controlled trials. *J Psychopharmacol.* 2007;21(1):102-111. doi: 10.1177/0269881106065102.

44. Xu W, Gray DL, Glase SA, Barta NS. Design and synthesis of reboxetine analogs morpholine derivatives as selective norepinephrine reuptake inhibitors. *Bioorganic Med Chem Lett.* 2008;18(20):5550-5553. doi:10.1016/j.bmcl.2008.09.007.

45. Montgomery SA. Tolerability of serotonin norepinephrine reuptake inhibitor antidepressants. *CNS Spectrums.* 2008;13(S11):27-33. doi:10.1017/S1092852900028297.

46. El Mansari M, Guiard BP, Chernoloz O, Ghanbari R, Katz N, Blier P. Relevance of norepinephrine–dopamine interactions in the treatment of major depressive disorder. *CNS Neurosci Therapeut.* 2010;16(3):e1-e17. doi:10.1111/j.1755-5949.2010.00146.x.

47. Fangmann P, Assion HJ, Juckel G, González CÁ, López-Muñoz F. Half a century of antidepressant drugs: on the clinical introduction of monoamine oxidase inhibitors, tricyclics, and tetracyclics. Part II: tricyclics and tetracyclics. *J Clin Psychopharmacol.* 2008;28(1):1-4. doi: 10.1097/jcp.0b013e3181627b60.

48. Zajecka JM, Zajecka AM. A clinical overview of monoamine oxidase inhibitors: pharmacological profile, efficacy, safety/tolerability, and strategies for successful outcomes in the management of major depressive disorders. *Psychiatr Ann.* 2014;44(11):513. doi:10.3928/00485713-20141106-07.

49. Swedo SE, Leonard HL, Garvey M, et al. Pediatric autoimmune neuropsychiatric disorders associated with streptococcal infections. *FOCUS.* 2014;2(3):496-506. doi:10.1176/foc.2.3.496.

50. Welter ML, Burbaud P, Fernandez-Vidal S, et al. Basal ganglia dysfunction in OCD: subthalamic neuronal activity correlates with symptoms severity and predicts high-frequency stimulation efficacy. *Translat Psychiatry.* 2011;1(5):e5. doi:10.1038/tp.2011.5.

51. Koran LM, Hackett E, Rubin A, Wolkow R, Robinson D. Efficacy of sertraline in the long-term treatment of obsessive-compulsive disorder. *Am J Psychiatry*. 2014;159(1):88-95. doi:10.1176/appi.ajp.159.1.88.

52. Marcourakis T, Bernik MA, Neto FL, Shavitt RG, Gorenstein C. Clomipramine demethylation rate is important on the outcome of obsessive–compulsive disorder treatment. *Int Clin Psychopharmacol*. 2015;30(1):43-48. doi: 10.1097/YIC.0000000000000050.

53. Mathew SJ, Coplan JD, Gorman JM. Neurobiological mechanisms of social anxiety disorder. *Am J Psychiatry*. 2014;158(10):1558-1567. doi:10.1176/appi.ajp.158.10.1558.

54. Offidani E, Guidi J, Tomba E, Fava GA. Efficacy and tolerability of benzodiazepines versus antidepressants in anxiety disorders: a systematic review and meta-analysis. *Psychother Psychosomat*. 2013;82(6):355-362. doi:10.1159/000353198.

55. Garakani A, Murrough JW, Iosifescu DV. Advances in psychopharmacology for anxiety disorders. *Psychopharmacology*. 2014;12(2):152-162. doi:10.1176/appi.focus.12.2.152.

56. Reinares M, Rosa AR, Franco C, et al. A systematic review on the role of anticonvulsants in the treatment of acute bipolar depression. *Int J Neuropsychopharmacol*. 2013;16(2):485-496. doi:10.1017/S1461145712000491.

57. Pollack MH, Matthews J, Scott EL. Gabapentin as a potential treatment for anxiety disorders. *Am J Psychiatry*. 2014;155(7):992-993. doi:10.1176/ajp.155.7.992.

58. Wang HR, Woo YS, Bahk WM. Anticonvulsants to treat post-traumatic stress disorder. *Hum Psychopharmacol Clin Exper*. 2014;29(5):427-433. doi: 10.1002/hup.2425.

59. Smink FR, van Hoeken D, Hoek HW. Epidemiology of eating disorders: incidence, prevalence and mortality rates. *Curr Psychiatr Rep*. 2012;14(4):406-414. doi: 10.1007/s11920-012-0282-y.

60. Bailer UF, Kaye WH. Serotonin: imaging findings in eating disorders. *Behav Neurobiol Eat Disord*. 2011;6:59-79. doi:10.1007/7854_2010_78.

61. Compan V, Laurent L, Jean A, Macary C, Bockaert J, Dumuis A. Serotonin signaling in eating disorders. *Wiley Interdiscip Rev Membr Transp Signal*. 2012;1(6):715-729. doi: 10.1002/wmts.45.

62. Mischoulon D, Eddy KT, Keshaviah A, et al. Depression and eating disorders: treatment and course. *J Affect Disord*. 2011;130(3):470-477. doi:10.1016/j.jad.2010.10.043.

63. Milano W, De Rosa M, Milano L, Riccio A, Sanseverino B, Capasso A. A comparative study between three different SSRIs in the treatment of bulimia nervosa. *Curr Neurobiol*. 2013;4(1&2):39-42.

64. Mas S, Plana MT, Castro-Fornieles J, et al. Common genetic background in anorexia nervosa and obsessive compulsive disorder: preliminary results from an association study. *J Psychiatr Res*. 2013;47(6):747-754. doi:10.1016/j.jpsychires.2012.12.015.

65. Perlstein WM, Carter CS, Noll DC, Cohen JD. Relation of prefrontal cortex dysfunction to working memory and symptoms in schizophrenia. *Am J Psychiatry*. 2001;158(7):1105-1113. doi:10.1176/appi.ajp.158.7.1105.

66. Karlsson P, Farde L, Halldin C, Sedvall G. PET study of D1 dopamine receptor binding in neuroleptic-naive patients with schizophrenia. *Am J Psychiatry*. 2002;159(5):761-767. doi:10.1176/appi.ajp.159.5.761.

67. Goff DC, Coyle JT. The emerging role of glutamate in the pathophysiology and treatment of schizophrenia. *Am J Psychiatry*. 2001;158(9):1367-1377. doi:10.1176/appi.ajp.158.9.1367.

68. Cannon TD, Huttunen MO, Dahlström M, Larmo I, Räsänen P, Juriloo A. Antipsychotic drug treatment in the prodromal phase of schizophrenia. *Am J Psychiatry*. 2002;159(7):1230-1232. doi:10.1176/appi.ajp.159.7.1230.

The Neurologic Substrates of Addiction

- Addiction is a neurobiological phenomenon that is rooted in genetic factors.
- The most recent research regarding the addiction process suggests the following:
  - A person's risk for addiction is influenced by genetic, neurochemical, and environmental factors.
  - Once the brain becomes addicted to a substance, it may always remain in an addicted state unless pharmaceutical and psychosocial intervention are obtained.
  - An addicted brain remains in this state despite years of abstinence.
- The course of addiction is characterized by repeated remission and relapse. Remission and relapse are largely regulated by neurological processes rather than indicative of weak moral character or poor volitional control.[1,2]

THE ADDICTION EXPERIENCE

- Initially, the high produced by alcohol or other substances is experienced as a pleasurable sensation by the user.
- Then, very quickly and after repeated exposure to the substance, the amount that initially produced feelings of euphoria is no longer effective.
- People find that they require more of the substance to produce the sensation of well-being.
- The euphoria of the initial high is never obtained again. Instead, people require greater and greater amounts of the substance just to feel normal. Without the substance, they become depressed, irritable, and often physically ill.
- At this point, addiction takes hold, and people commonly lose control over their intended use, often ingesting far more than anticipated and for longer amounts of time.
- The brain has now become addicted to the substance and begins to elicit the severe cravings that drive people to relapse. Such neurochemically driven cravings compel people to seek and use substances despite clear feedback that the addiction is harming their health, finances, and relationships.[3]

NEUROBIOLOGY OF THE ADDICTION PROCESS

The Brain's Reward System: The Mesolimbic Dopamine System

- The euphoria induced by substances of abuse occurs as a result of their effect on the brain's reward system.
- The brain's reward system is called the *mesocorticolimbic*, or *mesolimbic*, *system*. This system consists of a complex circuit of neurons that evolved to encourage people to repeat pleasurable behavior that supports survival. For example, eating, quenching thirst, and sexual behavior all produce surges of pleasurable neurochemicals in the mesolimbic system.
- Researchers have demonstrated that chronic substance use can cause changes in the structure and function of the mesolimbic system that can last for years after a person's last substance use experience.
- There are 3 primary changes in the brain's reward system:
  1. *Tolerance*: when the substance is used chronically, it no longer elicits the same pleasurable feelings.
  2. *Cravings*: the addicted brain produces intense cravings for the substance that cause an escalation in substance use.

Gutman SA. *Quick Reference Neuroscience for Rehabilitation Professionals: The Essential Neurologic Principles Underlying Rehabilitation Practice, Third Edition* (pp 354-364). © 2017 Taylor & Francis Group.

3. *Sensitization*: in a period of abstinence, the brain adapts to the lack of substance by becoming highly sensitized to the substance, so that ingestion of the substance after periods of abstinence is experienced with heightened pleasure. This often causes relapse.

- These changes in the mesolimbic system, in response to chronic substance use, trap people in a destructive spiral of escalating use, attempts at abstinence, and repeated relapse.[4]

Neuroanatomical Structures of the Mesolimbic System

- The mesolimbic system is a set of interrelated neuroanatomical structures of the cortex, midbrain, and limbic system.
- This system is able to interpret whether behavior is rewarding or aversive and sends this information to other brain areas that function in decision making and action.
- The primary neural pathway of the mesolimbic system originates in the ventral tegmental area of the midbrain. This area sends projections to the nucleus accumbens, which is located deep beneath the frontal cortex.
- The primary neurotransmitter used by this system is dopamine.
- Almost all drugs of abuse have the potential to become addictive because of their ability to increase dopamine levels in the brain's reward system.
- Drugs of abuse activate the system with an intensity and persistence that far exceed that of nonaddicting substances, which can also trigger the reward system (such as eating and sex).[5]
- The ventral tegmental area of the midbrain acts as a meter that measures reward. It sends signals to other brain regions with information about how pleasurable a specific substance or behavior is.[6]
- The amygdala is a limbic system structure that also has a role in the interpretation of whether a behavior is pleasurable or aversive. When the amygdala is lesioned, individuals no longer link pleasure to its cause.
- The amygdala has connections with the hippocampus, another limbic system structure. The hippocampus records and stores the memories of emotionally laden events, such as the euphoria of a drug-induced state or the extreme irritability and physical illness associated with withdrawal.[7]
- These subcortical structures send messages to the frontal lobes of the cortex, which processes this information on a conscious level and uses it to make decisions and initiate action.[5-7]

Addiction Also Involves Distorted Learning and Memory

- In addition to the neurochemical addiction of the brain, the process of addiction involves a distorted type of learning and memory.
- Researchers have shown that addiction is associated with alterations in the frontal lobe that produce the following[8]:
  ○ An overvaluing of the reward
  ○ An undervaluing of the risks associated with obtaining the reward
  ○ A diminished ability to connect addictive behaviors with their negative consequences

Priming

- Another cognitive distortion related to addiction is called *priming*.
- Priming is a phenomenon in which people learn to associate the euphoria of a drug-induced state with the objects and people involved in the process of drug use.[9]
- For example, the sight of white lines on a mirror can produce anticipatory pleasure that activates the same areas of the brain as actual consumption of the substance.
- Any sensory stimuli associated with drug seeking and obtaining can cause priming and relapse (ie, visual images of the substance, the paraphernalia used to ingest the substance, and the smell or taste of the substance).
- Researchers have shown that when cocaine addicts are shown videos of someone using cocaine, the structures of the mesolimbic system light up on functional magnetic resonance imaging (fMRI) and positron emission tomography (PET) scans.[10] The same regions respond similarly when compulsive gamblers are shown images of slot machines.[11] This finding suggests that the mesolimbic system responds similarly in nondrug addictions such as gambling, eating disorders, and compulsive shopping.

Dopamine

- All drugs of abuse cause the nucleus accumbens to receive a flood of dopamine. Repeatedly dosing the brain with addictive drugs is akin to a chemical assault that alters the structure of neurons in the brain's reward system.
- There is evidence that people with low levels of dopamine D2 receptors are at greater risk for addiction and substance abuse.
- People with low levels of D2 receptors may be less able to experience feelings of pleasure from activities that are commonly intrinsically rewarding, such as engaging in enjoyable hobbies or eating tasteful foods.
- Researchers have also shown that people with low D2 receptor levels are more likely to be obese or possess a binge-eating disorder. Low levels of D2 receptors may compel people to overeat to feel satiated and a sense of gratification from food.[12]
- Deficient levels of D2 receptors have also been linked to a range of compulsive behaviors, including excessive hand washing and checking disorders (as seen in obsessive-compulsive disorder [OCD]).[13]

Delta FosB

- Delta FosB is a gene transcription factor that has been identified in all forms of behavioral and substance addictions. Overexpression of Delta FosB in the D1 neurons of the nucleus accumbens results in neuroplastic changes in the brain's reward centers.
- Delta FosB increases a user's sensitivity to a substance and may be responsible for the experience of cravings and relapse.
- The genetic overexpression of Delta FosB can be used as a biomarker of addiction.[14]

Tolerance and Dependence

- Tolerance and dependence occur in the early stages of addiction. Tolerance occurs when a drug makes the brain less responsive to that drug. The reward response of the mesolimbic system becomes diminished and people experience depressed mood and motivation.
- Consuming more of the substance is the easiest and quickest way for people to feel normal again.
- Dependence involves the physical illness that occurs when the drug is not consumed.
- Both tolerance and dependence occur because chronic drug use suppresses the brain's reward circuits.
- Chronic drug use causes neural receptors in the mesolimbic system to adapt by resisting the drug, thereby increasing the need for higher doses just to feel normal.[15]
- The neurophysiologic mechanism that underlies tolerance and dependence involves a molecule known as *CREB* (cAMP [cyclic adenosine monophosphate] response element-binding protein).
- CREB is a protein that regulates the expression of genes. When drugs of abuse are consumed, dopamine levels increase in the nucleus accumbens, causing the eventual activation of CREB.
- Chronic drug use causes sustained activation of CREB, which eventually dampens the responsiveness of the brain's reward system.[16]

Sensitization

- Sensitization is a heightened response to a substance of abuse after a period of abstinence.
- After a period of abstinence from the substance, which could last for weeks, months, or even years, the brain responds to re-exposure to the substance with increased sensitivity.
- Sensitization is a neurobiological process that can cause relapse even after years of abstinence.
- Shortly after repeated exposure to a substance, CREB activity is high and tolerance to the substance increases. During this period, people need increasingly greater amounts of the drug to trigger the brain's reward pathways.
- However, if the person abstains from substance use, CREB activity declines. It is at this point that tolerance begins to lessen and sensitization becomes the dominant process, setting off the intense cravings that drive compulsive drug seeking.[17]

Glutamate's Role in Sensitization

- Glutamate is a neurotransmitter important in learning and the formation of memories.
- Substances of abuse alter the sensitivity of glutamate in the ventral tegmental area and the nucleus accumbens for extended periods of time.
- Researchers suggest that this state of prolonged heightened glutamate sensitivity strengthens the neural pathways of memories that link substance use with reward. This phenomenon appears to serve as the basis for the formation of memories that distort the substance abuse experience.
- People tend to remember their experience as more positive and enjoyable than it actually was. They also tend to undervalue the risks associated with substance abuse and appear unable to connect their addiction to real-life negative consequences.[18]

ADDICTION TO COMPULSIVE BEHAVIORS

- In addition to substances, people can develop addictions to compulsive behaviors.
- Addiction is any repeated behavior that produces a chemical change in the brain's reward system, thus compelling the individual to repeat the addicting behavior.[19]
- Addiction commonly involves the following:
  - Unsuccessful attempts to reduce, stop, or control one's use of the addictive substance or behavior
  - Neglect of major life role obligations and responsibilities
  - Increasingly greater time spent participating in addictive behaviors
  - Continued substance abuse or participation in behaviors despite health, financial, work, and family-related problems
- The addiction literature extends the definition of addiction to compulsive behaviors that meet these criteria. In addition to substance use, addiction also involves compulsive behaviors such as the following[20]:
  - Eating disorders (anorexia, bulimia, compulsive binge eating)
  - Work (workaholism)
  - Relationships/sex
  - Gambling
  - Shopping
  - Kleptomania
  - Exercise
  - Video gaming and Internet overuse
- These repeated behaviors cause a chemical change in the brain that produces a sense of well-being.[19]

Addictions Can Also Involve Obsessions

- Obsessions are recurrent ideas that invade consciousness.
- Obsessions are mediated by neural circuits that appear to originate in the basal ganglia.
- The abnormality in the neural pathway involves recurrent electrical brain waves that will not stop firing; in other words, the messages running in the pathway will not shut off.
- Researchers have long known that a link exists between obsessive thoughts and the need to act out compulsive behaviors. The basal ganglia appear to play an important role in this phenomenon.
- The basal ganglia are a part of the primitive survival centers in the brain.
- Obsessions involve ideas and behaviors that are often linked with survival and control (eg, food, money and possessions, and cleanliness and order).
- OCD is a component of all addictions.
- The etiology of OCD is believed to be rooted in the same dysfunction of the serotonin and dopamine systems that is believed to underlie the addiction process.[21]

- OCD often involves obsessions with the following[22]:
  - Symmetry of objects
  - Checking behaviors
  - Cleanliness
  - Orderliness
  - Counting
  - Invasive thoughts about sex, religion, or catastrophic events
  - Invasive music that runs through the mind repetitively

Serotonin as an Obsession Blocker

- Serotonin helps to shut off the neural circuits that cause obsessive-compulsive behaviors.
- The selective serotonin reuptake inhibitors (SSRIs) increase serotonin levels in the brain and have shown effectiveness in the treatment of OCD.[23]

Addictive Behaviors Can Be Cross-Addicting

- People with addictions often leave rehabilitation programs and remain abstinent from their former addictive behaviors only to switch to another addictive substance or compulsive behavior.
- For example, a person with a gambling disorder may remain free of gambling behaviors after rehabilitation but may begin to shop compulsively.
- Switching from one substance or compulsive behavior to another occurs because treatment did not address the neurochemical mechanisms maintaining the brain in an addicted state.
- The addicted brain activates cravings that compel the person to use a similar substance or engage in a comparable compulsive behavior that will positively affect the brain's reward circuits.
- Individuals often recover from one addiction only to go to another.[24]

Addictive Behaviors Are Heritable

- There is considerable evidence that addictive behaviors are genetically and neurochemically based.
- The same deficiency in the serotonin and dopamine systems that underlies addictive behaviors tends to run in families.
- While the neurophysiologic substrates of addiction may be similar in members of the same family, the type of addiction that emerges in individual members may be different.
- For example, it is common to observe that children of alcoholics often have OCD or eating disorders, and vice versa.
- As a result of cultural influences, environmental factors, and unique psychological makeup, people in the same biological family group may have similar deficiencies in the serotonin and dopamine systems that are expressed as distinctly different addictive behaviors.[25]

Treating the Addicted Brain

- Pharmaceutical advances in addiction treatment have largely addressed physical dependence and withdrawal.
- In contrast, it has been more difficult to develop effective medications that address craving and relapse, the actual processes that maintain addiction.
- Interventions that do not address craving and relapse are unable to treat the brain's addicted state. This is the main factor accounting for the ineffectiveness of most addiction treatment; intervention may address dependence, withdrawal, and environmental stressors but leaves the brain in an addicted state.
- People who have received intervention that leaves the brain in an addicted state have a high likelihood of relapse.[26]

Three Primary Approaches to Pharmaceutical Treatment

1. Medication that prevents a drug from reaching its neurologic target, thus rendering the drug's effects inert
2. Medication that mimics a drug's action without causing the deleterious effects of the addictive substance, thereby reducing cravings
3. Medication that stops the neurologic addiction process, thus eliminating cravings, sensitization, and relapse[27]

Blocking Drug Targets

- The most common pharmaceutical approach to treat addiction involves blocking the substance from reaching its neurologic target.
- Naltrexone is a narcotic antagonist used to treat opiate and alcohol addiction.
- Naltrexone was designed to block opiate receptors in the brain, thereby preventing opiate action.
- It also triggers a withdrawal reaction in people who are physically dependent upon opiates.
- Studies have shown that naltrexone can reduce the risk of relapse in the first 3 months after withdrawal by 36%.
- However, because naltrexone does not stop cravings, many people who begin its use eventually stop taking the medication.
- Polysubstance abuse is also problematic. While naltrexone blocks the effects of opiates, it has no effect on other illicit drugs.[28]

Mimicking Drug Action

- Medications that block drug targets do not address craving; thus, relapse is likely.
- In contrast, medications that attempt to mimic a drug's action in the brain can alleviate cravings that can cause relapse.
- Methadone is a long-acting opioid receptor agonist used in the treatment of heroin addiction.
- Because of methadone's long half-life, people taking the medication have a low level of sustained opioid receptor activation. This prevents cravings and enables people to return to a more stable employment and family life.
- Methadone maintenance is controversial, as some believe that it legally reinforces opiate addiction.
- However, methadone maintenance has a significant amount of research supporting its effectiveness.
- Studies show that people on methadone maintenance are less depressed, more likely to maintain stable employment and family lives, are less likely to commit crimes, and are less likely to contract HIV or hepatitis.
- Methadone and other long-acting opioid agonists, such as levo-alpha-acetylmethadol, are effective because they allow the brain to believe that it is receiving the addictive substance without causing the deleterious effects of that substance.[29,30]

Halting the Addiction Process

- To truly end the addiction process and relapse, medication must both alleviate cravings and stop sensitization.
- While medications have been developed that can block drug targets and mimic drug action, it has been more difficult to design medication that addresses both craving and sensitization, the primary factors that maintain addiction.
- To date, while such medications are in development, they remain untested in humans.[28-30]

REFERENCES

1. Kalivas PW, Volkow ND. The neural basis of addiction: a pathology of motivation and choice. *Am J Psychiatry.* 2005;162(8):1403-1413. doi:10.1176/appi.ajp.162.8.1403.

2. Koob GF, Volkow ND. Neurocircuitry of addiction. *Neuropsychopharmacology.* 2010;35(1):217-238. doi:10.1038/npp.2009.

3. Addolorato G, Abenavoli L, Leggio L, Gasbarrini G. How many cravings? Pharmacological aspects of craving treatment in alcohol addiction: a review. *Neuropsychobiology.* 2005;51(2):59-66. doi:10.1159/000084161.

4. Pitchers KK, Balfour ME, Lehman MN, Richtand NM, Yu L, Coolen LM. Neuroplasticity in the mesolimbic system induced by natural reward and subsequent reward abstinence. *Biol Psychiatry.* 2010;67(9):872-879. doi:10.1016/j.biopsych.2009.09.036.

5. Russo SJ, Dietz DM, Dumitriu D, Morrison JH, Malenka RC, Nestler EJ. The addicted synapse: mechanisms of synaptic and structural plasticity in nucleus accumbens. *Trends Neurosci.* 2010;33(6):267-276. doi:10.1016/j.tins.2010.02.002.

6. Niehaus JL, Murali M, Kauer JA. Drugs of abuse and stress impair LTP at inhibitory synapses in the ventral tegmental area. *Eur J Neurosci.* 2010;32(1):108-117. doi:10.1111/j.1460-9568.2010.07256.x.

7. Belujon P, Grace AA. Hippocampus, amygdala, and stress: interacting systems that affect susceptibility to addiction. *Ann N Y Acad Sci.* 2011;1216(1):114-121. doi:10.1111/j.1749-6632.2010.05896.x.

8. Torregrossa MM, Corlett PR, Taylor JR. Aberrant learning and memory in addiction. *Neurobiol Learn Mem.* 2011;96(4):609-623. doi:10.1016/j.nlm.2011.02.014.

9. Everitt BJ, Robbins TW. Neural systems of reinforcement for drug addiction: from actions to habits to compulsion. *Nat Neurosci.* 2005;8(11):1481-1489. doi:10.1038/nn1579.

10. Thomas MJ, Kalivas PW, Shaham Y. Neuroplasticity in the mesolimbic dopamine system and cocaine addiction. *Br J Pharmacol.* 2008;154(2):327-342. doi:10.1038/bjp.2008.77.

11. Potenza MN. The neurobiology of pathological gambling and drug addiction: an overview and new findings. *Phil Transact R Soc B Biol Sci.* 2008;363(1507):3181-3189. doi:10.1098/rstb.2008.0100.

12. Davis C, Levitan RD, Yilmaz Z, Kaplan AS, Carter JC, Kennedy JL. Binge eating disorder and the dopamine D2 receptor: genotypes and sub-phenotypes. *Prog Neuropsychopharmacol Biol Psychiatry.* 2012;38(2):328-335. doi:10.1016/j.pnpbp.2012.05.002.

13. Schneier FR, Martinez D, Abi-Dargham A, et al. Striatal dopamine D2 receptor availability in OCD with and without comorbid social anxiety disorder: preliminary findings. *Depression Anxiety.* 2008;25(1):1-7. doi: 10.1002/da.20268.

14. Vialou V, Robison AJ, LaPlant QC, et al. [Delta] FosB in brain reward circuits mediates resilience to stress and antidepressant responses. *Nat Neurosci.* 2010;13(6):745-752. doi:10.1038/nn.2551.

15. Hyman SE, Malenka RC, Nestler EJ. Neural mechanisms of addiction: the role of reward-related learning and memory. *Annu Rev Neurosci.* 2006;29:565-598. 10.1146/annurev.neuro.29.051605.113009.

16. McPherson CS, Lawrence AJ. The nuclear transcription factor CREB: involvement in addiction, deletion models and looking forward. *Curr Neuropharmacol.* 2007;5(3):202. doi:10.2174/157015907781695937.

17. Leao RM, Cruz FC, Marin MT, da Silva Planeta C. Stress induces behavioral sensitization, increases nicotine-seeking behavior and leads to a decrease of CREB in the nucleus accumbens. *Pharmacol Biochem Behav.* 2012;101(3):434-442. doi:10.1016/j.pbb.2012.01.025.

18. Kalivas PW, LaLumiere RT, Knackstedt L, Shen H. Glutamate transmission in addiction. *Neuropharmacology.* 2009;56:169-173. doi:10.1016/j.neuropharm.2008.07.011.

19. Voon V, Pessiglione M, Brezing C, et al. Mechanisms underlying dopamine-mediated reward bias in compulsive behaviors. *Neuron.* 2010;65(1):135-142. doi:10.1016/j.neuron.2009.12.027.

20. Frascella J, Potenza MN, Brown LL, Childress AR. Shared brain vulnerabilities open the way for nonsubstance addictions: carving addiction at a new joint?. *Ann N Y Acad Sci.* 2010;1187(1):294-315. doi:10.1111/j.1749-6632.2009.05420.x.

21. Fontenelle LF, Oostermeijer S, Harrison BJ, Pantelis C, Yücel M. Obsessive compulsive disorder, impulse control disorders and drug addiction. *Drugs.* 2011;71(7):827-840. doi:10.2165/11591790-000000000-00000.

22. American Psychiatric Association. *Diagnostic and Statistical Manual of Mental Disorders.* 5th ed. Arlington, VA: American Psychiatric Association; 2013.

23. Besiroglu L, Çetinkaya N, Selvi Y, Atli A. Effects of selective serotonin reuptake inhibitors on thought-action fusion, metacognitions, and thought suppression in obsessive-compulsive disorder. *Compr Psychiatry.* 2011;52(5):556-561. doi:10.1016/j.comppsych.2010.10.003.

24. Sussman S, Black DS. Substitute addiction: a concern for researchers and practitioners. *J Drug Educ.* 2008;38(2):167-180. doi: 10.2190/DE.38.2.e.

25. Agrawal A, Lynskey MT. Are there genetic influences on addiction: evidence from family, adoption and twin studies. *Addiction.* 2008;103(7):1069-1081. doi: 10.1111/j.1360-0443.2008.02213.x.

26. Spanagel R, Vengeliene V. New pharmacological treatment strategies for relapse prevention. *Addiction.* 2013;13:583-609. doi:10.1007/978-3-642-28720-6_205.

27. Lobmaier P, Gossop M, Waal H, Bramness J. The pharmacological treatment of opioid addiction—a clinical perspective. *Eur J Clin Pharmacol.* 2010;66(6):537-545. doi:10.1007/s00228-010-0793-6.

28. Krupitsky E, Nunes EV, Ling W, Illeperuma A, Gastfriend DR, Silverman BL. Injectable extended-release naltrexone for opioid dependence: a double-blind, placebo-controlled, multicentre randomised trial. *Lancet.* 2011;377(9776):1506-1513. doi:10.1016/S0140-6736(11)60358-9.

29. Kleber HD. Methadone maintenance 4 decades later. *JAMA.* 2008;300(19):2303-2305. doi:10.1001/jama.2008.648.

30. Anglin MD, Conner BT, Annon J, Longshore D. Levo-alpha-acetylmethadol (LAAM) versus methadone maintenance: 1-year treatment retention, outcomes and status. *Addiction.* 2007;102(9):1432-1442. doi: 10.1055/s-0028-1083818.

CLINICAL TEST QUESTIONS

Sections 28 to 30

1. After Joaquim's football accident in which he injured his brachial plexus, he has numbness, weakness, and paresthesias in his right forearm and hand. Joaquim's physician is sending him for a test that evaluates the presence of peripheral nerve disorder. This test involves the insertion of thin needles into specific muscles to detect electrical activity. This test is called:

   a. myelogram

   b. electroencephalogram

   c. electromyelogram

   d. computed tomography

2. Mateo's doctors ordered this test after he was admitted to the emergency room with an acute spinal cord injury. This test uses magnets and radio waves to detect subtle electromagnetic fields in soft tissue. This test can provide high resolution images of Mateo's injury level and is called:

   a. positron emission tomography

   b. magnetic resonance imaging

   c. single photon emission tomography

   d. computed tomography

3. Mr. Polito has been diagnosed with myasthenia gravis. This disease is caused when the body inappropriately produces antibodies against a specific neurotransmitter receptor site. This neurotransmitter is stored in the neuromuscular junction and is responsible for musculoskeletal movement. When this neurotransmitter is inhibited, muscle weakness and fatigue occur. This neurotransmitter is called:

   a. GABA

   b. dopamine

   c. norepinephrine

   d. acetylcholine

4. Mrs. Marrero has been diagnosed with Parkinson disease. The loss of this neurotransmitter from the substantia nigra and the nigrostriatal pathway is a primary cause of Parkinson disease, causing movement paucity, festinating gait, and masked face. This neurotransmitter is called:

   a. dopamine

   b. serotonin

   c. norepinephrine

   d. glutamate

5. Adelphi has obsessive compulsive disorder (OCD) and depression. One primary neurotransmitter that has been shown to be associated with disruption in sleep-wake cycles, eating disorders, OCD, depression, and aggression is:

   a. norepinephrine

   b. serotonin

   c. substance P

   d. glutamate

6. This neuropeptide acts as a neurotransmitter in the nociceptive pathway and is involved in the transmission of pain sensation.

   a. glutamate

   b. dopamine

   c. substance P

   d. endorphins

7. While the previous neurotransmitter is responsible for pain sensation, the neuropeptide called _____ is responsible for the inhibition of pain and is referred to as *the body's natural painkiller*.
   a. dopamine
   b. GABA
   c. serotonin
   d. opioid (endorphin, enkephalin, dynorphin)

8. Johnson is addicted to cocaine use. When this neurotransmitter reaches heightened levels in the brain's mesolimbic system (the reward center), the brain becomes addicted to a substance and induces cravings that compel a person to engage in substance use again.
   a. dopamine
   b. serotonin
   c. glutamate
   d. GABA

9. _____ occurs when a drug makes the brain less responsive to that specific substance. The reward response of the mesolimbic system becomes diminished, and people need greater amounts of the substance to feel pleasure.
   a. tolerance
   b. priming
   c. cravings
   d. sensitization

10. _____ is a heightened response to a substance after a period of abstinence. The brain responds to re-exposure of the substance with increased pleasure. This phenomenon is the mechanism that commonly causes relapse after periods of abstinence.
    a. tolerance
    b. priming
    c. cravings
    d. sensitization

Answers

1. c
2. b
3. d
4. a
5. b
6. c
7. d
8. a
9. a
10. d

Neurologic Mechanisms of Memory

EARLY THEORIES ABOUT MEMORY

- Early theories describing memory were based on a computer model.
- Memories were compared to computer files that could be placed in storage and pulled up into consciousness when needed.
- Today, more is known about how memory works. Information has been gained through experimental research and research on patients with cerebral damage.

MEMORY IS NOT A FACTUAL-BASED RECORD OF REALITY

- Our memories are not passive or literal recordings of reality.
- Instead, our memories are recreations of specific events that become distorted and lose accuracy over time.
- For example, members of one family commonly find that each person's memory of a specific event differs significantly from the way that other family members recall that event. Some members have forgotten the memory entirely, while others adamantly recall the event's occurrence. Some family members insist that the sequence of events occurred differently from the way others recall it.
- People rarely recall all of the details in an event accurately.
- We often recall occurrences that made general sense or fit our expectations of what should have happened but were not actually part of the original event.[1]
- False memories have become highly debated in recent years as reports of early childhood abuse are questioned. Some have asked if false memories are the product of psychological techniques that induce memories of events that never occurred.[2]

MEMORIES ARE ENCODED BY BRAIN NETWORKS

- A person's experience is encoded by brain networks involving multiple cerebral structures. There is no single anatomical structure that alone deals with memory functions.
- PET scans have enabled researchers to observe the brain in action while people remember specific events.
- Memories are encoded by brain networks whose connections have already been shaped by previous encounters with the world.
- This pre-existing structure powerfully influences how individuals encode and store new memories. It influences what an individual will remember and why.
- Memories that have a strong emotional significance appear to be more readily remembered. This may occur because the hippocampus and the amygdala (both limbic system emotional centers) play an important role in the storage of long-term memories (LTM) that have a strong emotional component.[3]

Gutman SA. *Quick Reference Neuroscience for Rehabilitation Professionals:*
The Essential Neurologic Principles Underlying Rehabilitation Practice,
Third Edition (pp 366-375).
© 2017 Taylor & Francis Group.

- LTMs that have emotional significance are also subject to distortion based on an individual's psychological interpretation of an event.
- Human memory is thus predisposed to corruption by suggestive influences. Memories more likely involve distortions of reality rather than being factual snapshots or video.[2]

TYPES OF MEMORY

Short-Term Memory

- Short-term memory (STM) is the ability to remember others and events encountered less than 1 hour ago.
- STM is limited by capacity, or the amount of information that can be held at any given time.
- STM is also limited by duration, the length of time items can be held before decay occurs. This time limit is considered by many researchers to be roughly seconds. Clinically, when patients cannot remember events that occurred several minutes or hours ago, they are said to exhibit STM deficits.[4]

Working Memory

- Working memory is a subcomponent of STM and involves moment-to-moment awareness.
- Working memory also plays a role in the search and retrieval of archived information. We use working memory in the temporary storage and use of information.[5]

Long-Term Memory

- LTM is the ability to remember one's past, familiar others, and events encountered more than several hours ago.
- LTM is dependent on the ability to encode items from STM into LTM storage, as well as the ability to search for and retrieve items from LTM so that they can be used in the moment by working memory processes.[6]

Recent Memory

- Recent memory is considered to be a component of LTM. Recent memory refers to the ability to recall events/information that occurred hours to weeks ago.[7,8]

Remote Memory

- Remote memory is a component of LTM and refers to the ability to recall events/information that occurred in the distant past (eg, several years ago).[7,8]

Prospective Memory

- Prospective memory is the ability to remember to carry out an event in the future (eg, remembering to attend an appointment with your primary care physician).[7,8]

Semantic Memory

- Semantic memory involves the recall of facts (eg, dates of people's birthdays, state capitals, the names of presidents).
- Semantic memory includes the definitions of words and how to use the rules of grammar.[9]

Episodic Memory

- Episodic memory involves significant events that happened to an individual (eg, the first day of school, one's wedding, the birth of a child).[10]

Flashbulb Memory

- Flashbulb memories are a type of episodic memory in which the images and sensory experiences of a highly emotional event are remembered with heightened clarity. Many people have flashbulb memories of the moment in which they became aware of such events as the Kennedy assassination, the first moon landing, and 9/11.[11]

Procedural Memory

- Procedural memory involves the recall of steps involved in specific tasks (eg, knowing the steps involved in fabricating a wrist cock-up splint or knowing the steps involved in changing a flat tire).[12]

Explicit Memory

- Explicit memory involves the conscious, intentional recall of information.
- This type of memory requires effortful recollection of information needed throughout a day (eg, remembering the steps of an unfamiliar recipe or the directions to drive to a new job location).
- Explicit memory also involves knowledge that an individual consciously knows he or she has acquired (eg, a pianist knows that she has received extensive training to master piano playing).[13]

Implicit Memory

- Implicit memory involves the unconscious, unintentional recall of previously learned information needed to complete a task in the present moment.
- In implicit memory, previously learned information aids in task performance without conscious awareness of past experience (eg, mastery of basketball skills may aid an individual's performance the first time she plays soccer).
- Implicit memory also involves knowledge that the individual does not consciously know he or she has acquired. For example, someone with amnesia may not consciously know she has acquired knowledge of how to play the piano, but when seated at the piano, she can play fluently.[13]

Source Memory

- Source memory involves the recall of how, where, and when information was learned. For example, an anatomist may recall that he learned specific information about the human shoulder joint from a specific dissection class.
- Often, people remember facts but cannot recall how they came to learn those facts. An example involves the rehearsal of legal witnesses by lawyers. If lawyers over-rehearse a witness, the witness may confuse rehearsed information with the events that they actually observed.[14]

PERCEPTUAL MEMORY

- Memory can also be categorized by sensation and perception.

Visual Memory

- Visual memory is the ability to accurately identify objects and people by recalling their unique visual characteristics.[15]

Olfactory Memory

- Olfactory memory is the ability to accurately identify animate and inanimate objects by recalling their unique olfactory characteristics.[16]

Gustatory Memory

- Gustatory memory is the ability to accurately identify objects by recalling their unique gustatory characteristics.[17]

Somatosensory Memory

- Somatosensory memory is the ability to accurately identify animate and inanimate objects by recalling their unique somatosensory characteristics.[18]

Auditory Memory

- Auditory memory is the ability to accurately identify objects, animals, and people by recalling their unique auditory characteristics.[19]

FIELD MEMORIES VS OBSERVER MEMORIES

- Field and observer memories refer to a person's own perspective of him- or herself within the remembered event.

Field Memory

- In a field memory, people do not see themselves in the memory. The memory is remembered as though the individual is seeing it through his or her own eyes.[20]

Observer Memory

- In an observer memory, the person has incorporated his or her own image into the remembered event. The individual has altered the original scene because the original perspective of an event is always viewed from a field perspective. The person is now able to visualize him- or herself within the remembered event.[20]

Field and Observer Memories Are a Factor of Time

- More recent memories are remembered from a field perspective, while older memories are remembered from an observer perspective.
- This is a phenomenon of time. People tend to incorporate themselves into the remembered event as time goes by.[20]

AMNESIA

Retrograde Amnesia

- Retrograde amnesia is a common consequence of brain damage.
- This type of memory problem involves the loss of one's entire personal past and occurs after the injury or trauma.
- Memory of one's past is often recovered at some point after injury.
- LTM often returns to patients as their brain injury resolves. This may be due to neurogenesis (the birth of new brain cells), which has been found to occur in the hippocampus throughout life, until old age (ie, the seventh decade of life).
- If retrograde amnesia resulted after an accident or traumatic event in which the individual lost consciousness, the accident is usually never remembered. It is suggested that this phenomenon occurs because the memory of the accident was never transferred from STM to LTM before the individual lost consciousness.
- The most commonly involved neural areas in retrograde amnesia are the hippocampus, diencephalon, and temporal lobes; all structures involved in the encoding of information from STM to LTM storage.[21]

Anterograde Amnesia

- Anterograde amnesia is a memory dysfunction resulting from brain damage in which, after the injury or disease process, the person cannot remember ongoing day-to-day events, although memory of one's personal past remains intact.
- Anterograde amnesia is a dysfunction of the encoding process; the individual cannot transfer STMs into LTM storage. In effect, the individual cannot develop any new LTMs.
- Neurological areas of impairment include the hippocampus, diencephalon, and temporal lobes. Also commonly impaired are the pathways that connect these neural structures to the frontal cortex and function in the encoding of STM into LTM storage.[22]

Transient Global Amnesia

- Transient global amnesia (TGA) involves a loss of memory of one's past and an inability to remember ongoing day-to-day occurrences.
- Patients with TGA generally do not display other cognitive dysfunction and are commonly alert and lucid.
- They recall only the last seconds of consciousness and deeply encoded personal information such as their names and family members.
- The onset of TGA is rapid, does not appear to result from identifiable neurological impairment (such as traumatic brain injury or cerebrovascular accident), and usually clears within 24 hours or less.
- Although the etiology of TGA is unclear, researchers suggest that possible causes include an epileptic event, migraine-like aura, or rapidly resolving occlusion of oxygenated blood to a specific brain region.
- Possible psychological causes include heightened levels of anxiety and/or depression and trauma.[23]

THE ENCODING PROCESS

- The encoding process involves the actual steps that the brain uses to turn an event into a stored memory that can be recalled.
- Items in STM can only be remembered for seconds unless they are encoded and stored.
- Encoding information involves moving it from STM to LTM storage. It also involves associating novel information with information that has already been learned.
- The encoding process must involve the formation of neural circuits that can be easily accessed in order to retrieve stored information. Otherwise, newly learned information could not be recalled.
- Being able to retrieve information involves a subcomponent of STM called *working memory*. Working memory is a function of the prefrontal cortex and consists of moment-to-moment awareness. Working memory also plays a role in the search and retrieval of archived information.[4,5]
- LTM is the brain's archival system. It is a collaborative function of the hippocampus and other cortical areas that are only beginning to be understood.[24]

How the Brain Stores Information

- Memories of single objects appear to be fragmented into pieces that are stored in different regions of the brain.[25,26]
- For example, storage of the names of tools is a function of the medial temporal lobe and the left premotor area.
    - Humans name tools through the association of the sounds that they make. This is a function of audition and the temporal lobe.
    - We also name tools by their actions. This is a function of the premotor area.
- The storage for the names of animals is primarily a function of the medial occipital lobe.
    - Humans categorize animals primarily by their appearance (a function of the occipital lobe).
    - We also categorize animals by the sounds they make (a function of the temporal lobe).
    - The way the animal feels to one's touch is a function of the parietal lobe.
    - Storage for the movement characteristics of animals appears to be a function of the premotor area.
- When patients have difficulty naming actions (eg, swimming, driving), it usually indicates prefrontal lobe damage. The prefrontal lobe is where words of action are processed and where motor plans are stored.

Establishing a Durable Memory

- Incoming information must be encoded thoroughly, or deeply, by associating it with meaningful knowledge that already exists in memory storage.
- The human memory system is built so that individuals are more likely to remember what is most important to them and what has great emotional significance.
- The amygdala and hippocampus play an important role in encoding memories that have emotional significance.[27]

Frontal Lobe Memory Functions

- The prefrontal lobe is the seat of STM and is largely responsible for the following[28]:
  - Moment-to-moment awareness
  - Encoding STMs into LTM storage
  - Searching for and retrieving archived information
  - Recalling the source of information
- The premotor area specifically stores information about the motor actions of objects and people.

Parietal, Occipital, and Temporal Memory Functions

- The parietal, occipital, and temporal lobes participate in the storage of various attributes of objects and people.
- For example, the parietal lobe stores information about the somatosensory and visuospatial properties of an object or person.[29] The occipital lobe stores information about the visual characteristics of an object or person.[30]
- The temporal lobe stores information about the auditory properties of an object or person.[31]

Hippocampus and Amygdala

- The hippocampus and amygdala are responsible for the storage and gating of LTMs that have great emotional significance.
- Some researchers have suggested that pathology in these structures may account for the symptoms of post-traumatic stress disorder in which people cannot stop flooding of images of the traumatic event.
- Researchers have also suggested that the amygdala may act as a gate, preventing the retrieval of specific LTMs that have become repressed.[32]

MNEMONIC AND ENCODING DEVICES

- Mnemonic devices are techniques that facilitate learning and the recall of learned material.
- Encoding is the process of moving STMs to LTM storage by attaching newly learned or experienced information to archived material that is similar.

Method of Loci

- The method of loci is a mnemonic device involving the creation of a visual map of one's house.[33]
- For example, if one wanted to remember to buy soda, potato chips, and soap, one would use the rooms of one's house and visualize the kitchen with spilled soda on the floor, the bedroom with potato chips scattered on the bed sheets, and the bathroom tub filled with soap bubbles.
- At the store, one would then take a mental walk around one's house and recall which object is in each room.
- The cognitive act of creating a visual image and linking it to a mental location is a form of deep elaborative encoding.

Acronyms

- Acronyms are another form of mnemonic device in which the first letter of each word is chained to form a meaningful sentence.[34]
- For example, a common acronym used to remember the Classification of Living Systems (kingdom, phylum, class, order, family, genus, species) is "King Phyl came over for good spaghetti."
- A common acronym for remembering the order of the planets (Mercury, Venus, Earth, Mars, Jupiter, Saturn, Uranus, Neptune, Pluto) is "Mary's very extravagant mother just sold us ninety parrots."
- There are acronyms that students use to remember the cranial nerves and the bones of the skeleton.

Rhymes

- Rhymes are another form of mnemonic device that facilitate learning and memory.[35]
- The familiar rhyme to remember the number of days of each month illustrates the effectiveness of using rhymes to enhance learning and memory: "Thirty days has September, April, June, and November. All the rest have 31. February is great with 28. Leap year is fine with 29."

DAMAGE TO FRONTAL LOBE REGIONS AND ENCODING PROBLEMS

- The prefrontal cortex plays an important role in deep or elaborative encoding.
- Patients who have sustained damage to the frontal lobe regions often have encoding problems. In other words, they cannot move information from STM to LTM storage.
- Such patients fail to organize and categorize new information as it comes into STM. They have difficulty associating novel information with similar archived information in order to store and retrieve it.
- The problem lies in the processes of working memory rather than LTM storage. LTMs that were established prior to frontal lobe damage can easily be retrieved. This is why patients with frontal lobe damage can often recall events that occurred in their distant past, while they cannot remember events that occurred in the past 24 hours; because events that occurred recently can no longer be moved from STM to LTM storage, they cannot become LTMs.[36]
- LTM may remain intact in brain injury because of the process of neurogenesis. Neurogenesis is the birth of new brain cells. Researchers have found that neurogenesis occurs in the hippocampus (the seat of LTM) throughout life.[37]
- The hippocampal region becomes activated when people encode novel events.
- The brain activates the hippocampus in response to a novel stimulus to determine whether it has already developed associations to that stimulus.
- When associations are found (or if none are found), the prefrontal cortex then becomes activated in preparation to encode the novel stimulus.
- Patients with frontal lobe damage often lose the ability to encode new memories.

RECONSTRUCTION OF MEMORY

- The brain engages in an act of reconstruction during the retrieval process.
- Theorists once believed that engrams, or single neural pathways, existed for each stored memory. Today, researchers understand that the reconstruction of a past memory involves a series of neural pathways and structures.
- Retrieved memories are a temporary construction of information from several distinct brain regions, a reconstruction that has many anatomic contributors.
- We reconstruct our memories in a similar fashion to a jigsaw puzzle. Pieces of the puzzle are reconstructed until we have enough to remember an event. Fragments of the memory may be left out, just as pieces of the puzzle may be lost. Other pieces may be inaccurately borrowed from a similar memory and confused with the event we are attempting to recall.[38]
- In the reconstruction of a memory, the perceptual regions of the brain that are concerned with sight and sound merge with the posterior multimodal association area (or convergence zone).
- The posterior multimodal association area contains codes that bind sensory fragments to one another and to pre-existing information.
- The limbic association area contains codes that bind emotions to sensory fragments and to archived information.
- Researchers believe that the limbic and posterior multimodal association areas contain a type of index that indicates the location of information stored in separate cortical areas.
- The index is initially needed to keep track of all sights, sounds, emotions, and thoughts that compose an event until the memory can be held together by direct connections between the cortical regions themselves. Once direct connections between the cortical regions are established, the index is then no longer needed to recall a specific event.[39]

THE CONSOLIDATION PROCESS

- Consolidation is the process of forming strong and stable neural networks that can be used to efficiently search for and retrieve archived information.
- LTM consolidation occurs, in part, because people talk and think about their past experiences.
- The older the memory, the greater the opportunity for such past event rehearsal.
- Thinking and talking about a past experience promotes the direct connections between cortical storage areas.
- Once an experience has been repeatedly retrieved, it becomes consolidated and no longer depends upon the integrity of the multimodal association areas to act as an index.
- Sleep also plays a role in the consolidation process, particularly rapid eye movement (REM) sleep.
- During sleep, the hippocampus plays back a recent experience to areas of the cortex where it will eventually be stored.[40]

The Passage of Time and Decreasing Memory

- As time passes, humans encode and store new experiences that interfere with the ability to recall previous ones.
- For about 1 year after the occurrence of an event, it can be readily accessed with virtually any cue.
- As more time elapses, the memory becomes blurry, and the range of cues that elicit a specific event progressively narrows.
- This means that when an individual suddenly and unexpectedly recovers a forgotten memory, it may be because he or she has stumbled upon a retrieval cue that easily elicits the faded memory.[41]

REFERENCES

1. Schacter DL, Guerin SA, Jacques PLS. Memory distortion: an adaptive perspective. *Trends Cogn Sci.* 2011;15(10):467-474. doi:10.1016/j.tics.2011.08.004.

2. Ramirez S, Liu X, Lin PA, et al. Creating a false memory in the hippocampus. *Science.* 2013;341(6144):387-391. doi:10.1126/science.1239073.

3. Roozendaal B, McGaugh JL. Memory modulation. *Behav Neurosci.* 2011;125(6):797-824. doi.org/10.1037/a0026187.

4. Kamiński J, Brzezicka A, Wróbel A. Short-term memory capacity (7±2) predicted by theta to gamma cycle length ratio. *Neurobiol Learn Mem.* 2011;95(1):19-23. doi:10.1016/j.nlm.2010.10.001.

5. Baddeley A. Working memory. *Curr Biol.* 2010;20(4):R136-R140. doi:10.1016/j.cub.2009.12.014.

6. Konkle T, Brady TF, Alvarez GA, Oliva A. Scene memory is more detailed than you think: the role of categories in visual long-term memory. *Psychol Sci.* 2010;21(11):1551-1556. doi:10.1177/0956797610385359.

7. Schacter DL, Addis DR, Hassabis D, Martin VC, Spreng RN, Szpunar KK. The future of memory: remembering, imagining, and the brain. *Neuron.* 2012;76(4):677-694. doi:10.1016/j.neuron.2012.11.001.

8. Schacter DL, Addis DR, Buckner RL. Remembering the past to imagine the future: the prospective brain. *Nat Rev Neurosci.* 2007;8(9):657-661. doi:10.1038/nrn2213.

9. Binder JR, Desai RH. The neurobiology of semantic memory. *Trends Cogn Sci.* 2011;15(11):527-536. doi:10.1016/j.tics.2011.10.001.

10. Chadwick MJ, Hassabis D, Weiskopf N, Maguire EA. Decoding individual episodic memory traces in the human hippocampus. *Curr Biol.* 2010;20(6):544-547. doi:10.1016/j.cub.2010.01.053.

11. Lanciano T, Curci A, Mastandrea S, Sartori G. Do automatic mental associations detect a flashbulb memory? *Memory.* 2013;21(4):482-493. doi:10.1080/09658211.2012.740050.

12. Lum J, Kidd E, Davis S, Conti-Ramsden G. Longitudinal study of declarative and procedural memory in primary school-aged children. *Aust J Psychol.* 2010;62(3):139-148. doi:10.1080/00049530903150547.

13. Kantak SS, Mummidisetty CK, Stinear JW. Primary motor and premotor cortex in implicit sequence learning—evidence for competition between implicit and explicit human motor memory systems. *Eur J Neurosci.* 2012;36(5):2710-2715. doi:10.1111/j.1460-9568.2012.08175.x.

14. Duarte A, Henson RN, Graham KS. Stimulus content and the neural correlates of source memory. *Brain Res.* 2011;1373:110-123. doi:10.1016/j.brainres.2010.11.086.

15. Brady TF, Konkle T, Alvarez GA. A review of visual memory capacity: beyond individual items and toward structured representations. *J Vision.* 2011;11(5):4. doi:10.1167/11.5.4.

16. Sultan S, Mandairon N, Kermen F, Garcia S, Sacquet J, Didier A. Learning-dependent neurogenesis in the olfactory bulb determines long-term olfactory memory. *J Fed Am Soc Exper Biol.* 2010;24(7):2355-2363. doi:10.1096/fj.09-151456.

17. Miranda MI. Taste and odor recognition memory: the emotional flavor of life. *Rev Neurosci.* 2012;23(5-6):481-499. doi:10.1515/revneuro-2012-0064.

18. Haegens S, Osipova D, Oostenveld R, Jensen O. Somatosensory working memory performance in humans depends on both engagement and disengagement of regions in a distributed network. *Hum Brain Mapp.* 2010;31(1):26-35. doi:10.1002/hbm.20842.

19. Cohen MA, Evans KK, Horowitz TS, Wolfe JM. Auditory and visual memory in musicians and nonmusicians. *Psychon Bull Rev.* 2011;18(3):586-591. doi:10.3758/s13423-011-0074-0.

20. Sutton J. Observer perspective and a centred memory: some puzzles about point of view in personal memory. *Philos Stud.* 2010;148(1):27-37. doi:10.1007/s11098-010-9498-z.

21. McCarthy RA, Pengas G. Transient retrograde amnesia: a focal and selective (but temporary) loss of memory for autobiographical events. *Cortex.* 2015;64:426-428. doi:10.1016/j.cortex.2014.12.012.

22. Aggleton JP. Understanding anterograde amnesia: disconnections and hidden lesions. *Q J Exper Psychol.* 2008;61(10):1441-1471. doi:10.1080/17470210802215335.

23. Bartsch T, Deuschl G. Transient global amnesia: functional anatomy and clinical implications. *Lancet Neurol.* 2010;9(2):205-214. doi:10.1016/S1474-4422(09)70344-8.

24. Murty VP, Ritchey M, Adcock RA, LaBar KS. fMRI studies of successful emotional memory encoding: a quantitative meta-analysis. *Neuropsychologia.* 2010;48(12):3459-3469. doi:10.1016/j.neuropsychologia.2010.07.030.

25. Schacter DL. *Searching for Memory: The Brain, the Mind, and the Past.* New York, NY: Basic Books; 2008.

26. Nadel L, Samsonovich A, Ryan L, Moscovitch M. Multiple trace theory of human memory: computational, neuroimaging, and neuropsychological results. *Hippocampus.* 2000;10(4):352-368. doi: 10.1002/1098-1063(2000).

27. Phelps EA. Human emotion and memory: interactions of the amygdala and hippocampal complex. *Curr Opin Neurobiol.* 2004;14(2):198-202. doi:10.1016/j.conb.2004.03.015.

28. Warden MR, Miller EK. Task-dependent changes in short-term memory in the prefrontal cortex. *J Neurosci.* 2010;30(47):15801-15810. doi: 10.1523/JNEUROSCI.1569-10.2010.

29. Olson IR, Berryhill M. Some surprising findings on the involvement of the parietal lobe in human memory. *Neurobiol Learn Mem.* 2009;91(2):155-165. doi:10.1016/j.nlm.2008.09.006.

30. Harrison SA, Tong F. Decoding reveals the contents of visual working memory in early visual areas. *Nature.* 2009;458(7238):632-635. doi:10.1038/nature07832.

31. Wixted JT, Squire LR. The medial temporal lobe and the attributes of memory. *Trends Cogn Sci.* 2011;15(5):210-217. doi:10.1016/j.tics.2011.03.005.

32. Roozendaal B, McEwen BS, Chattarji S. Stress, memory and the amygdala. *Nat Rev Neurosci.* 2009;10(6):423-433. doi:10.1038/nrn2651.

33. Dalgleish T, Navrady L, Bird E, Hill E, Dunn BD, Golden AM. Method-of-loci as a mnemonic device to facilitate access to self-affirming personal memories for individuals with depression [published online February 12, 2013]. *Clin Psychol Sci.* doi:10.1177/2167702612468111.

34. Izura C, Playfoot D. A normative study of acronyms and acronym naming. *Behav Res Meth.* 2012;44(3):862-889. doi:10.3758/s13428-011-0175-8.

35. Taconnat L, Baudouin A, Fay S, et al. Aging and implementation of encoding strategies in the generation of rhymes: the role of executive functions. *Neuropsychology.* 2006;20(6):658. doi:10.1037/0894-4105.20.6.658.

36. Blumenfeld RS, Ranganath C. Prefrontal cortex and long-term memory encoding: an integrative review of findings from neuropsychology and neuroimaging. *Neuroscientist.* 2007;13(3):280-291. doi: 10.1177/1073858407299290.

37. Deng W, Aimone JB, Gage FH. New neurons and new memories: how does adult hippocampal neurogenesis affect learning and memory? *Nat Rev Neurosci.* 2010;11(5):339-350. doi:10.1038/nrn2822.

38. Hassabis D, Maguire EA. The construction system of the brain. *Phil Transact R Soc B Biol Sci.* 2009;364(1521):1263-1271. doi:10.1098/rstb.2008.0296.

39. Klingberg T. Training and plasticity of working memory. *Trends Cogn Sci.* 2010;14(7):317-324. doi:10.1016/j.tics.2010.05.002.

40. Fogel SM, Smith CT. The function of the sleep spindle: A physiological index of intelligence and a mechanism for sleep-dependent memory consolidation. *Neurosci Biobehav Rev.* 2011;35(5):1154-1165. doi:10.1016/j.neubiorev.2010.12.003.

41. Inda MC, Muravieva EV, Alberini CM. Memory retrieval and the passage of time: from reconsolidation and strengthening to extinction. *J Neurosci.* 2011;31(5):1635-1643. doi:10.1523/JNEUROSCI.4736-10.2011.

The Neurologic Substrates of Emotion

- Research regarding how the brain processes emotion has been advanced in recent years by functional magnetic resonance imaging (fMRI) and positron emission tomography (PET) scans. Imaging scans have enabled researchers to identify which brain regions become activated when people experience specific emotions.
- Much like memory, researchers used to believe that emotion was processed by one single cerebral system, largely the limbic system. Today, researchers believe that emotions are processed by multiple cerebral networks.

MAJOR NEUROANATOMICAL STRUCTURES INVOLVED IN EMOTION

- The primary neuroanatomical structures involved in the processing of emotion include the following:
  - Prefrontal cortex (in both the left and right hemispheres)
  - Limbic system (including the amygdala, hippocampus, and cingulate gyrus)
- Secondary structures in the processing of emotion include the following:
  - Thalamus
  - Anterior insular region (of the temporal lobe)
  - Septum pellucidum[1,2]

ROLE OF THE LEFT VS THE RIGHT HEMISPHERE IN EMOTION

- The left and right hemispheres have different roles in the processing of emotion.
- Both hemispheres act in a mutual cross-modulatory relationship, a relationship much like reciprocal inhibition, in which each hemisphere keeps the other's innate emotional response in check.
- The 2 hemispheres are specialized for the processing of different kinds of emotions, just as they are specialized for different kinds of cognitive, sensory, perceptual, and motor skills.[3]

PREFRONTAL AREAS OF THE LEFT VS THE RIGHT HEMISPHERE

- Imaging scans have revealed that activation of the left prefrontal area coincides with positive emotions and a sense of well-being.
- Activation of the right prefrontal area coincides with emotions of agitation, nervousness, distress, anxiety, sadness, and depression.[4]
- Stimulation of the left prefrontal area through repeated transcranial magnetic stimulation (rTMS) appears to enhance one's mood.
- Stimulation of the right prefrontal area by rTMS produces saddened moods in subjects.[5]

Gutman SA. *Quick Reference Neuroscience for Rehabilitation Professionals: The Essential Neurologic Principles Underlying Rehabilitation Practice, Third Edition* (pp 376-387).
© 2017 Taylor & Francis Group.

RIGHT AND LEFT HEMISPHERES MAY DIVIDE NEGATIVE AND POSITIVE EMOTIONS

- Reported feelings of sadness, depression, and anxiety are accompanied by increased electrical activity of the right prefrontal lobe, using single photon emission computed tomography (SPECT) scans.
- Emotional states of happiness and enjoyment are reported to increase the electrical activity in the left prefrontal lobe using SPECT.[6,7]
- Infants who are prone to distress when separated from their mothers show increased activity in the right prefrontal lobe. People who identify themselves as pessimists also show increased activity in the right prefrontal lobe.[8]
- People who were at one time depressed (but who do not report feelings of depression in the present) show decreased left prefrontal lobe activity when compared with people who never experienced depression.[9] This finding supports Kramer's Kindling Theory of Depression[10]; each depressive episode produces permanent changes in the brain's structure and chemical balance. Such changes tend to make the recurrence of depressive episodes more likely.

TWO SYNDROMES RELATED TO THE SITE OF BRAIN INJURY

Left Prefrontal Lobe Damage

- When brain damage occurs to the left hemisphere, the intact right hemisphere assumes control of emotional regulation.
- Left brain damage appears to release the right hemisphere's predisposition toward anxiousness and depression.
- Patients with left prefrontal lobe damage tend to be emotionally labile, depressed, and despondent. This is sometimes referred to as *catastrophic reaction*. Catastrophic reaction tends to occur during the acute stages of brain damage.[11-13]

Right Prefrontal Lobe Damage

- Right prefrontal lobe damage often leaves patients with an indifference to their impairment (referred to as *anosognosia*). Patients commonly report states of euphoria and well-being.
- This may occur because right hemisphere brain damage allows the left hemisphere to assume control of emotional regulation.
- The left hemisphere appears to have an innate emotional bias toward experiences of optimism and well-being.
- This may account for the optimistic denial of disability and a disowning of impaired appendages that is clinically observed in the acute stages of right brain damage.[14]

LEFT HEMISPHERE REGULATES THE EMOTIONAL RESPONSES OF BOTH HEMISPHERES

- In the absence of pathology, it appears that the left hemisphere may regulate the emotional responses of both hemispheres.
- When pathology occurs to both hemispheres, however, patients tend to become depressed, similar to cases of unilateral left hemisphere damage.
- In bilateral hemisphere damage, it is as though the coexisting right hemisphere injury had not occurred. The left hemisphere is unable to alleviate the right brain's negative emotional response, and patients tend to become depressed.
- It appears that the left hemisphere may play a role in balancing a person's emotional equanimity; therefore, under normal circumstances, the right brain's propensity toward depression does not take over.[15]
- In patients with chronic episodic depression, the left brain's ability to mitigate right brain emotional negativity appears to become decreased with each depressive episode.[16]

THERAPEUTIC SIGNIFICANCE

- If depressed patients exhibit heightened activity in the right hemisphere, one way to enhance mood may be to provide activity that stimulates left brain function.
- This may account for the effectiveness of cognitive therapy with depressed patients. Research has shown that cognitive therapy, concomitantly administered with drug therapy, has been found to be more effective than drug therapy alone.[17]
- Cognitive therapy challenges patients to assess their cognitive mindset in order to determine whether their thought patterns are reality-based. If one's thought patterns are found to be non–reality-based, the therapist challenges the patient to make needed mental set changes. These activities require left brain cognitive functions.
- Occupational therapy that provides depressed patients with activity that stimulates left brain function may also be an effective treatment for depression (if administered conjointly with drug therapy).
- It is also likely that workaholism has the same effect as stimulating left brain functions. People who are workaholics may use work as an attempt to self-medicate an underlying depression.

ORBITOFRONTAL VS DORSOLATERAL FRONTAL LOBE LESIONS

- There are 2 further emotional syndromes related to the site of brain injury/disease.

Orbitofrontal Lobe Lesions

- Patients with orbitofrontal lobe lesions exhibit impulsiveness and disinhibition.
- The orbitofrontal region mediates the brain's executive functions. When the orbitofrontal region is lesioned, the executive functions become impaired.
- Patients exhibit poor judgment, risk-taking behaviors, rowdiness, and socially inappropriate behaviors.
- Patients may also more easily become irritated, agitated, aggressive, and angry.[18,19]

Dorsolateral Frontal Lobe Lesions

- Patients with dorsolateral frontal lobe lesions exhibit decreased drive and motivation, lethargy, and a flat affect.
- Such patients rarely initiate activity or display emotion. It is as though their emotional center has become blunted.[20,21]

THE AMYGDALA'S ROLE IN EMOTION

- The amygdala has several roles in the processing of emotion.
- The amygdala is part of the mesolimbic dopamine system, or the pleasure center of the brain.
- Patients with lesions to the amygdala do not experience pleasure from people and activities that once provided them with an internal sense of happiness (referred to as *anhedonia*).
- Patients who have bilateral lesions to the amygdala no longer experience the emotion of fear.
- Such patients have difficulty recognizing dangerous situations and often engage in risk-taking behavior as a result.
- The amygdala works cooperatively with the anterior cingulate gyrus, prefrontal lobe regions, and the right hemisphere to assess whether situations are dangerous.
- This circuit generates a response that is transmitted along 2 pathways for feedback about the internal and external environment.[22]
  - One pathway travels to the sympathetic nervous system to check the body's sympathetic response to a stimulus. Messages from the sympathetic nervous system are then sent to the secondary somatosensory area (SS2).
  - In the second pathway, SS2 sends the information to the thalamus and the prefrontal lobe for cognitive decisions regarding the appropriate response to the stimulus in question. Example:
    - An individual hears the roar of a lion.
    - Her sympathetic nervous system becomes activated.
    - The sympathetic nervous system information travels to SS2.
    - SS2 then sends this information back to the thalamus and prefrontal cortex.
    - The prefrontal cortex, observing that the lion is in a confined zoo area, overrides the amygdala's initial fear response.

PATIENTS WITH LESIONED AMYGDALAE CANNOT RECOGNIZE FEAR IN OTHERS

- When presented with a chart of faces with different emotions, patients with lesioned amygdalae are unable to recognize the emotion of fear on the observed faces. However, they can identify expressions of happiness, sadness, and anger.
- They are also unable to produce the facial expression of fear when asked to do so.[23]

THE AMYGDALA MAY PLAY A ROLE IN THE RECOGNITION OF SOCIAL AND EMOTIONAL CUES

- There is evidence that individuals with autism spectrum disorder (ASD) have impairment within the limbic structures, particularly the amygdala.
- The inability to interpret social cues and generate an appropriate emotional response (eg, empathy, sadness, or happiness for others) is commonly impaired in people with ASD.
- The anterior insular region, the amygdala, and the hippocampus appear to be involved in attaching emotional significance to thoughts and memories. If any of these brain regions are lesioned, the individual has difficulty identifying important and meaningful experiences.
- Such individuals also have difficulty recognizing meaningful events for others and tend to react without emotion in response to another's discussion of emotionally significant experiences. This, too, is a common characteristic of ASD.[24]

THE AMYGDALA AND POST-TRAUMATIC STRESS DISORDER

- In PET scans of people who experience post-traumatic stress disorder (PTSD), the amygdala becomes highly activated, perhaps overactive.
- People with PTSD report feeling that the traumatic event is vividly occurring all over again, as though the amygdala and other limbic system structures are flooding the visual, auditory, and somatosensory cortices with the painful memories.
- Another phenomenon of PTSD is that the language areas of the brain shut down during the PTSD experience. People experiencing PTSD episodes report that they cannot transfer their emotions regarding the event into words (referred to as *alexithymia*).
- Without the ability to use language to describe their emotions, they cannot integrate the right hemisphere's emotional response to the event with the left hemisphere's ability to cognitively analyze the event.
- The traumatic event continues to be experienced as an overwhelming somatic experience that has a life of its own and that invades one's consciousness without modulation from the left hemisphere.
- Treatment for PTSD has not been significantly effective. This may be related to the finding that emotional memories involving extreme fear are permanently encoded into limbic structures. While such memories can be suppressed, they may never be fully erased.
- The goal of treatment is to mitigate flooding experiences and help the individual use cognitive and emotional strategies to subdue PTSD when it occurs.[25]

The Limbic System's Role in Anxiety, Panic Attacks, Phobias, and Obsessive-Compulsive Disorder

- PET scans of individuals with anxiety, panic attacks, phobias, and obsessive-compulsive disorder (OCD) reveal heightened activity in limbic system structures, particularly the anterior cingulate gyrus, amygdala, and anterior temporal cortex (the location of the parahippocampal gyrus). Other structures include the insula and the posterior orbitofrontal cortex.
- This circuit is sometimes called the *worry circuit*.
- The locus ceruleus (part of the brainstem that rouses the body to action by secreting norepinephrine) also becomes activated during anxiety, panic attacks, phobias, and OCD.
- There is evidence that pathways leading from the amygdala to the cortex are far greater in number than pathways traveling from the cortex back to the amygdala.
- This suggests that the amygdala structures are designed to alert the cortex to threatening situations and danger.
- Such cerebral architecture may serve as the brain's attempt to ensure that danger is consciously recognized and addressed.
- In a modern world, however, in which threats to one's survival may be ongoing and without clear end (eg, fear of losing employment), the amygdala's alerting system may go into overdrive and become dysfunctional.
- In such situations, the lesser number of pathways leading from the cortex to the amygdala may mean that the conscious mind is unable to shut off the amygdala's fear signals through cognitive self-talk.
- What was once an adaptive cytoarchitectural design ensuring safety may now become a maladaptive strategy.[26]

The Septal Area and Anger

- Another brain region that appears to mediate anger is the septal area, a region in both cerebral hemispheres comprising the subcallosal area and the septum pellucidum. The area has olfactory, hypothalamic, and hippocampal connections.
- The role of the septal area is to provide a means of communication between the limbic structures and the diencephalon (particularly the thalamus and hypothalamus).
- If the septal area is stimulated with an electrode in a cat, the cat lashes out with rage.
- PET scans reveal heightened activity in the septal area when people experience anger.
- A lesion to the septal area in animals produces rage and hyper-emotionality.
- In humans, destruction of the septal area gives rise to emotional overreactions to stimuli in the environment.[27]

Differences in the Neurologic Substrates of Emotion Between Male and Female Brains

- The brains of men and women generate specific emotions using different patterns of brain activity.
- When women and girls feel sadness, they experience greater activity in the anterior limbic system than do men and boys.
- According to some research studies, women also tend to experience a more profound sadness than do men. This tends to support the research finding that women experience twice the risk of depression than men.
- Because women activate both hemispheres during the experience of significant emotions (as observed in PET scans), they may be more able to describe their emotions using words, a process requiring the use of both left and right hemisphere language areas. The ability to integrate left and right language areas facilitates the association between words and emotions. As a result, women may be more aware of their emotions than men.
- Men do not as readily integrate both hemispheres during the experience of significant emotions. This may predispose men to greater difficulty attaching words to their emotions.[28,29]

Depression

- Depression affects approximately 16% of the population at least once throughout the lifespan.
- The mean age of onset is in the late 20s.
- Twice as many women as men report experiencing depression, although this disparity appears to be decreasing in recent decades.
- Male/female differences in incidence disappear roughly after age 55 years (after most women have experienced menopause).
- The World Health Organization has reported that major depression is currently the leading cause of disability in the United States and is expected to become the second leading cause of disability worldwide by 2020.
- Primary symptoms of depression are as follows:
  - Feelings of extreme sadness
  - Anhedonia, or an inability to experience pleasure from previously enjoyed activities
  - Changes in appetite (loss of or increased appetite)
  - Changes in sleep patterns (insomnia, hypersomnia, or disrupted sleep)
  - Psychomotor agitation or retardation
  - Mental and/or physical fatigue and loss of energy
  - Feelings of guilt, helplessness, and/or hopelessness
  - Decreased concentration and a general slowing of mental functions
  - Recurrent thoughts of death, suicidal ideation with or without specific plans, suicide attempt
- Anxiety and debilitating fear commonly accompany depression.[30]
- Neurologic substrates of depression have been identified as follows:
  - Decreased activation of the prefrontal cortex (primarily in the left hemisphere)
  - Decreased activation of the anterior cingulate gyrus
  - Increased activity of the amygdala and hippocampus (researchers have suggested that increased activity of the amygdala and hippocampus may represent an alerting system for the cortex. In other words, in depressive states, the amygdala and hippocampus may become highly sensitive to negative stimuli. These structures initiate messages to the cortex that facilitate the cognitive processes of worrying and ruminating over negative thoughts.)
- Additionally, neurotransmitter systems that are believed to be involved in states of depression include serotonin, norepinephrine, and dopamine. Such neurochemicals may become imbalanced, causing a dysregulation of emotions and mood.[31]

Mirror Neurons and Emotional Perception

- Mirror neurons are specialized cells designed to facilitate learning.
- The discovery that specialized neurons have a mirroring function was made by researchers who found that groups of neurons fire whenever humans observe novel behaviors and then imitate such actions.
- The existence of mirror neurons suggests that humans mentally rehearse all motor actions, language, and emotions prior to imitation.
- Mirror neurons may underlie the very basics of how we learn, from imitating facial expressions to replicating complex athletic movements. The presence of mirror neurons may shed light on how humans develop elaborate social interaction skills and social support systems.
- Mirror neurons have been found in the following neural regions:
  - Premotor cortex (motor planning and speech)
  - Parietal lobe (perception of oneself and one's relationship to the external environment; comprehension of language)
  - Temporal lobe and insula (comprehension of emotions and the ability to feel empathy; expression of language)
- In addition to using mirror neurons to imitate and learn novel actions, it appears that humans also use mirror neurons to understand the intention behind others' actions. One type of mirror neuron fires in response to observing novel behaviors, language, emotions, facial expressions, and body gestures. A second type fires when we attempt to understand the intention behind the actions just observed. Understanding intention is a key component in the development of empathy and social bonding.
- Other studies have demonstrated that mirror neurons may enable humans to share others' emotions by mirroring their facial expressions and verbal tone. For example, when observing the emotion of disgust on others' faces, the same set of mirror neurons will be triggered in the viewer's insula, causing similar feelings. This process may serve as one neurologic basis of empathy.[32]
- Some researchers have suggested that pathology in the mirror neuron system may, in part, underlie disorders such as ASD, in which the ability to learn and feel empathy by mirroring others is impaired. When researchers showed photos of people with distinctive facial expressions to 2 groups of adolescents (one group consisting of highly functioning adolescents with ASD; the other group without ASD), both groups could imitate the expressions and state which emotions they represented. However, while the group without ASD displayed heightened activity in their mirror neurons (in regions that corresponded to the emotions they observed), the adolescents with ASD showed no mirror neuron activity. The group with ASD stated that they had learned to cognitively understand the emotions represented by distinct facial expressions but felt no empathy in response to observing such emotions.[33]

REFERENCES

1. Kohn N, Eickhoff SB, Scheller M, Laird AR, Fox PT, Habel U. Neural network of cognitive emotion regulation—an ALE meta-analysis and MACM analysis. *Neuroimage.* 2014;87:345-355. doi:10.1016/j.neuroimage.2013.11.001.

2. Frank DW, Dewitt M, Hudgens-Haney M, et al. Emotion regulation: quantitative meta-analysis of functional activation and deactivation. *Neurosci Biobehav Rev.* 2014;45:202-211. doi:10.1016/j.neubiorev.2014.06.010.

3. Costanzo EY, Villarreal M, Drucaroff LJ, et al. Hemispheric specialization in affective responses, cerebral dominance for language, and handedness: lateralization of emotion, language, and dexterity. *Behav Brain Res.* 2015;288:11-19. doi:10.1016/j.bbr.2015.04.006.

4. Etkin A, Egner T, Kalisch R. Emotional processing in anterior cingulate and medial prefrontal cortex. *Trends Cogn Sci.* 2011;15(2):85-93. doi:10.1016/j.tics.2010.11.004.

5. Fitzgerald PB, Benitez J, de Castella A, Daskalakis ZJ, Brown TL, Kulkarni J. A randomized, controlled trial of sequential bilateral repetitive transcranial magnetic stimulation for treatment-resistant depression. *Am J Psychiatry.* 2014;163(1): 88-94. doi:10.1176/appi.ajp.163.1.88.

6. Herrington JD, Heller W, Mohanty A, et al. Localization of asymmetric brain function in emotion and depression. *Psychophysiology.* 2010;47(3):442-454. doi: 10.1111/j.1469-8986.2009.00958.x.

7. Colibazzi T, Posner J, Wang Z, et al. Neural systems subserving valence and arousal during the experience of induced emotions. *Emotion.* 2010;10(3):377. doi:10.1037/a0018484.

8. Dawson G, Klinger LG, Panagiotides H, Hill D, Spieker S. Frontal lobe activity and affective behavior of infants of mothers with depressive symptoms. *Child Dev.* 1992;63(3):725-737. doi: 10.1111/j.1467-8624.1992.tb01657.x.

9. Liao Y, Huang X, Wu Q, et al. Is depression a disconnection syndrome? Meta-analysis of diffusion tensor imaging studies in patients with MDD. *J Psychiatry Neurosci.* 2013;38(1):49-56. doi:10.1503/jpn.110180.

10. Kramer D. *Listening to Prozac.* New York, NY: Penguin Books; 1997.

11. Tranel D, Bechara A, Denburg NL. Asymmetric functional roles of right and left ventromedial prefrontal cortices in social conduct, decision-making, and emotional processing. *Cortex.* 2002;38(4):589-612. doi:10.1016/S0010-9452(08)70024-8.

12. Alfano KM, Cimino CR. Alteration of expected hemispheric asymmetries: valence and arousal effects in neuropsychological models of emotion. *Brain Cogn.* 2008;66(3):213-220. doi:10.1016/j.bandc.2007.08.002.

13. Vataja R, Leppävuori A, Pohjasvaara T, et al. Poststroke depression and lesion location revisited. *J Neuropsychiatry Clin Neurosci.* 2004;16(2):156-162.

14. Vossel S, Weiss PH, Eschenbeck P, Saliger J, Karbe H, Fink GR. The neural basis of anosognosia for spatial neglect after stroke. *Stroke.* 2012;43(7):1954-1956. doi:10.1161/STROKEAHA.112.657288.

15. Lisiecka DM, Carballedo A, Fagan AJ, Ferguson Y, Meaney J, Frodl T. Recruitment of the left hemispheric emotional attention neural network in risk for and protection from depression. *J Psychiatry Neurosci.* 2013;38(2):117-128. doi: 10.1503/jpn.110188.

16. Bremner JD, Narayan M, Anderson ER, Staib LH, Miller HL, Charney DS. Hippocampal volume reduction in major depression. *Am J Psychiatry.* 2004;157(1):115-118. doi.org/10.1176/ajp.157.1.115.

17. Hofmann SG, Asnaani A, Vonk IJ, Sawyer AT, Fang A. The efficacy of cognitive behavioral therapy: a review of meta-analyses. *Cogn Ther Res.* 2012;36(5):427-440. doi:10.1007/s10608-012-9476-1.

18. Bechara A, Damasio H, Damasio AR. Emotion, decision making and the orbitofrontal cortex. *Cereb Cortex.* 2000;10(3): 295-307. doi: 10.1093/cercor/10.3.295.

19. Studer B, Manes F, Humphreys G, Robbins TW, Clark L. Risk-sensitive decision-making in patients with posterior parietal and ventromedial prefrontal cortex injury. *Cereb Cortex.* 2015;25(1):1-9. doi: 10.1093/cercor/bht197.

20. Fellows LK, Farah MJ. Different underlying impairments in decision-making following ventromedial and dorsolateral frontal lobe damage in humans. *Cereb Cortex.* 2005;15(1):58-63. doi: 10.1093/cercor/bhh108.

21. Szczepanski SM, Knight RT. Insights into human behavior from lesions to the prefrontal cortex. *Neuron.* 2014;83(5): 1002-1018. doi:10.1016/j.neuron.2014.08.011.

22. Kim MJ, Loucks RA, Palmer AL, et al. The structural and functional connectivity of the amygdala: from normal emotion to pathological anxiety. *Behav Brain Res.* 2011;223(2):403-410. doi:10.1016/j.bbr.2011.04.025.

23. Brotman MA, Rich BA, Guyer AE. Amygdala activation during emotion processing of neutral faces in children with severe mood dysregulation versus ADHD or bipolar disorder. *Am J Psychiatry.* 2014;167(1):61-69. doi:10.1176/appi.ajp.2009.09010043.

24. Bellani M, Calderoni S, Muratori F, Brambilla P. Brain anatomy of autism spectrum disorders II. Focus on amygdala. *Epidemiol Psychiatr Sci.* 2013;22(04):309-312. doi:10.1017/S2045796013000346.

25. Hayes JP, LaBar KS, McCarthy G, et al. Reduced hippocampal and amygdala activity predicts memory distortions for trauma reminders in combat-related PTSD. *J Psychiatr Res.* 2011;45(5):660-669. doi:10.1016/j.jpsychires.2010.10.007.

26. Etkin A, Prater KE, Hoeft F, Menon V, Schatzberg AF. Failure of anterior cingulate activation and connectivity with the amygdala during implicit regulation of emotional processing in generalized anxiety disorder. *Am J Psychiatry.* 2014;167(5):545-554. doi.org/10.1176/appi.ajp.2009.09070931.

27. Schutter DJ, Harmon-Jones E. The corpus callosum: a commissural road to anger and aggression. *Neurosci Biobehav Rev.* 2013;37(10):2481-2488. doi:10.1016/j.neubiorev.2013.07.013.

28. Kret ME, De Gelder B. A review on sex differences in processing emotional signals. *Neuropsychologia.* 2012;50(7): 1211-1221. doi:10.1016/j.neuropsychologia.2011.12.022.

29. Whittle S, Yücel M, Yap MB, Allen NB. Sex differences in the neural correlates of emotion: evidence from neuroimaging. *Biol Psychol.* 2011;87(3):319-333. doi:10.1016/j.biopsycho.2011.05.003.

30. American Psychiatric Association. *Diagnostic and Statistical Manual of Mental Disorders.* 5th ed. Arlington, VA: American Psychiatric Association; 2013.

31. Willner P, Scheel-Krüger J, Belzung C. The neurobiology of depression and antidepressant action. *Neurosci Biobehav Rev.* 2013;37(10):2331-2371. doi:10.1016/j.neubiorev.2012.12.007.

32. Cook R, Bird G, Catmur C, Press C, Heyes C. Mirror neurons: from origin to function. *Behav Brain Sci.* 2014;37(02): 177-192. doi.org/10.1017/S0140525X13000903.

33. Gallese V, Rochat MJ, Berchio C. The mirror mechanism and its potential role in autism spectrum disorder. *Dev Med Child Neurol.* 2013;55(1):15-22. doi: 10.1111/j.1469-8749.2012.04398.x.

CLINICAL TEST QUESTIONS

Sections 31 to 32

1. Franklin sustained a brain injury in a motor vehicle accident 3 years ago. Since that time, Franklin has difficulty remembering people and events encountered less than 1 hour ago. Franklin's brain is now unable to encode new memories into long-term storage. The type of memory that Franklin has lost is referred to as:
   a. short-term memory
   b. long-term memory
   c. recent memory
   d. remote memory

2. After Zachariah's car accident 24 hours ago, he can no longer remember his personal past. He is unable to remember his name, address, and family members. Despite losing his long-term memories of his personal past, Zachariah is able to proficiently play the piano and guitar. He cannot, however, remember how and where he learned these skills. Knowledge of the steps involved in specific activities is referred to as _____ memory.
   a. semantic
   b. episodic
   c. procedural
   d. source memory

3. After 2 more days in the hospital, Zachariah begins to recover his long-term memory. When individuals temporarily lose memory of their entire personal past as a result of brain injury, this condition is known as:
   a. temporary remote memory dysfunction
   b. transient global amnesia
   c. anterograde amnesia
   d. retrograde amnesia

4. Elijah is in the same brain injury unit as Zachariah due to a fall and resultant head injury. Unlike Zachariah, Elijah can remember his entire personal past but can no longer remember day-to-day, ongoing events occurring since his head injury. Elijah is now unable to encode short-term memories into long-term storage. It is likely that Elijah will not regain this ability. This clinical condition is known as:
   a. temporary remote memory dysfunction
   b. transient global amnesia
   c. anterograde amnesia
   d. retrograde amnesia

5. Miriam was admitted to the hospital yesterday after her husband noticed that she could no longer remember her past history or day-to-day ongoing events. Miriam reports that she can remember her name and those of her husband and children but cannot remember where she lives or works. She is alert and displays no other cognitive problems. Miriam recovers both her short- and long-term memories in approximately 24 hours, and it is unclear what event caused this memory loss. This clinical condition is known as:
   a. temporary remote memory dysfunction
   b. transient global amnesia
   c. anterograde amnesia
   d. retrograde amnesia

6. Two days after Mr. Sutton's stroke, he has become uncharacteristically labile and despondent. This clinical emotional syndrome tends to occur in the acute stages of neurologic insult. This syndrome is referred to as _____ and frequently results from _____ prefrontal lobe damage.
   1. catastrophic reaction
   2. euphoric reaction
   3. left
   4. right
   a. 1, 3
   b. 1, 4
   c. 2, 3
   d. 2, 4

7. Mrs. Konkle sustained a severe stroke, causing her anosognosia, in which she is unaware of her left-sided hemiplegia and appears cheerful and positive. She does not recognize her left side as her own and believes that she has no impairment. This dissociated emotional state, which commonly occurs in the acute stages of neurologic insult, is referred to as _____ and most frequently results from _____ prefrontal lobe damage.
   1. catastrophic reaction
   2. euphoric reaction
   3. right
   4. left
   a. 1, 3
   b. 2, 3
   c. 1, 4
   d. 2, 4

8. After his traumatic brain injury (TBI), Jonah has become impulsive, disinhibited, rowdy, and aggressive. This emotional syndrome, which appears long-lasting, commonly results from damage to the:
   a. dorsolateral frontal lobe
   b. parietotemporal lobe
   c. limbic lobe
   d. orbitofrontal lobe

9. Sawyer is Jonah's roommate in the TBI unit and has also sustained a brain injury. However, Sawyer's injury has resulted in an emotional syndrome in which he has become lethargic and displays decreased drive and a flat affect. This emotional syndrome, which is also long-lasting, commonly results from damage to the:
   a. dorsolateral frontal lobe
   b. parietotemporal lobe
   c. limbic lobe
   d. orbitofrontal lobe

10. Which type of neuron is specialized to facilitate human understanding of (a) the intention underlying others' actions and (b) the association between body language, facial expression, and emotional meaning?
    a. nociceptive neurons
    b. vestibular neurons
    c. mirror neurons
    d. proprioceptive neurons

Answers

1. a
2. c
3. d
4. c
5. b
6. a
7. b
8. d
9. a
10. c

The Aging Brain

EPIDEMIOLOGY

- In developed nations, the leading cause of senile dementia (loss of memory and reason in the elderly) is Alzheimer disease (AD).[1]
- Other diseases of high incidence in the elderly include Parkinson disease and multiple cerebrovascular accidents (CVA).[2,3]

POSITRON EMISSION TOMOGRAPHY SCANS OF AGED BRAINS

- Positron emission tomography (PET) scans of aged brains reveal the following:
  - Cortical atrophy
  - Broadening of the sulci
  - Decrease in the size of the gyri
  - Widening of ventricular cavities
- Brain weight and volume also decrease with age. Approximately 5% to 10% of brain volume is lost between the ages of 30 and 90 years.[4]

AGE-RELATED DAMAGE

- Age-related damage depends upon the following:
  - Age of onset when damage occurred
  - Type and extent of physical brain alterations
  - Past and current medical history
  - Genetic history
  - Use of brain structures throughout the lifespan
- Most age-related structural and chemical changes become apparent in late middle life (the 50s and 60s).
- Some age-related changes become pronounced after age 70 years.[5]

AGE-RELATED DAMAGE IN THE DIENCEPHALON AND BRAINSTEM

- Certain cells and brain areas are more susceptible to age-related damage than others.
- Scientists used to believe that as people aged, their overall number of neurons decreased. Recent research involving neurologic imaging suggests that most of the brain's neurons remain intact throughout life unless pathology or disease exists.
- Areas of the brain where neurons do appear to be lost include the substantia nigra and locus ceruleus (both located in the brainstem). Such neuronal loss in these areas may account for the slowing of motor skills seen in the elderly.[6] Parkinson disease can destroy 70% or more of the neurons in the substantia nigra and locus ceruleus.[7]
- In the healthy elderly, only 20% to 40% of neurons are lost from the substantia nigra and locus ceruleus.[6]

Gutman SA. *Quick Reference Neuroscience for Rehabilitation Professionals: The Essential Neurologic Principles Underlying Rehabilitation Practice, Third Edition* (pp 388-393).
© 2017 Taylor & Francis Group.

AGE-RELATED DAMAGE IN THE LIMBIC SYSTEM

- The hippocampus can lose 5% of neurons each decade in the second half of life. Twenty percent of hippocampal neurons can be lost as a result of the normal aging process.
- Large neurons tend to be more affected than short neurons. It has been found that large neurons in the hippocampus and cortex have a greater tendency than shorter neurons to shrink.
- Cell bodies and axons also degenerate in certain acetylcholine-secreting neurons. These types of neurons project from the forebrain to the hippocampus.
- Some neuronal changes may represent attempts by surviving neurons to compensate for loss or shrinkage of other neurons and their projections.
- Studies have found an increase in the net growth of dendrites in the hippocampus and some areas of the cortex occurring in the 40s and 50s.
- In late life (the 80s and 90s), the net growth of dendrites in the hippocampus decreases.
- This suggests that certain areas of the brain are capable of dynamically remodeling their neuronal connections.
- This may also suggest that therapy can augment this type of age-related neuronal plasticity.[8,9]

AGE-RELATED CHANGES IN NEURONS, CELL BODIES, AND EXTRACELLULAR SPACES

- In the normal aging process, the cytoplasm of cells in the hippocampus and the cortex (both critical for learning and memory) begin to fill with protein filaments known as *neurofibrillary tangles*.
- An abundance of these tangles was once believed to contribute to AD.
- Recent research instead suggests that the formation of neurofibrillary tangles occurs in normal aging rather than from a disease process.
- Additionally, the extracellular spaces between neurons in the hippocampus and certain cortical areas accumulate moderate numbers of deposits known as *plaques*.
- Plaques, or amyloid bodies, develop very slowly in the presence of inflammation in the brain.
- While such amyloid proteins are now thought to form as a normal part of aging, research also suggests that amyloid proteins develop in brain regions that are particularly affected by AD (eg, the hippocampus).
- Once formed, amyloid proteins appear to interfere with the hippocampus's ability to encode short-term memories into long-term memory storage.[10,11]

DNA DAMAGE AND THE AGING PROCESS

- Predominant theories suggest that the body ages as a result of DNA damage in the cells.
- The enzymatic mechanisms that are designed to repair faulty DNA in cellular structures become less efficient as we age, particularly in late life (70s+).
- The DNA in mitochondria (the energy provider of the cells) slowly become defective.[12]

OXIDATION OF CELLS AND THE AGING PROCESS

- The levels of oxidized proteins in human cells also progressively increase with age.
- Cells from young adults with progeria (a syndrome of premature aging) contain levels of oxidized proteins that approach those found in healthy 80-year-old persons.
- There is evidence to suggest that such oxidation of proteins may lead to a loss of mental function.[13]

DEGENERATION OF MYELIN AND THE AGING PROCESS

- Age-related changes occur in the myelin that sheathes and insulates axons.
- Alterations of myelin can have a measurable effect on the speed and efficiency with which neurons propagate electrical impulses.
- Functionally, this may translate into decreased speed of movement and thought.[14]

REPRESSOR ELEMENT 1-SILENCING TRANSCRIPTION FACTOR

- Repressor element 1-silencing transcription factor (REST) is a transcriptional regulator, or a switch-like mechanism that turns genes on and off in the brain.

- REST activity first occurs during prenatal development, when it acts to keep essential genes deactivated until progenitor cells are developmentally ready to differentiate into specific neurons.
- Although REST stays active in the human body throughout life and protects against various diseases, it was thought that, after prenatal development, REST becomes deactivated in the human brain.
- Research has now demonstrated that REST reactivates during aging in the hippocampus and cortex to counter oxidative stress and dysfunctional protein synthesis responsible for amyloid plaques and neurofibrillary tangles.
- Researchers have demonstrated that REST becomes activated in normal aging brains. In contrast, REST activity begins to decline in people with mild cognitive impairment and becomes severely deficient in people with dementia.
- REST levels were found to be highest in the brains of people who lived well into their 90s and 100s without cognitive impairment.[15]

The Healthy Elderly

- In the healthy elderly, the extent of anatomic and physiologic alterations tends to be modest.
- The degree of neuronal loss, the accumulation of plaques, and the deficiency of enzymatic activity range from 5% to 30% above those of young adults.
- Such gradual declines often appear to have little functional effect on mental faculties.
- PET scans of the healthy elderly have shown that the brains of healthy people in their 80s were almost as active as those of people in their 20s.
- The brain appears to have considerable physiologic reserve and the ability to tolerate small losses of neuronal function.
- Epidemiological studies show that, as a group, almost 90% of all people older than 65 are free of dementia. Fewer than 5% of people aged 65 to 75 years exhibit symptoms of dementia.
- In people aged 75 to 84 years, 20% are found to exhibit some symptoms of dementia. The percentage then jumps to 50% in people older than age 85 years.
- Studies have found that when people in their 70s and 80s remain in good health, they show only a subtle decline in performance on tests of memory, perception, and language.
- The speed of processing, however, significantly declines.
- While the healthy elderly may be unable to retrieve certain details of events or information (eg, dates, places, names) as quickly, they are nevertheless often able to recall the information minutes or hours later.
- Given enough time and a stress-reduced environment, most healthy elderly score about as well as young or middle-aged adults on tests of mental performance.
- The more complex a task is (eg, a multiple-step math problem), however, the more likely a healthy elder will perform less well than a young adult.
- While one may not learn or remember quite as rapidly during healthy late life, the ability to learn and remember declines only minimally.[16-18]

Protecting the Aging Brain

- Researchers suggest that remaining physically fit and mentally active may lessen age-related cognitive deficits. Older people who consistently exercise and read perform better on cognitive tests than do sedentary individuals of the same age and health status.[19]
- Physicians also must be cautious about the type and mix of medications they prescribe for elderly patients. One research study suggested that the average person aged 65 years and older takes approximately 8 to 10 different prescription or over-the-counter medications. People over age 60 years are particularly sensitive to benzodiazepines (sedatives such as Valium [diazepam]) and other depressants and stimulants of the central nervous system. Compared with young adults, older people experience a greater decline in reasoning while such drugs are in their system. The elderly are affected longer and react to lower doses more strongly. Drug interactions can also have serious side effects that impair mental function.[20]
- The same is true of anesthesia used during surgical procedures. General anesthesia has a greater effect and lasts longer in the elderly, causing disorientation and confusion.[21]
- Health care professionals must also be aware that nutritional deficiencies can mask as dementia. A common cause of memory loss is an insufficient supply of nutrients to the brain. Deficiencies in amino acids and B vitamins (particularly B_6 and B_{12}) can produce dementia-like symptoms, which can be reversed with nutritional supplements.[22]

Age-Related Dementia and Alzheimer Disease

- Approximately 4 million people in the United States are diagnosed with AD. The World Health Organization projects this number to increase 4 times by 2040.
- AD is a degenerative disease characterized by a progressive loss of memory and cognitive function.
- Related symptoms include depression, disorientation, decreased concentration, difficulty communicating, loss of bowel and bladder control, personality change, and severe mood swings.
- One of the strongest indicators of AD and age-related dementia involves difficulty carrying out daily activities that were once easily mastered (eg, difficulty understanding how to dress or carry out other self-care tasks, difficulty remembering the route to a familiar store, or difficulty remembering how to prepare a simple meal).
- Death from AD or age-related dementia usually occurs within 5 to 10 years after diagnosis.
- The average age of onset is in the eighth decade of life; however, the disease can occur as early as the 40s, 50s, or 60s.
- AD and dementia are genetically based. Approximately 50% of people who have a parent or sibling with AD will also develop the disease by age 87 years.
- Early-onset AD has been linked to mutations in 3 genes encoding amyloid precursor protein and presenilins 1 and 2. Mutations in these genes increase the production of the protein $A\beta 42$, a primary component of senile plaque.
- Late-onset AD has been linked with apolipoprotein E.
- Mutations in the TREM2 gene have also been linked with a greater likelihood of AD development.
- Early detection involves assessment of cerebrospinal fluid for beta-amyloid or tau proteins. This analysis can predict AD onset with a sensitivity ranging from 94% to 100%.[23-26]

The Benefits of Cognitively Stimulating and Leisure Activities

- There is growing evidence that cognitively stimulating activity reduces the risk of AD and other forms of age-related dementia.
- Some of the strongest research supporting the protective factors of mentally stimulating activities have emerged from the Nun Studies, a body of research demonstrating that nuns who remained intellectually active throughout life and displayed high linguistic and verbal reasoning skills were significantly less likely to develop AD in later life. Maintaining intellectually stimulating activities into old age and mastering verbal reasoning were significantly associated with higher brain weight, less cerebral atrophy, and reduced neurofibrillary pathology.[27]
- Similarly, researchers have found that participation in mentally stimulating leisure and social activities can significantly decrease one's risk for AD and related dementia. Although the exact mechanism of this protection is unknown, some researchers have suggested that synaptic complexity and neuronal reserve, which both result from participation in intellectually stimulating activities, may play a role.[28]
- Synaptic complexity occurs when neurons build greater connections with each other as the brain learns new skills and associates newly learned skills with mastered ones that have existing neural pathways. Neuronal reserve involves the preservation of functioning neurons that are silent or nonactive.
- In the event of brain damage, silent neurons can take over the functions of damaged neurons. Neuronal reserve allows the brain to remain plastic and flexibly adapt to change, whether from the natural aging process, illness, or accident. The more a person builds new neural connections and preserves existing neurons, the less likely it is that neurodegeneration will occur.
- Conversely, participation in mentally passive activities has been found to significantly increase one's risk for the development of AD and related dementia. Several studies have shown that television viewing actually heightens one's risk for dementia. In one study, the risk for developing AD increased 1.3 times for each daily hour of television viewing a person engaged in. In contrast, for each hour spent engaged in intellectual activities per day, the risk of developing AD decreased by 16%.[29]
- Gerontologists suggest that participation in intellectually and socially stimulating activities throughout the lifespan provides protection against age-related dementia. Intellectually stimulating activities include reading, completing crossword puzzles, playing a musical instrument, engaging in crafts and fine arts, writing, playing cards and board games, participating in needlework, and completing handy work and home repairs. Researchers suggest that, in addition to these activities, people can participate in intellectually stimulating activities by learning new skills and hobbies, taking educational courses, participating in book clubs, and traveling to new places.[30]

REFERENCES

1. Reitz C, Mayeux R. Alzheimer disease: epidemiology, diagnostic criteria, risk factors and biomarkers. *Biochem Pharmacol.* 2014;88(4):640-651. doi:10.1016/j.bcp.2013.12.024.

2. Williams-Gray CH, Mason SL, Evans JR, et al. The CamPaIGN study of Parkinson's disease: 10-year outlook in an incident population-based cohort. *J Neurol Neurosurg Psychiatry.* 2013;84(11):1258-1264. doi:10.1136/jnnp-2013-305277.

3. Mozaffarian D, Benjamin EJ, Go AS, et al. Heart disease and stroke statistics—2015 update: a report from the American Heart Association. *Circulation.* 2015;131(24):e535.

4. Fjell AM, Walhovd KB. Structural brain changes in aging: courses, causes and cognitive consequences. *Rev Neurosci.* 2010;21(3):187-222. doi: 10.1515/REVNEURO.2010.21.3.187.

5. Giorgio A, Santelli L, Tomassini V, et al. Age-related changes in grey and white matter structure throughout adulthood. *Neuroimage.* 2010;51(3):943-951. doi:10.1016/j.neuroimage.2010.03.004.

6. Chan CS, Gertler TS, Surmeier DJ. A molecular basis for the increased vulnerability of substantia nigra dopamine neurons in aging and Parkinson's disease. *Mov Disord.* 2010;25(S1):S63-S70. doi: 10.1002/mds.22801.

7. Ohtsuka C, Sasaki M, Konno K, et al. Changes in substantia nigra and locus coeruleus in patients with early-stage Parkinson's disease using neuromelanin-sensitive MR imaging. *Neurosci Lett.* 2013;541:93-98. doi:10.1016/j.neulet.2013.02.012.

8. Woodruff-Pak DS, Foy MR, Akopian GG, et al. Differential effects and rates of normal aging in cerebellum and hippocampus. *Proc Natl Acad Sci U S A.* 2010;107(4):1624-1629. doi: 10.1073/pnas.0914207107.

9. Persson J, Kalpouzos G, Nilsson LG, Ryberg M, Nyberg L. Preserved hippocampus activation in normal aging as revealed by fMRI. *Hippocampus.* 2011;21(7):753-766. doi: 10.1002/hipo.20794.

10. Braskie MN, Klunder AD, Hayashi KM, et al. Plaque and tangle imaging and cognition in normal aging and Alzheimer's disease. *Neurobiol Aging.* 2010;31(10):1669-1678. doi:10.1016/j.neurobiolaging.2008.09.012.

11. Lesné SE, Sherman MA, Grant M, et al. Brain amyloid-β oligomers in ageing and Alzheimer's disease. *Brain.* 2013;136(Pt 5):1383-1398. doi.org/10.1093/brain/awt062.

12. Park CB, Larsson NG. Mitochondrial DNA mutations in disease and aging. *J Cell Biol.* 2011;193(5):809-818. doi: 10.1083/jcb.201010024.

13. López-Otín C, Blasco MA, Partridge L, Serrano M, Kroemer G. The hallmarks of aging. *Cell.* 2013;153(6):1194-1217. doi:10.1016/j.cell.2013.05.039.

14. Bartzokis G, Lu PH, Heydari P, et al. Multimodal magnetic resonance imaging assessment of white matter aging trajectories over the lifespan of healthy individuals. *Biol Psychiatry.* 2012;72(12):1026-1034. doi:10.1016/j.biopsych.2012.07.010.

15. Lu T, Aron L, Zullo J, et al. REST and stress resistance in ageing and Alzheimer's disease. *Nature.* 2014;507:448-454. doi: 10.1038/nature13163.

16. La Rue A. Healthy brain aging: role of cognitive reserve, cognitive stimulation, and cognitive exercises. *Clin Geriatr Med.* 2010;26(1):99-111. doi:10.1016/j.cger.2009.11.003.

17. Bennett IJ, Madden DJ, Vaidya CJ, Howard DV, Howard JH. Age-related differences in multiple measures of white matter integrity: a diffusion tensor imaging study of healthy aging. *Hum Brain Mapp.* 2010;31(3):378-390. doi: 10.1002/hbm.20872.

18. Pascual-Leone A, Freitas C, Oberman L, et al. Characterizing brain cortical plasticity and network dynamics across the age-span in health and disease with TMS-EEG and TMS-fMRI. *Brain Topography.* 2011;24(3-4):302-315. doi: 10.1007/s10548-011-0196-8.

19. Liu-Ambrose T, Nagamatsu LS, Voss MW, Khan KM, Handy TC. Resistance training and functional plasticity of the aging brain: a 12-month randomized controlled trial. *Neurobiol Aging.* 2012;33(8):1690-1698. doi:10.1016/j.neurobiolaging.2011.05.010.

20. Maher RL, Hanlon J, Hajjar ER. Clinical consequences of polypharmacy in elderly. *Expert Opin Drug Safety.* 2014;13(1):57-65. doi:10.1517/14740338.2013.827660.

21. Neufeld KJ, Leoutsakos JMS, Sieber FE, et al. Outcomes of early delirium diagnosis after general anesthesia in the elderly. *Anesth Analg.* 2013;117(2):471-478. doi: 10.1213/ANE.0b013e3182973650.

22. Lachner C, Steinle NI, Regenold WT. The neuropsychiatry of vitamin B12 deficiency in elderly patients. *J Neuropsychiatry Clin Neurosci.* 2014;24(1):5-15. doi.org/10.1176/appi.neuropsych.11020052.

23. Alzheimer's Association. 2013 Alzheimer's disease facts and figures. *Alzheimers Dement.* 2013;9(2):208-245. doi:10.1016/j.jalz.2013.02.003.

24. Jack CR, Knopman DS, Jagust WJ, et al. Tracking pathophysiological processes in Alzheimer's disease: an updated hypothetical model of dynamic biomarkers. *Lancet Neurol.* 2013;12(2):207-216. doi:10.1016/S1474-4422(12)70291-0.

25. Stern Y. Cognitive reserve in ageing and Alzheimer's disease. *Lancet Neurol.* 2012;11(11):1006-1012. doi:10.1016/S1474-4422(12)70191-6.

26. Villemagne VL, Burnham S, Bourgeat P, et al. Amyloid β deposition, neurodegeneration, and cognitive decline in sporadic Alzheimer's disease: a prospective cohort study. *Lancet Neurol.* 2013;12(4):357-367. doi:10.1016/S1474-4422(13)70044-9.

27. Riley KP, Snowdon DA, Desrosiers MF, Markesbery WR. Early life linguistic ability, late life cognitive function, and neuropathology: findings from the Nun Study. *Neurobiol Aging.* 2005;26(3):341-347. doi:10.1016/j.neurobiolaging.2004.06.019.

28. Tucker AM, Stern Y. Cognitive reserve in aging. *Curr Alzheimer Res.* 2011;8(4):354-360. doi.org/10.2174/156720511795745320.

29. Lindstrom HA, Fritsch T, Petot G. The relationships between television viewing in midlife and the development of Alzheimer's disease in a case-control study. *Brain Cognition.* 2005;58(2):157-165. doi:10.1016/j.bandc.2004.09.020.

30. Fratiglioni L, Paillard-Borg S, Winblad B. An active and socially integrated lifestyle in late life might protect against dementia. *Lancet Neurol.* 2004;3(6):343-353. doi:10.1016/S1474-4422(04)00767-7.

SECTION 34

Sex Differences in Male and Female Brains

RESEARCH REGARDING SEX-BASED BRAIN DIFFERENCES

- Findings regarding the differences between male and female brains have largely come from the following:
  - Positron emission tomography (PET), single photon emission computed tomography (SPECT), and magnetic resonance imaging (MRI) scans
  - Research regarding noninjured and brain-injured patients
  - Research regarding sex-based hormonal differences in fetal development
- It is important, as with any research that is in the early stages of development, that findings are not misinterpreted and that false generalizations are not extrapolated from the data.

OVERLAP BETWEEN THE MALE AND FEMALE BRAIN

- Despite male and female brain differences found through research, there is still greater overlap of brain similarity than dissimilarity.
- In both men and women, there is a substantial range of abilities within each sex.
- While men as a group may perform better on tasks of spatial skills than women, there are women who perform equally or better than men on spatial skill tasks, and vice versa.

THE EFFECTS OF SEX HORMONES ON BRAIN ORGANIZATION IN UTERO

- Differing patterns of ability between men and women likely reflect different hormonal influences upon fetal development of each sex.
- The action of estrogen (female hormone) and androgens (male hormones, chief of which is testosterone) establish sexual differentiation in utero.
- All mammal embryos, including human ones, have the potential to develop into a male or female in the first weeks of life.
- Humans have 46 chromosomes: XX (female) and XY (male)
- If a Y chromosome is present, testes or male gonads form. This is the critical first step toward becoming male.[1]

Female Default System

- If gonads do not produce male hormones, or if the hormones cannot act on the fetal tissue, the XY embryo defaults into the form of a female organism. This is called the *female default system*.
- There are many abnormalities that can occur regarding the release of specific hormones necessary to differentiate the unisex embryo into a male. The female default system is an evolutionary safeguard to maintain the life of the fetus.
- If testes are formed, they produce substances that facilitate the development of a male. One such substance, testosterone, causes masculinization by promoting the male or Wolffian ducts to convert to the external appearance of a scrotum and penis. Wolffian ducts in the male embryo develop into the vas deferens and seminal vesicles.
- The Mullerian ducts cause the female gonads to regress physically. In a female embryo, the Mullerian ducts develop into the uterus, fallopian tubes, and vagina.[1]

Gutman SA. *Quick Reference Neuroscience for Rehabilitation Professionals: The Essential Neurologic Principles Underlying Rehabilitation Practice, Third Edition* (pp 394-405).
© 2017 Taylor & Francis Group.

Adam Plan

- Like the female default system, there is an evolutionary safeguard that maintains fetal life if a prenatal anomaly prevents the XX organism from developing into a female. This is called the *Adam plan*, and it involves a defeminization process of the female template. The Adam plan stops the embryonic development of the female sex anatomy and instead facilitates the masculinization of embryonic structures through Mullerian inhibiting hormone, dihydrotestosterone, and testosterone.[1,2]

Gender-Based Brain Differences: Established in Utero by Sex Hormones

- Gender-based brain differences begin in the womb. The hormones responsible for transforming embryonic tissue into male or female anatomy act on brain development early in the gestational period.
- The most current research regarding brain development suggests that the human brain is permanently and irreversibly transformed into male or female by the 18th week of pregnancy.[1-3]

Abnormalities That Occur in Utero

Turner Syndrome

- Chromosomal anomaly of 45 XO. The female is missing one sex chromosome.
- Causes the absence of ovaries. The female is infertile.
- Other signs and symptoms include short stature and webbed neck.
- Girls require sex hormone treatment in puberty to induce secondary sex characteristics and menstruation.[4]

Klinefelter Syndrome

- Chromosomal anomaly in male humans. The male has an extra sex chromosome: 47 XXY.
- Signs and symptoms include small penis, small testes, sterility (no sperm production), tall and thin body type, and male gynecomastia (development of male breasts). Secondary male sex characteristics are often weakly developed and do not respond well to hormonal therapy.[5]

Dihydrotestosterone Deficiency Syndrome

- Dihydrotestosterone (DHT) deficiency syndrome; also called *deficiency of 5-alpha reductase*
- DHT is a powerful androgen converted from testosterone (through the enzymatic action of 5-alpha reductase).
- This directs the differentiation of the penis and scrotum (in utero).
- DHT is converted from testosterone, but in DHT deficiency syndrome, DHT cannot be produced.
- DHT is necessary for the development of male external sexual anatomy.
- The fetus possesses the normal 46 XY chromosomes.
- However, the external anatomy remains female because testosterone cannot convert into DHT, which directs the differentiation of the penis and scrotum.
- The testes develop in the second month of pregnancy but do not descend.
- Mullerian inhibiting hormone is present and negates the development of the fallopian tubes, uterus, and vagina.
- At puberty, the common testosterone surge (occurring at this stage of life) may trigger the transformation of a clitoral-like phallus into a small penis.
- Weak secondary male sexual characteristics may develop at this time.
- It appears that the little girl, at puberty, turns into a boy.
- This anomaly has been reported commonly in the Dominican Republic.[6]

Testicular Feminizing Syndrome

- Also called *androgen insensitivity syndrome*
- The embryo possesses the normal 46 XY chromosomes.
- However, the cells of the embryo are not able to respond to testosterone.
- The internal anatomy is male but is incomplete.
- The female default plan is attempted by the organism but cannot be carried out fully. Because of the presence of testosterone, the development of internal female anatomy is prevented; the development of ovaries cannot occur, and the individual is infertile.
- The external anatomy appears to be that of a normal female.[7]

Persistent Mullerian Duct Syndrome

- This disorder results in a type of intersex.
- Internal female sex organs are present.
- External male sex organs are also present.[8]

In Addition to Differentiating Male/Female Sex Organs, Sex Hormones May Also Organize Male/Female Behavior in Animals and Humans

Animal Studies

- If a rodent with functional male genitals is deprived of androgens immediately after birth, male sexual behavior, such as mounting, will be reduced.
- Instead, female behaviors, such as lordosis (arching of the back to receive intercourse), will be increased.
- Similarly, if androgens are administered to female rodents directly after birth, the female rodent displays more male sexual behavior and less female behavior.[9]

Congenital Adrenal Hyperplasia in Humans

- Congenital adrenal hyperplasia (CAH) occurs as a result of a genetic anomaly that causes large amounts of adrenal androgens to be produced in the XX embryo.
- These are female embryos that were exposed to an excess of androgens in the prenatal stage.
- Although the consequent masculinization of genitals can be surgically corrected in early life and drug therapy can stop the overproduction of androgens, the effects of prenatal exposure on the brain cannot be reversed.
- Females who were exposed to prenatal androgens grow up to be self-reported tomboys and prefer typically masculine toys more than their unaffected biological sisters.
- Researchers also found that the CAH females performed better than their unaffected biological sisters on spatial manipulation tasks.[10]

Differences in the Anatomy of the Male vs Female Brain

- Anatomical differences between male and female human brains exist.
- Men generally have about 4% more brain cells and approximately 100 grams more brain tissue than women.
- Women have more dendritic connections between cells.
- While the male brain is somewhat larger than the female brain, specific regions of each brain have been found to have differing sizes.[11]

Frontal Cortex

- Certain regions of the frontal cortex have been found to be larger in women than in men. One such area is the region where higher level executive functions are mediated (ie, skills including judgment, problem solving, and regulating raw emotions).[12]

Parietal Cortex

- The inferior parietal lobule is a bilateral region in the parietal lobes that has been linked to higher level, abstract mathematical skills. This region was shown to be enlarged in the brain of Albert Einstein and in other mathematicians and physicists.
- The inferior parietal lobule (IPL) has been found to be significantly larger in men than in women.
- The right IPL has been correlated with the ability to manipulate objects in space.
- The left IPL appears to be associated with the perception of time and speed and the ability to rotate 3-dimensional figures.
- Research regarding gender-based skills have shown that men are generally more adept at rotating objects in space, abstract mathematical reasoning skills, route navigation, and targeted motor skills (such as intercepting projectiles like a ball tossed in the air).
- Researchers have also shown that the brain regions responsible for these skills appear to mature approximately 4 years earlier in boys than in girls.[13]

Corpus Callosum

- PET scans have shown that the corpus callosum is more extensive in women than in men. Women have 11% more neurons in the corpus callosum, thus creating more neural fibers that connect the 2 hemispheres.
- This may suggest that women are more able to integrate both hemispheres in activities than men.

- In language skills, women activate both hemispheres to interpret the literal meaning of the words (left brain function) as well as the emotional tone of the words (right brain function).
- Men activate only the left hemisphere in language skills and have greater difficulty interpreting the subtle emotional tone of a conversation.
- The incidence of language disorders (aphasia) is higher in men than in women after damage to the left hemisphere.
- Research has also shown that women typically recover from aphasia after cerebrovascular accident more readily than do men. This may relate to a woman's greater ability to integrate both hemispheres during language tasks.[14]

Broca Area and Wernicke Area

- Broca area is located in the left frontal lobe (beneath the premotor area) and has been associated with expressive communication.
- The Wernicke area is located in the left parietal lobe in the superior temporal gyrus and has been associated with receptive communication.
- Both areas have been found to be significantly larger in women than in men, which may account for women's greater performance in tests of language-based skills. Women have approximately 23% more volume in Broca area and 13% more volume in the Wernicke area than men.
- Researchers have also found that the brain regions involved in language and fine motor skills appear to mature 6 years earlier in girls than in boys.[15]

The Amygdala and Limbic System: Emotion

- Research has found that men generally possess larger amygdala structures than women.
- Women, conversely, have more dendritic connections between the amygdala and the cortex.
- The amygdala is a structure in the limbic system that is believed to be responsible for the feelings of anger and fear.
- The connections between the amygdala and the cortex may be used to alert the cortex to the threat of danger.
- Researchers have suggested that, because women possess greater connections between the amygdala and cortex, they may be better at modulating their anger and using symbolic signals to de-escalate a potentially threatening situation.
- Because of this anatomical difference, men may have greater difficulty modulating anger and may respond with more overt displays of aggression.
- PET scans have also shown that men exhibit greater brain activity in the more ancient regions of the limbic system, the regions that mediate action in response to emotion.
- Women exhibit greater activity in the phylogenetically newer and more complex regions of the limbic system that mediate symbolic action in response to emotion.
- One researcher explained that, if a dog is angry and jumps and bites, that is an active response to the emotion of anger. If the dog bears its teeth and growls, that is a symbolic response to the emotion of anger.
- The implication may be that women are more predisposed to a symbolic display of their emotions, while men react with action to their emotions.
- Women are also more adept at recognizing symbolic expressions of emotions in others than are men. Men seem to need an overt reaction that clearly demonstrates emotion; otherwise they miss emotions that are symbolically or subtly displayed.
- Studies have shown that women are more sensitive at recognizing subtle facial expressions than are men (a limbic system function).
- In studies, both men and women were equally adept at recognizing happiness in the photos of faces of both men and women.
- However, women were more adept at determining whether a man or woman was sad. A woman's face had to be tearful for men to recognize the emotion of sadness. Subtle expressions of sadness were not recognized.
- Researchers have also found that emotional activity appears to be localized in the amygdala. At 6 years of age, the connections to the cortex have not been fully established, and thus, the lack of connections between the amygdala and cortex may account for a child's difficulty regulating emotions and attaching words to feelings.
- Such connections between the amygdala and cortex begin to more fully develop in adolescence, although predominately in girls.[16]

NATURE VS NURTURE

- Researchers have suggested that the effects of sex hormones on brain organization occur so early in development that from birth, the environment is acting on differently wired male and female brains.
- One study found that 3-year-old boys perform better at physical targeting skills (guiding or intercepting projectiles) than girls of the same age.
- Other studies have shown that the extent of experience playing sports does not account for sex differences in targeting skills exhibited by young adults.
- Some researchers have argued that sex differences in spatial rotation performance are present before puberty.[17]

SKILLS FOR WHICH MEN SHOW GREATER PROFICIENCY

- Skills that men perform more proficiently than women include the following. It should be noted that this finding considers men as a group, without considering differences occurring in both sexes.[15]
  - Spatial tasks requiring the individual to imagine rotating an object or visually manipulating it in some way
  - Mathematical reasoning
  - Navigating through a route
  - Target-directed motor skills (guiding or intercepting projectiles)

SKILLS FOR WHICH WOMEN SHOW GREATER PROFICIENCY

- Skills that women perform more proficiently than men include the following. It should be noted that this finding considers women as a group, without considering differences occurring in both sexes.[15]
  - Rapidly identifying matching items (called *perceptual speed*)
  - Verbal fluency (including the ability to find words that begin with a specific letter or fulfill some other constraint)
  - Arithmetic calculation
  - Recalling landmarks from a route
  - Precision fine motor skills

ROUTE NAVIGATION

- In studies, men learned a route in fewer trials than women and made fewer errors.
- Once learned, however, women remembered more of the landmarks than did men.
- Women appear to use landmarks as a strategy to orient themselves.
- Men appear to navigate using the spatial relationships of routes as depicted on maps.[18]

THE RECALL OF OBJECTS AND THEIR LOCATIONS

- In studies that tested the ability of men and women to recall objects and their locations in a confined space (a room or tabletop), it was found that women were better able to remember whether an item had been displaced or not.
- Women were also better able to replace objects in their original locations after they had been moved.[18]

POSSIBLE EVOLUTIONARY SIGNIFICANCE

- Some theorists suggest that the previously mentioned sex-based differences may have evolutionary roots.
- Such theorists suggest that, for thousands of years during which human brain characteristics evolved, humans lived in relatively small hunter-gatherer groups.
- The division of labor between the sexes in such societies was probably distinct, as it is in existing hunter-gatherer societies.
- Men were believed to be responsible for large game hunting, requiring long-distance travel.
- Women were believed to gather food near the campsite, prepare food and clothing, and care for children.
- Theorists argue that such specializations placed different evolutionary selection pressures on men and women.
- Men would require long-distance route-finding abilities to recognize a geographic area from varying locations. They would also need targeting skills for hunting.
- Women would require short-range navigation using landmarks, fine motor capabilities carried out within a circumscribed space, and perceptual discrimination skills sensitive to small changes in the environment or in children's appearance and behavior.[19]

GENDER IDENTITY AND SEXUAL ORIENTATION

- Gender identity is the internal feeling of being male or female and does not necessarily correlate with one's sex-based genotype (sex-based genetic code) or phenotype (sex-based reproductive organs).
- Sexual orientation is the internal feeling of being attracted to a particular sex-based phenotype (men, women, or intersex people [individuals with both male and female sex-based chromosomes and/or reproductive organs]).
- Sex classification is determined by genetic chromosomal pattern and phenotypic reproductive organs. The dualistic view that gender identity exists as a dichotomy (male or female) is increasingly reconsidered, as Western society has grown more aware and accepting of people who do not fit into such dimorphic classifications. Some researchers suggest that gender identity and sexual orientation exist on a spectrum, rather than dualistic poles.
- A growing body of research indicates that gender identity and sexual orientation are strongly influenced by neurochemical and neuroanatomical characteristics that impact the organism as early as fetal development, when exposure to prenatal hormones (eg, androgen, testosterone, estrogen) begin to shape fetal differentiation.
- Brain structures have also been implicated in the formation of gender identify and sexual orientation. The hypothalamus has long been known to regulate reproductive behaviors; however, in 1991, Simon LeVay demonstrated that the interstitial nucleus of the anterior hypothalamus is highly associated with sexual orientation.[20] Other researchers similarly identified the suprachiasmatic nucleus of the hypothalamus as having a critical role in the development of sexual orientation.
- In 1992, Allen and Gorski found that the anterior commissure was larger in homosexual men than in heterosexual men or women.[21] In 2008, Savic and Lindstrom found that the volume of both hemispheres was symmetrical in homosexual men and heterosexual women but asymmetrical (in the right hemisphere) in heterosexual men and homosexual men.[22]
- Ragini Verma and colleagues, in 2014, found greater neural connectivity extending from rostral to caudal regions within one hemisphere in men. Conversely, in women, greater connectivity runs between hemispheres. This finding suggests that typical female brains may be structured to facilitate communication between language, emotion, and perception, while the typical male brain may be more adept at spatial skills and coordinated action. This finding was reversed in the cerebellum, where men had greater interhemispheric connection and women had greater intrahemispheric connection.[15]

The Empathizing vs Systematizing Brain

- Simon Baron-Cohen developed the idea that male and female brains are specialized for either empathizing or systematizing.
- Baron-Cohen suggests that the female brain is predominantly hard-wired for empathy, identifying the meanings of facial expression, decoding nonverbal communication, detecting subtle nuances of tone and gesture, analyzing contextual social cues, and responding in emotionally appropriate ways that foster cooperation and well-being of a group as a whole.
- He suggests that the male brain is predominantly hard-wired for constructing rule-based analyses of the external world, particularly of inanimate objects and events. They seek to understand and build systems, whether mechanical, governmental, or gaming systems.
- The greater spatial skill of men, and the greater language and emotional skills of women, seem to serve the basic differences of empathizing and systematizing.
- Baron-Cohen suggests that this neural difference appears in children's preferences for toys (mechanical trucks vs humanlike dolls), styles of interaction (ordering vs negotiating), and methods of navigation (women appear to personalize space through landmarks; men more commonly visualize space as a geometric system).[23]

Joining and Hosting Groups

- To better examine empathizing versus systematizing skills, researchers have developed tests that assess the differences between the sexes in various scenarios.
- In one scenario, children are tested to determine the differences between girls and boys in the way each joins a new group. This has been investigated by introducing a new child to a group that has already formed.
- As a newcomer to an established play group, female children tend to stand back and observe for a while before joining. They evaluate what is happening in the group and attempt to fit into the ongoing activity.
- Male children, as newcomers, are more likely to attempt to take over the game, try to change its rules, and direct everyone's attention onto them.
- Another scenario involves investigating differences between boys and girls as they attempt to host a group. Female children are more attentive to the newcomer and offer ways through which the newcomer can become part of the group activities.
- Male children, as hosts, more commonly ignore the newcomer's attempt to join in and are more likely to continue the activities in which they were already engaged.[23]

Eye Contact and Language

- Sex differences can be found as early as birth. Researchers have shown that 1-day-old female infants look longer at a face, while 1-day-old male infants look longer at a suspended mechanical mobile.
- The amount of eye contact that children make is in part determined by prenatal testosterone.
- At the age of 1 year, male toddlers show a stronger preference for watching video games of cars. One-year-old female toddlers show a greater preference for watching videos of human faces demonstrating a range of emotions.
- Testosterone level during fetal development also influences language skills. The higher the prenatal testosterone level, the smaller a child's vocabulary was measured to be at 18 and 24 months.[24,25]

Asperger Syndrome

- Baron-Cohen also suggests that autism, particularly Asperger syndrome, may reflect a brain that has been too highly systematized by gestational hormones in utero.
- Asperger syndrome is a form of autism in which intelligence is average or higher but social communication is highly impaired. Asperger syndrome predominantly affects men, at a 10:1 ratio.
- Baron-Cohen's theory is similar to one that Geschwind and Galaburda had proposed years earlier: that the male hormone testosterone slows the growth of the brain's left hemisphere and accelerates growth on the right. Some have suggested that when too much testosterone tilts this maturational process to one extreme, a range of problems can potentially occur, including learning disability, attention-deficit disorder (ADD), attention-deficit hyperactivity disorder (ADHD), and autism. All of these disorders disproportionately affect men.
- Lack of eye contact and poor language skills are early signs of autism. Other characteristics include difficulty developing social relationships, difficulty interpreting and responding to social cues, narrow interests, and a strong adherence to routines.
- Baron-Cohen suggests that Asperger syndrome may be indicative of an extreme male brain, particularly talented at systemizing and deficient in the skill of empathy.[1,26-28]

REFERENCES

1. Bao AM, Swaab DF. Sexual differentiation of the human brain: relation to gender identity, sexual orientation and neuropsychiatric disorders. *Front Neuroendocrinol.* 2011;32(2):214-226. doi:10.1016/j.yfrne.2011.02.007.

2. Flück CE, Meyer-Böni M, Pandey AV, et al. Why boys will be boys: two pathways of fetal testicular androgen biosynthesis are needed for male sexual differentiation. *Am J Hum Genet.* 2011;89(2):201-218. doi:10.1016/j.ajhg.2011.06.009.

3. Hines M. Sex-related variation in human behavior and the brain. *Trends Cogn Sci.* 2010;14(10):448-456. doi:10.1016/j.tics.2010.07.005.

4. Pinsker JE. Turner syndrome: Updating the paradigm of clinical care. *J Clin Endocrinol Metab.* 2012;97(6):E994-E1003. doi.org/10.1210/jc.2012-1245.

5. Groth KA, Skakkebæk A, Høst C, Gravholt CH, Bojesen A. Klinefelter syndrome—a clinical update. *J Clin Endocrinol Metab.* 2012;98(1):20-30. doi.org/10.1210/jc.2012-2382.

6. Bhasin S, Cunningham GR, Hayes FJ, et al. Testosterone therapy in adult men with androgen deficiency syndromes: an endocrine society clinical practice guideline. *J Clin Endocrinol Metab.* 2006;91(6):1995-2010. doi.org/10.1210/jc.2005-2847.

7. Hughes IA, Davies JD, Bunch TI, Pasterski V, Mastroyannopoulou K, MacDougall J. Androgen insensitivity syndrome. *Lancet.* 2012;380(9851):1419-1428. doi:10.1016/S0140-6736(12)60071-3.

8. Chamrajan S, Vala NH, Desai JR, Bhatt NN. Persistent Mullerian duct syndrome in a patient with bilateral cryptorchid testes with seminoma. *J Hum Reproduct Sci.* 2012;5(2):215-217. doi: 10.4103/0974-1208.101025.

9. Lenz KM, Nugent BM, McCarthy MM. Sexual differentiation of the rodent brain: dogma and beyond. *Front Neurosci.* 2012;6:26. doi: 10.3389/fnins.2012.00026.

10. Hines M. Prenatal endocrine influences on sexual orientation and on sexually differentiated childhood behavior. *Front Neuroendocrinol.* 2011;32(2):170-182. doi:10.1016/j.yfrne.2011.02.006.

11. Ruigrok ANV, Salimi-Khorshidi G, Lai MC, et al. A meta-analysis of sex differences in human brain structure. *Neurosci Behav Rev.* 2014;39:34-50. doi: 10.1016/j.neubiorev.2013.12.004.

12. Valera EM, Brown A, Biederman J, et al. Sex differences in the functional neuroanatomy of working memory in adults with ADHD. *Am J Psychiatry.* 2014;167:86-94. doi.org/10.1176/appi.ajp.2009.09020249.

13. Salinas J, Mills ED, Conrad AL, Koscik T, Andreasen NC, Nopoulos P. Sex differences in parietal lobe structure and development. *Gender Med.* 2012;9(1):44-55. doi:10.1016/j.genm.2012.01.003.

14. Luders E, Toga AW, Thompson PM. Why size matters. Differences in brain volume account for apparent sex differences in callosal anatomy: the sexual dimorphism of the corpus callosum. *Neuroimage.* 2014;84:820-824. doi:10.1016/j.neuroimage.2013.09.040.

15. Ingalhalikar M, Smith A, Parker D, et al. Sex differences in the structural connectome of the human brain. *Proc Natl Acad Sci U S A.* 2014;111(2):823-828. doi:10.1073/pnas.1316909110.

16. Cooke BM, Woolley CS. Sexually dimorphic synaptic organization of the medial amygdala. *J Neurosci.* 2005;25(46):10759-10767. doi:10.1523/JNEUROSCI.2919-05.2005.

17. Wu MV, Manoli DS, Fraser EJ, et al. Estrogen masculinizes neural pathways and sex-specific behaviors. *Cell.* 2009;139(1):61-72. doi:10.1016/j.cell.2009.07.036.

18. Persson J, Herlitz A, Engman J, et al. Remembering our origin: gender differences in spatial memory are reflected in gender differences in hippocampal lateralization. *Behav Brain Res.* 2013;256:219-228. doi:10.1016/j.bbr.2013.07.050.

19. Eagly AH, Wood W. The origins of sex differences in human behavior: evolved dispositions versus social roles. *Am Psychologist.* 1999;54(6):408. doi.org/10.1037/0003-066X.54.6.408.

20. LeVay S. A difference in hypothalamic structure between heterosexual and homosexual men. *Science.* 1991;253(5023):1034-1037.

21. Allen LS, Gorski RA. Sexual orientation and the size of the anterior commissure in the human brain. *Proc Natl Acad Sci U S A.* 1992;89:7199-7202.

22. Savic I, Lindstrom P. PET and MRI show differences in cerebral asymmetry and functional connectivity between homo- and heterosexual subjects. *Proc Natl Acad Sci U S A.* 2008;105:9403-9408.

23. Baron-Cohen S, Wheelwright S. The empathy quotient: an investigation of adults with Asperger syndrome or high functioning autism, and normal sex differences. *J Autism Dev Disord.* 2004;34(2):163-175. doi: 10.1023/B:JADD.0000022607.19833.00.

24. Alexander GM, Wilcox T, Woods R. Sex differences in infants' visual interest in toys. *Arch Sex Behav*. 2009;38(3):427-433. doi:10.1007/s10508-008-9430-1.

25. Auyeung B, Baron-Cohen S, Ashwin E, et al. Fetal testosterone predicts sexually differentiated childhood behavior in girls and in boys. *Psychol Sci*. 2009;20(2):144-148. doi:10.1111/j.1467-9280.2009.02279.x.

26. Baron-Cohen S. The extreme male brain theory of autism. *Trends Cogn Sci*. 2002;6(6):248-254. doi:10.1016/S1364-6613(02)01904-6.

27. Geschwind N, Galaburda AM. Cerebral lateralization: biological mechanisms, associations, and pathology: I. A hypothesis and a program for research. *Arch Neurol*. 1985;42(5):428-459. doi:10.1001/archneur.1985.04060050026008.

28. Wakabayashi A, Baron-Cohen S, Uchiyama T, Yoshida Y, Kuroda M, Wheelwright S. Empathizing and systemizing in adults with and without autism spectrum conditions: cross-cultural stability. *J Autism Dev Disord*. 2007;37(10): 1823-1832. doi: 10.1007/s10803-006-0316-6.

CLINICAL TEST QUESTIONS

Sections 33 to 34

1. Normal, healthy aging commonly involves all of the following except for which one?
   a. widening of the ventricular cavities
   b. increased production of CSF in the ventricles
   c. cortical atrophy
   d. decreased size of the gyri and broadening of the sulci

2. Research demonstrates that most of the brain's neurons remain intact throughout life unless pathology or disease exists. However, neurons do appear to significantly degenerate in a specific area of the brain in normal, healthy aging and may account for the slowing of motor skills seen in the elderly. This area is the:
   a. primary motor area
   b. thalamus
   c. substantia nigra and locus ceruleus
   d. cerebellum

3. This area of the brain experiences an increase in the net growth of dendrites in mid to late life and may account for why long-term memories (particularly those with an emotional component) remain intact while short-term memories easily fade in normal, healthy aging.
   a. hippocampus
   b. brainstem
   c. cingulate gyrus
   d. cerebellar vermis

4. All of the following occur in normal, healthy aging except for which one?
   a. Moderate amounts of neurofibrillary tangles (protein filaments) and plaque deposits (amyloid proteins) begin to form in the brain.
   b. Enzymatic mechanisms designed to repair faulty DNA in cellular structures become less efficient.
   c. REST (a transcriptional gene regulator) becomes reactivated in mid to late life in the hippocampus and cortex to counter the effects of oxidation and dysfunctional protein synthesis.
   d. Genetic mutations begin to occur with regularity and rapidity in the frontal lobes and limbic system.

5. Martha's occupational therapist recommended that she engage in which of the following to enhance healthy and productive aging?
   1. Engage in regular and frequent cognitively stimulating activities to build new neuronal connections and preserve already existing ones.
   2. Monitor the interaction of prescribed and over-the-counter medications that can have serious side effects on mental function.
   3. Be cautious of elective surgical procedures, as anesthesia can cause disorientation and confusion in the elderly.
   4. Be aware of nutritional deficiencies that can mask as dementia.
   5. Regularly engage in exercise that maintains joint range and moderately elevates heart rate.
   a. 1, 2, 3
   b. 1, 3, 4
   c. 2, 3, 4, 5
   d. all of the above

6. When Luciano and his wife consulted a fertility specialist because they had difficulty conceiving a child, the doctor performed genetic testing on Luciano and found that he has a chromosomal pattern of 47 XXY, with one additional sex chromosome than normal. In his teenage years and adulthood, Luciano was tall and thin, had small external reproductive organs, and had developed fat deposits in his chest area (gynecomastia). It is likely that Luciano has:
   a. androgen insensitivity syndrome (testicular feminizing syndrome)
   b. dihydrotestosterone deficiency syndrome
   c. Klinefelter syndrome
   d. Turner syndrome

7. When Maria was born, she was assigned the sex of female and was raised as a little girl. At puberty, when this stage of development triggered a naturally occurring testosterone surge, Maria's clitoris developed into a small penis and she developed weak secondary sex characteristics (eg, facial and chest hair, deepening voice, broadened shoulders). Maria was found to have a normal 46 XY male chromosomal pattern but has a hormonal deficiency syndrome that prevented fetal development of a penis and scrotum. This hormonal deficiency is called:
   a. androgen insensitivity syndrome (testicular feminizing syndrome)
   b. dihydrotestosterone deficiency syndrome
   c. Klinefelter syndrome
   d. Turner syndrome

8. Andrea was also born and raised as a little girl. At 15, when menstruation had not as yet occurred, her parents accompanied her to a physician who found that Andrea had a normal 46 XY chromosomal pattern. Because her embryonic cells were unable to respond to testosterone during fetal development, Andrea's internal anatomy developed as male, but incompletely. The presence of testosterone during fetal development prevented the development of female internal anatomy (causing infertility). External anatomy developed as female. This syndrome is referred to as:
   a. androgen insensitivity syndrome (testicular feminizing syndrome)
   b. dihydrotestosterone deficiency syndrome
   c. Klinefelter syndrome
   d. Turner syndrome

9. Research has shown that when women sustain stroke in the left hemisphere language centers, the resultant aphasia tends to be less severe than that experienced by men and tends to resolve more quickly. The reasons accounting for this sex-based difference include which of the below?
   1. Female cortical language centers appear to have higher volumes of dendritic connections than do male cortical language centers.
   2. Women tend to more commonly use both hemispheres in language production than do men (who use the left side language centers more commonly).
   3. The cortical language centers have been shown to mature approximately 6 years earlier in girls than in boys.
   a. 1, 2
   b. 1, 3
   c. 2, 3
   d. 1, 2, 3

10. Although men typically possess larger amygdala volumes than do women (because of their overall larger body size), women have been found to possess greater numbers of dendritic connections between the amygdala and cortex. Some researchers have suggested that such connections allow women to be better modulators of anger than men. This emotional modulation skill may allow women to be better at which of the below skills?
   1. use of symbolic signals to de-escalate potentially threatening situations
   2. recognition of subtle expressions of emotions in other humans
   3. response to potential threats with overt displays of physical aggression
   4. attachment of words to emotions during communication
   a. 1, 2
   b. 2, 3
   c. 1, 2, 4
   d. all of the above

Answers

1. b
2. c
3. a
4. d
5. d
6. c
7. b
8. a
9. d
10. c

Glossary

A1: See *Primary Auditory Area.*

Abarognosis: The inability to accurately estimate the weight of objects, particularly in comparison with each other.

Abducens Nerve: Cranial nerve (CN) 6. Responsible for extraocular eye movements. Lesion symptoms include medial strabismus, diplopia, and nystagmus.

Acalculia: A type of expressive aphasia that involves the inability to calculate mathematical problems.

Accessory Nerve: CN 11. Responsible for elevation of the larynx during swallowing, innervation of the sternocleidomastoid muscle (for head rotation and flexion/extension), and innervation of the upper trapezius muscle (for shoulder elevation and flexion above 90 degrees).

Accommodation: The ability of the eye to focus images of near or distant objects on the retina. The ciliary muscles are responsible for changing the thickness of the lens to focus images on the retina.

Acetylcholine (ACh): A neurotransmitter that acts at the neuromuscular junction to facilitate muscle movement.

Acetylcholinesterase (AChE): The enzyme that destroys ACh soon after it is released from its terminal boutons, thus terminating the postsynaptic potential.

ACh: See *Acetylcholine.*

AChE: See *Acetylcholinesterase.*

Achromatopsia: A condition that occurs when V4 is lost and the world appears in shades of gray. The memory of color is erased.

Action Potential: The brief electrical impulse that provides the basis for conduction of nerve signals along the axon. It results from the brief changes in the cell's membrane permeability to sodium and potassium ions. A strong enough action potential will cause the neuron to become excited and start the conduction process.

Adiadochokinesia: Inability to perform rapid alternating movements—as in supinating and pronating one's forearms and hands quickly and synchronously. Sign of cerebellar pathology.

Agnosia: Literally "not to know." **Tactile Agnosia:** An inability to interpret sensations through touch. **Auditory Agnosia:** An inability to interpret sounds. **Visual Agnosia:** An inability to interpret visual stimuli. All of these agnosias result from lesions to the cortex; the sensory receptor anatomy remains intact.

Agraphesthesia: Loss of the ability to interpret letters written on the contralateral hand. Indicates damage to SS2.

Agraphia: A type of expressive aphasia resulting in the inability to write intelligible words and sentences.

Agrammation: A type of expressive aphasia that involves the inability to arrange words sequentially so that they form intelligible sentences.

Ahylognosia: The inability to discriminate between different types of materials by touch alone.

Akathisia: An inability to remain still, caused by an intense urge to move or fidget.

Akinesia: An inability to perform voluntary movement. Commonly seen in the late stages of Parkinson disease. Patients report that a tremendous amount of mental concentration is required to perform basic motor tasks.

Akinetopsia: A cortical visual disorder in which people neither see nor understand the world in motion. Occurs as a result of lesions to V5.

Alexia: A type of receptive aphasia resulting in the inability to read and interpret written words. See also *Dyslexia* (difficulty interpreting the written word).

Alexithymia: A type of expressive aphasia. Inability to attach words to one's emotions; inability to express one's emotions using words. *Dyslexithymia* is difficulty attaching words to one's emotions.

Allodynia: A condition in which nonpainful stimuli now produce pain.

Amorphognosia: The inability to discriminate between different forms/shapes by touch alone.

Amygdala: An almond-shaped nucleus in the anterior temporal lobe that attaches to the caudate nucleus. May have roles in the mediation of fear and anger and the perception of social cues.

Gutman SA. *Quick Reference Neuroscience for Rehabilitation Professionals: The Essential Neurologic Principles Underlying Rehabilitation Practice, Third Edition* (pp 406-423). © 2017 Taylor & Francis Group.

Analgesia: Loss of pain sensation.

Anhedonia: An inability to experience pleasure. Often accompanies states of depression.

Anomia: A type of expressive aphasia that involves the inability to remember and express the names of people and objects.

Anosmia: Loss of smell (olfaction).

Anosognosia: Extensive neglect and failure to recognize one's own body paralysis. Results from lesions to the right hemisphere.

ANS: See *Autonomic Nervous System*.

Anterior: Also referred to as *ventral*. Refers to the front of an organism. Ventral means the belly of a 4-legged animal.

Anterior Commissure: Located in the anterior thalamus; allows information to travel between both thalamic lobes.

Anterior Median Fissure: Divides the medulla into equal left and right halves. The fissure continues all the way down the spinal cord.

Anterior Spinocerebellar Tract: Ascending sensory spinal cord tract. Carries unconscious information from the lower extremities to the cerebellum regarding proprioception.

Anterior Spinothalamic Tract: Ascending sensory spinal cord tract. Carries conscious information about crude and light touch.

Anterograde Amnesia: A memory dysfunction resulting from brain damage, in which—after the injury or disease process—the person cannot remember ongoing day-to-day events, although memory of one's personal past remains intact. Anterograde amnesia is a dysfunction of the encoding process—the individual cannot transfer short-term memories into long-term memory storage. In effect, the individual cannot develop any new long-term memories.

Antitransmitter: A chemical substance that breaks down a neurotransmitter so that the postsynaptic neuron can repolarize in order to fire again. Antitransmitters terminate the postsynaptic neuron's response.

Aphagia: Inability to swallow. See also *Dysphagia* (difficulty swallowing).

Aphasia: Impairment in the expression and/or comprehension of language. Receptive aphasia (Wernicke aphasia) is impairment in the comprehension of language. Expressive aphasia (Broca aphasia) is impairment in the expression of language.

Aphonia: An inability to make sounds. *Hypophonia* refers to reduced vocal force.

Aphrenia: Stoppage of thought. The individual experiences poverty of thought.

Apnea: Arrest of breathing.

Apraxia: Inability or difficulty (dyspraxia) executing motor plans. Results from lesions to the motor cortices in the frontal lobe. Ideational apraxia involves an inability to cognitively understand the motor demands of the task. Ideomotor apraxia involves the loss of motor plans for specific activities; or the motor plan may be intact, but the individual cannot access it.

Aprosodia: A receptive aphasia that involves difficulty comprehending tonal inflections used in conversation. Results from lesions to the right hemisphere language centers.

Arachnoid Mater: The middle meningeal layer located just below the subdural space. Has the appearance of a spider web.

Arachnoid Villi: Projections of the arachnoid mater into the dura mater. Cerebrospinal fluid (CSF) is reabsorbed in the arachnoid villi.

Associated Reactions: Stereotyped movements in which effortful use of one extremity influences the posture and tone of another extremity (usually the opposite extremity). Can occur as a result of neurologic pathology or as part of normal movement (as a result of reflex stimulation). Associated reactions result from an overflow of activity into the opposite limb. This occurs because of an inability to selectively inhibit the interneurons that synapse with the motor cell bodies of the opposite limb.

Astereognosis: The inability to identify objects by touch alone. Results from damage to SS2.

Asthenia: Muscle weakness. A sign of cerebellar damage.

Asymbolia: A receptive aphasia that involves difficulty comprehending gestures and symbols.

Ataxia: Uncoordinated movements resulting from cerebellar lesions.

Atopognosia: The inability to accurately perceive the exact location of a sensation.

Audition: The detection and perception of sound.

Auditory Agnosia: The umbrella term for the inability to attach meaning to non-language sounds.

Auditory Association Areas: Responsible for the interpretation of auditory data. There are several auditory association areas located throughout the cortex. These areas have not as yet been mapped as precisely as the visual association areas.

Autonomic Nervous System (ANS): Composed of the parasympathetic nervous system and the sympathetic nervous system. Responsible for the innervation of visceral muscles, regulates glandular secretion, and controls vegetative functions (eg, temperature, digestion, heart rate).

Axon: Fiber emerging from the axon hillock and extending to the terminal boutons of a neuron. Axons transmit action potentials, or nerve signals, to the terminal boutons.

Axon Collaterals: Project from the main axon structure of a neuron and serve to transmit nerve signals to several parts of the nervous system simultaneously.

Axon Hillock: The region where a neuron's cell body and axon attach.

Basal Ganglia: An unconscious motor system that mediates stereotypic or automatic motor patterns, such as those involved in walking, riding a bike, and writing. Composed of 3 primary structures: caudate nucleus, putamen, and globus pallidus. Some sources now include the subthalamus and substantia nigra as part of the basal ganglia system. Disorders of the basal ganglia often result in dystonia and dyskinesia.

Bitemporal Hemianopia: Occurs when the temporal fields in both eyes have been lost. Results from a lesion to the central optic chiasm. Results in tunnel vision.

Blood-Brain Barrier: Consists of the meninges, the protective glial cells, and the capillary beds of the brain. Responsible for the exchange of nutrients between the CNS and the vascular system. Some molecules can cross the membrane, while others cannot. This accounts for the inability of many pharmaceuticals to cross the blood-brain barrier.

Body Schema Perceptual Dysfunction: Body schema is a neural perception of one's body in space—formed by a synthesis of tactile, proprioceptive, and pressure sensory data about the body. Dysfunction occurs when there is a severe discrepancy between body schema and reality. Includes finger agnosia, unilateral neglect, anosognosia, and extinction of simultaneous stimulation.

Brachial Plexus: A network of peripheral spinal nerves that supply the upper extremities. Includes C5, C6, C7, C8, and T1. Common site of compression injuries.

Bradykinesia: Slowness of voluntary movement. Seen commonly in Parkinson disease. Also seen in depression.

Bradyphrenia: Slowness of thought. Seen commonly in Parkinson disease and depression.

Brainstem: Composed of the midbrain, pons, and medulla. Controls vegetative functions (eg, respiration, cough and gag reflex, pupillary response, swallowing reflex).

Broca Aphasia: An expressive language disorder in which patients can understand what is spoken to them, but they cannot express their ideas in an understandable way.

Broca Area: Located only in the left hemisphere, just above the lateral fissure in the premotor area. Mediates the motoric functions of speech and is responsible for the verbal expression of language.

Callosal Sulcus: Sulcus separating the corpus callosum and the cingulate gyrus.

Catastrophic Reaction: An acute emotional syndrome related to the site of brain injury. Patients with left prefrontal lobe damage tend to be emotionally labile, depressed, and despondent. Catastrophic reaction tends to occur during the acute stages of brain damage.

Cauda Equina: At the end of the spinal cord—the conus medullaris—the spinal cord sends off the remaining spinal nerves that have not yet exited the vertebral column. This mass of spinal nerves is called the *cauda equina* because it resembles a horse's tail.

Caudal: Refers to the tail of the organism. Also refers to structures that are below others.

Caudate Nucleus: A basal ganglial structure involved in the planning and execution of automatic movement patterns. The caudate acts like a brake on certain motor activities. When the brake is not working, extraneous, purposeless movements appear (eg, tics, dyskinesias).

Causalgia: An intense burning pain accompanied by trophic skin changes.

Cell Body: Contains the nucleus of the neuron, which stores the genetic code of the organism.

Central Canal: Passageway through which CSF flows. Begins in the caudal medulla and descends throughout the entire length of the spinal cord.

Central Nervous System (CNS): Composed of the brain and spinal cord.

Central Sulcus: (Also called the *sulcus of Rolando.*) Separates the primary motor cortex from the primary somatosensory cortex.

Cerebellar Peduncle: Carries sensorimotor information about the body's position in space from the pons to the cerebellum. There are 3 pairs of cerebellar peduncles: middle, inferior, and superior cerebellar peduncles.

Cerebellum: Responsible for proprioception, or the unconscious awareness of the body's position in space. The cerebellum is a sensorimotor system; it receives sensory information from joint and muscle receptors concerning the body's position. The cerebellum uses this information to make decisions about how to adjust the body for the coordinated, precision control of movement and balance.

Cerebral Achromatopsia: A condition that occurs when V4 is lost and the world appears in shades of gray. The memory of color is erased.

Cerebral Aqueduct: Part of the ventricular system. A narrow channel that connects the third and fourth ventricles, allowing CSF to flow through.

Cerebral Peduncles: Large fiber bundles located on the anterior surface of the midbrain. Carry descending motor tracts from the cerebrum to the brainstem. Have an inner coat (consisting of the red nucleus and substantia nigra—collectively called the *tegmentum*) and an outer coat (consisting of the crus cerebri).

Cerebromedullary Cistern: (Also called *cisterna magna.*) Largest cistern in the subarachnoid space; allows CSF to flow from the fourth ventricle to the subarachnoid space. Located between the medulla and the cerebellum. Often used as a shunt placement.

Cerebrospinal Fluid (CSF): A clear and colorless fluid that bathes and nourishes the brain and spinal cord. The composition of CSF is used for diagnostic purposes to identify disease processes.

Chemoreceptors: Sensory receptors that respond to the presence of a particular chemical; involved in olfaction and gustation.

Choroid Plexus: Vascular structures in the brain that protrude into the ventricles and produce CSF.

Cingulate Gyrus: Most medial and deepest gyrus in the frontal and parietal lobes. Sits right above the corpus callosum. Shares vast connections with limbic system structures.

Cingulate Sulcus: The sulcus that separates the cingulate gyrus from other gyri in the frontoparietal regions; located on the medial aspect of each hemisphere.

Circle of Willis: A circuit of 5 interconnecting arteries that function to prevent lack of blood flow to the brain due to occlusion.

Clasp Knife Phenomenon: Involves severe spasticity at a joint. A sustained stretch will relax the muscle group, and the spasticity will suddenly give way.

Claustrum: A group of nuclei located just lateral to the extreme capsule and just medial to the insula.

Clonus: An uncontrolled oscillation of a spastic muscle group that results from a quick muscle stretch. Occurs in upper motor neuron (UMN) lesions.

CN: See *Cranial Nerves.*

CNS: See *Central Nervous System.*

Cogwheel Rigidity: Cogwheel rigidity is characterized by a pattern of release/resistance in a quick, jerky movement. Commonly seen in Parkinson disease.

Color Agnosia: A visual perceptual disorder in which individuals appear to forget the concept of color. They do not appear to know the color of common objects.

Color Anomia: A visual perceptual disorder in which individuals have lost the names for colors. However, they would still recognize that a blue banana was strange.

Commissure: Any collection of axons that connect one side of the nervous system to the other. An example is the corpus callosum.

Contractures: Limitation in joint movement due to shortening of muscles, tendons, and ligaments. Results from inactivity at a joint.

Contralateral Homonymous Hemianopia: A loss of the visual field on the opposite side of the lesion. A left visual field cut, or left contralateral homonymous hemianopsia, results from a lesion in the right optic tract. A right visual field cut, or right contralateral homonymous hemianopsia, results from a lesion in the left optic tract.

Conus Medullaris: The end of the spinal cord at the L1-L2 vertebral area.

Convolutions: The collective name for the gyri and sulci located on the surface of the cerebral hemispheres.

Coronal Plane: (Also called *frontal* or *transverse plane.*) The coronal planes run perpendicular to the sagittal planes. Coronal planes divide the anterior aspect of the brain from the posterior aspect.

Coronal Suture: The suture lines are areas where cranial bones have fused. The coronal suture runs along the coronal plane and connects the frontal bone with the parietal bones.

Corpus Callosum: Largest commissure in the brain. Allows the right and left cerebral hemispheres to communicate with each other.

Corpus Striatum: Collective name for the caudate, putamen, and globus pallidus (structures of the basal ganglia).

Cortex: A cortex is a layer of gray matter that contains nuclei, or nerve cell bodies. Humans have a cerebral cortex and a cerebellar cortex. The cortex sits on the surface of the cerebrum and cerebellum—underneath which is white matter, or axons.

Corticobulbar Tract: Spinal cord tract that descends from the corticospinal tract and projects to CN nuclei having a motor component.

Corticospinal Tracts: Descending motor tracts originating from the primary motor cortex. Responsible for voluntary movement on the contralateral side of the body.

Cranial Nerves (CN): The CNs are 12 pairs of nerves that are considered to be part of the peripheral nervous system (PNS). Their nuclei are located in the brainstem and are considered to be within the CNS. CNs carry sensory and motor information to and from the receptors of the head, face, and neck.

CSF: See *Cerebrospinal Fluid.*

Cunctation: Resisting or hindering; the opposite of festination, which means *quickened.* Together, the cunctating-festinating gait—characteristic of Parkinson disease—describes difficulty initiating movement and inability to stop movement once started.

Cuneocerebellar Tract: Ascending sensory spinal cord tract. Carries unconscious information from the trunk and upper extremities to the cerebellum regarding proprioception.

Cutaneous Receptors: Respond to pain, temperature, pressure, vibration, and discriminative touch. Found in the layers of the skin.

DA: See *Dopamine.*

Decerebrate Rigidity: Damage to any tract that originates in the brainstem may result in decerebrate rigidity. Involves spastic extension of both the upper and lower extremities. The occurrence of decerebrate rigidity indicates a much poorer prognosis than does decorticate rigidity.

Decorticate Rigidity: Results from damage to the corticospinal tracts. Decorticate rigidity presents as spastic flexion of the upper extremities; spastic extension of the lower extremities.

Deep Tendon Reflexes: A reflex arc in which a muscle contracts when its tendon is percussed. Deep tendon reflexes work on the principle of the spinal reflex arc. In an UMN injury, deep tendon reflexes become hyperreflexive because the spinal reflex arc remains intact below the lesion level, causing the reflex arc to run unmodified by cortical input. In a lower motor neuron (LMN) injury, deep tendon reflexes become hyporeflexive because the reflex arc is lost.

Dendrites: The treelike processes that attach to the cell body and receive messages from the terminal boutons of a presynaptic neuron. Dendrites can bifurcate, or produce additional dendritic branches. Bifurcation increases the neuron's receptor sites.

Dentate Nuclei: One of 4 pairs of cerebellar nuclei.

Denticulate Ligaments: A projection of the pia mater of the spinal cord. The denticulate ligaments are a series of 22 triangular bodies that anchor the spinal cord.

Depth Perception Dysfunction: Involves difficulty determining whether one object is closer to the individual than another object. Also referred to as *stereopsis.*

Dermatome: Skin segment innervated by a specific peripheral nerve.

Diencephalon: Collective name for the thalamus, hypothalamus, epithalamus, and subthalamus.

Diplopia: Double vision.

Dopamine (DA): The DA system has major effects on the motor system and on cognition and motivation. Loss of DA from the substantia nigra is the primary cause of Parkinson disease. Too much DA has been implicated in schizophrenia. The DA system also plays a role in addictive behaviors.

Dorsal: (Also referred to as *posterior.*) The back of an organism.

Dorsal Column: Ascending sensory spinal cord tract. Carries conscious information about discriminative touch, pressure, vibration, proprioception, and kinesthesia.

Dorsal Horn: The dorsal horn is considered to be part of the CNS. It contains the cell bodies of the sensory spinal cord tracts. In the dorsal horn, the dorsal rootlets may synapse on interneurons. These interneurons then synapse with spinal cord tracts, or the dorsal rootlets may synapse directly on the cell bodies of spinal cord tracts.

Dorsal Intermediate Sulcus: Sulci that are located just lateral to the dorsal median sulcus.

Dorsal Median Sulcus: A sulcus that divides the posterior medulla into equal left and right halves.

Dorsal Root and Rootlets: Dorsal roots are axon bundles that emerge from an ascending spinal nerve. The dorsal root leads into the dorsal rootlets—thin, stringlike axons that emerge from the dorsal root and synapse in the dorsal horn of the spinal cord. The dorsal root and rootlets are considered to be part of the PNS.

Dorsal Root Ganglion: Contains the cell bodies of sensory nerves that are part of the somatic PNS. Each sensory nerve has its own dorsal root ganglion. The dorsal root emerges from the dorsal ganglia.

Double Simultaneous Extinction: The inability to determine that one has been touched on both the involved side and the uninvolved side—the neural sensation of the uninvolved side overrides the ability to perceive touch on the involved side. Also called *extinction of simultaneous stimulation.*

Downregulation: A decrease in the number of receptors for a neurotransmitter on the postsynaptic neuron, often due to long-term exposure to the neurotransmitter.

Dressing Apraxia: A form of ideomotor apraxia involving an inability to dress oneself due to impairment in either (a) body schema perception or (b) perceptual motor functions. Example: a patient may attempt to put his or her arm through pant legs or dress only one half of his or her body.

Dura Mater: The outermost meningeal layer. The dura has 2 projections that extend into the brain: falx cerebri and tentorium.

Dural Sinuses: Openings for blood vessels and nerves in the dura. Located above the frontal and parietal lobes. The sinuses function as a circulatory system: cerebral veins empty into the sinuses; they also receive CSF from the subarachnoid space.

Dysarthria: Difficulty articulating words clearly. Slurring words.

Dysesthesia: Unpleasant sensation, such as burning.

Dyslexia: The impaired ability to read. Dyslexia is a language problem in which the ability to break down words into their most basic units—phonemes—is impaired. See also *Alexia.*

Dysmetria: Inability to judge distance. Past-pointing or overshooting one's reach for objects. Occurs as a result of cerebellar lesions.

Dysphagia: Difficulty swallowing.

Dysphonia: Difficulty projecting one's voice audibly.

Dystonia: Also sometimes used interchangeably with *dyskinesia.* Both terms refer to abnormalities in muscle tone and movement. Includes athetosis, chorea, Parkinson disease, and idiopathic torsion dystonia.

Emboliform Nuclei: One of 4 pairs of cerebellar nuclei.

Endorphins: Work conjointly with Substance P to act as pain modulators. The primary action of endorphin is the inhibition of nociceptive information.

Enteric Nervous System: An independent circuit that is loosely connected to the CNS but can function alone without instruction from the CNS. Located in sheaths of tissue that line the esophagus, stomach, small intestines, and colon. Composed of a network of neurons, neurotransmitters, and proteins.

Epicritic Sensory Receptors: Can detect sensation with precision, accuracy, and acuteness. Discriminative touch, sharp pain, exact joint position, and the exact localization of a stimulus are within the functions of the epicritic system. Evolutionary function: allows the organism to explore the environment with precise detail, thus allowing the ability to detect imminent danger.

Episodic Memory: A type of memory involving significant events that happened to an individual—the first day of school, one's wedding, the birth of a child.

Epithalamus: Very small structure located just posterior to the thalamus and just anterior to the pineal gland. A principal structure of the epithalamus is the habenula—a nucleus at the posterior of the epithalamus.

Esotropia: Internal or medial strabismus. Results from lesions to the abducens nerve (CN 6).

Euphoric Reaction: An acute emotional syndrome related to the site of brain injury. Right prefrontal lobe damage often leaves patients with an indifference to their impairment (referred to as *anosognosia*). Patients commonly report states of euphoria and well-being despite severe impairment. Euphoric reaction tends to occur during the acute stages of brain damage.

Exotropia: External or lateral strabismus. Results from lesions to the oculomotor nerve (CN 3).

Explicit Memory: A type of memory involving knowledge that an individual consciously knows she has acquired. For example, an anatomist knows that he or she has acquired knowledge of the human body's musculoskeletal system.

Expressive Aphasia: A language perceptual problem involving difficulty expressing clear, meaningful language.

External Capsule: White matter located just lateral to the putamen (of the basal ganglia) and medial to the claustrum.

Exteroceptor: A sensory receptor that is adapted for the reception of stimuli from the external world (eg, visual, auditory, tactile, olfactory, and gustatory receptors).

Extinction of Simultaneous Stimulation: The inability to determine that one has been touched on both the involved side and the uninvolved side. The neural sensation of the uninvolved side overrides the ability to perceive touch on the involved side. Also called *double simultaneous extinction*.

Extrapyramidal System: Motor structures and spinal cord tracts that do not use the pyramids to send motor messages to the skeletal muscles.

Extreme Capsule: White matter located just lateral to the claustrum and medial to the insula.

Facial Nerve: CN 7. Responsible for taste on the anterior of the tongue. Also responsible for innervating the muscles of facial expression and eyelid closing.

Falx Cerebri: A projection of dura mater that extends into the medial longitudinal fissure.

Fasciculations: Brief contractions of motor units; can be observed in skeletal muscle and detected on clinical examination.

Fastigial Nuclei: One of 4 pairs of cerebellar nuclei.

Festinating: Quickened. Festinating is the opposite of cunctation—resisting or hindering. Together, the cunctating-festinating gait, characteristic of Parkinson disease, describes difficulty initiating movement and inability to stop movement once started.

Fibrillations: Fine twitches of single muscle fibers that usually cannot be detected on clinical examination but can be identified on an electromyogram.

Figure-Ground Discrimination Dysfunction: Involves difficulty distinguishing the foreground from the background.

Filum Terminale: A projection of the pia mater of the spinal cord. The filum terminale is a slender median fibrous thread that attaches the conus medullaris to the coccyx. It anchors the end of the spinal cord to the vertebral column.

Finger Agnosia: Involves an impaired perception concerning the relationship of the fingers to each other. It also involves an impaired identification and localization of one's own fingers.

Fissure: A deep groove in the surface of the brain—deeper than a sulcus.

Flaccidity: Loss of muscle tone resulting from denervation of specific peripheral nerves. Flaccidity occurs in LMN injuries. In an UMN injury, flaccidity occurs only at the lesion level; spasticity occurs below the lesion level.

Fontanels: Nonossified spaces or soft spots located between the cranial bones of fetuses and newborns. These allow the skull to expand to accommodate the growing brain (anterior, posterior, sphenoid, and mastoid fontanels).

Foramen Magnum: The largest foramina in the skull—specifically, the occipital bone. The opening through which the brainstem connects with the spinal cord.

Foramen of Luschka: (Also called *lateral aperture*.) Opening in the fourth ventricle through which CSF flows into the subarachnoid space. There are 2 foramen of Luschka in the fourth ventricle, located in the pons. Often a site of CSF blockage.

Foramen of Magendie: (Also called *median aperture*.) Opening in the fourth ventricle through which CSF flows into the subarachnoid space; located in the rostral medulla. Often a site of CSF blockage.

Foramen of Monro: A channel located in the ventricular system; allows CSF to flow from the lateral ventricles to the third ventricle. Often a site of CSF blockage.

Foramina: Openings in the skull for the passage of blood vessels and nerves.

Form Constancy Dysfunction: Involves difficulty attending to subtle variations in form or changes in form, such as size variation of the same object.

Fornix: The fornix bodies are a pair of arch-shaped fibers that begin in the uncus and wrap around to the mammillary bodies. The fornix is a relay system for messages generated by the limbic system.

Fossa (or *cranial fossa*): The undersurface of the brain sits in 3 cranial sections, or *fossa*. The anterior cranial fossa primarily supports the frontal lobes. The middle cranial fossa supports the anterior-inferior temporal lobes and the diencephalon. The posterior cranial fossa supports the cerebellum.

Fourth Ventricle: Region of the ventricular system through which CSF flows. Located between the pons and the cerebellum. Connected to the third ventricle via the cerebral aqueduct. The fourth ventricle connects to the spinal cord via the central canal.

Frontal Eye Field: Located in the middle frontal gyrus, anterior to the premotor area. Responsible for visual saccades.

Frontal Lobe: Responsible for cognition, expressive language, motor planning, mathematical calculations, and working memory.

Frontal Plane: (Also called *coronal* or *transverse plane*.) The frontal planes run perpendicular to the sagittal planes. Frontal planes divide the anterior aspect of the brain from the posterior aspect.

GABA: See *Gamma-Aminobutyric Acid.*

Gamma-Aminobutyric Acid (GABA): A major inhibitory neurotransmitter that turns off the function of cells. GABA deficiency is implicated in anxiety disorders, insomnia, and epilepsy. GABA excess is implicated in memory loss and the inability to learn new things.

Ganglia: A collection of neural cell bodies (or nuclei) usually located outside the CNS.

Globose Nuclei: One of 4 pairs of cerebellar nuclei.

Globus Pallidus: A basal ganglia structure involved in stereotypic or automatic movement patterns. While the caudate nucleus works like a brake on motor activity, the globus pallidus is an excitatory structure.

Glossopharyngeal Nerve: CN 9. Responsible for taste on the posterior of the tongue. Also innervates muscles of swallowing.

GLU: See *Glutamate.*

Glutamate (GLU): One of the major excitatory neurotransmitters of the CNS. Responsible for cell death when the brain experiences a major traumatic event. May also play a role in learning and memory.

Golgi Tendon Organ: Proprioceptors that are embedded in the tendons, close to the skeletal muscle insertion. Detect tension in the tendon of a contracting muscle.

Gray Matter: Sits on the surface of the cerebrum and cerebellum. Consists of nerve cell bodies.

Gustation: The detection and perception of taste.

Gyri (s., Gyrus): The wrinkles or folds on the surface of the cerebral hemispheres.

Hemianopia: Field cut. See also *Contralateral Homonymous Hemianopia* and *Bitemporal Hemianopia.*

Hemiparesis: Partial paralysis or muscular weakness of limbs on one side of the body. Occurs on the contralateral side (or opposite side) of the lesion site.

Hemiparesthesia: Loss of sensation of limbs on one side of the body. Occurs on the contralateral side (or opposite side) of the lesion site.

Hemiplegia: Complete paralysis of limbs on one side of the body. Occurs on the contralateral side (or opposite side) of the lesion site.

Hippocampus: Located within the parahippocampal gyrus. One of the major storehouses in the brain for long-term memory.

Homunculus: Cortical representation for each body part's motor and sensory function. See also *Motor Homunculus* and *Sensory Homunculus.*

Horizontal Plane: The horizontal planes divide the superior aspect of the brain from the inferior aspect.

Hypalgesia: A decrease in the ability to perceive pain.

Hyperalgesia: An increase in the ability to perceive pain (ie, pain sensation becomes heightened).

Hyperesthesia: An increase in sensory perception. Heightened perception of pain and temperature.

Hyperkinesia: Disorders involving speeded movement (eg, chorea, athetosis). Opposite of hypokinesia.

Hyperreflexia: An increase in deep tendon reflexes.

Hypertonia: Excessive muscle tone due to spasticity or rigidity. Opposite of hypotonia.

Hypoesthesia: A decrease in sensory perception.

Hypoglossal Nerve: CN 12. Responsible for innervating the tongue muscles.

Hypokinesia: The slowing of movement just short of complete loss of movement or akinesia.

Hyporeflexia: Decreased deep tendon reflexes.

Hypothalamus: Two lobes (one in each hemisphere) that contain nuclei responsible for the regulation of the autonomic nervous system, release of hormones from the pituitary gland, temperature regulation, hunger and thirst, and sleep/wake cycles.

Hypotonia: A lack of muscle tone. Opposite of hypertonia.

Ideational Praxis: The ability to cognitively understand the motor demands of a task. For example, a patient must understand that shirts are articles of clothing to be worn on the torso. This type of praxis is largely a function of the motor association area.

Ideomotor Planning I: The ability to access the appropriate motor plan. For example, this would involve the ability to sort through all stored motor plans and identify the specific one for shirt donning. Such motor plans are commonly stored in the premotor area.

Ideomotor Planning II: The ability to implement the appropriate motor plan or put it into action. For example, after identifying the appropriate motor plan for donning a shirt, the patient must put that plan into action. Implementing motor plans commonly involves M1.

Implicit Memory: A type of memory involving knowledge that the individual does not consciously know he has acquired. For example, someone with amnesia may not consciously know she has acquired knowledge of how to play the piano, but when seated at the piano, she can play fluently.

Inferior: Refers to the direction "below."

Inferior Colliculi: A pair of relay centers for audition that communicate directly with the medial geniculate nuclei of the thalamus. Located on the posterior region of the midbrain.

Inferior Olives (or *Olivary Nuclei*): Relay nuclei that carry ascending sensory information to the cerebellum. The sensory data pertain to the body's position in space.

Infundibulum: The stalk that extends from the hypothalamus and holds the pituitary gland.

Insula: A portion of the cerebral cortex that lies deep in the lateral fissure; covered from view by the frontal, parietal, and temporal lobes. Possible roles in (a) the perceptual processing of gustatory information and (b) the interpretation of music.

Intention Tremor: Occurs during voluntary movement of a limb and tends to increase as the limb nears its intended goal. Tremor is the rhythmic oscillation of joints caused by alternating contractions of opposing muscle groups. Intention tremors tend to diminish or stop when the patient's limbs are at rest. A sign of cerebellar damage.

Internal Capsule: A large fiber bundle that connects the cerebral cortex with the diencephalon. All descending motor messages from the cortex travel through the internal capsule to the thalamus, brainstem, spinal cord, and to the skeletal muscles. All sensory information travels through the internal capsule before reaching the cortex.

Interoceptors: Receive sensory information from inside the body, such as stomach pain, pinched spinal nerves, or inflammatory processes in the viscera.

Interpeduncular Fossa: The indentation between the pair of cerebral peduncles (on the anterior of the midbrain) that contains the mammillary bodies.

Interthalamic Adhesion: A commissure that connects the 2 thalamic lobes. Runs through the third ventricle.

Intervertebral Discs: Dense cushion-like structures that lie between each vertebrae. Each disc consists of the nucleus pulposus (a soft, pulpy, highly elastic tissue in the center of the disc) and the annulus fibrosus (the more fibrous outer-covering of the disc).

Joint Receptors: Proprioceptors that are located in the connective tissue of a joint capsule. Respond to mechanical deformation occurring in the joint capsule and ligaments.

Kinesthesia: The ability to sense one's body movement in space.

Lambdoid Suture: The suture lines are areas where cranial bones have fused. The lambdoid suture connects the 2 parietal bones to the occipital bone.

Lateral: Refers to structures that are further from the midline of the body.

Lateral Fissure: (Also called *fissure of Sylvius*.) Separates the temporal lobe from the frontal lobe.

Lateral Spinothalamic Tract: Ascending sensory spinal cord tract. Carries conscious information about pain and temperature.

Lateral Ventricle: One of 4 ventricles that contain cerebrospinal fluid. There are 2 lateral ventricles, 1 in each hemisphere. The lateral ventricle is an arch-shaped structure that has its anterior horn located in the frontal lobe, its body located in the parietal lobe, its posterior horn located in the occipital lobe, and its inferior horn located in the temporal lobe.

Lead Pipe Rigidity: Characterized by a uniform and continuous resistance to passive movement as the extremity is moved through its range of motion (in all planes).

Lenticular Nucleus: Collective name for the globus pallidus and putamen (of the basal ganglia). Also called *lentiform nucleus*.

Limbic System: Located deep within the core of the brain, the limbic system appears to be the source of human emotions before they are modulated by the frontal lobes. The limbic system is also a storehouse for long-term memory, particularly memories that have strong emotional significance.

LMN: See *Lower Motor Neuron*.

Locus Ceruleus: Located on the floor of the fourth ventricle in the brainstem. Secretes NE.

Long-Term Memory: The ability to remember one's past, familiar others, and events encountered more than several hours ago. Believed to be a function of the hippocampus and temporal lobe.

Lower Motor Neuron (LMN): Carries motor messages from the motor cell bodies in the ventral horn to the skeletal muscles in the periphery. A LMN is considered to be part of the PNS. Includes the CNs, peripheral spinal nerves, conus medullaris, cauda equina, and the ventral horn. Lesions to these structures will cause LMN signs.

Lumbar Plexus: A network of peripheral spinal nerves that supply the lower extremities. Includes L1, L2, L3, L4, and L5. Common site of compression injuries.

M1: See *Primary Motor Area*.

Mammillary Bodies: Two protrusions that sit within the interpeduncular fossa on the anterior surface of the midbrain. The mammillary bodies are nuclei groups that form attachments with the hypothalamus and fornix and may play a role in the processing of emotion.

Mechanoreceptors: Sensory receptors that are stimulated by mechanical deformity (eg, hair cell receptors of the skin).

Medial: Refers to structures that are close to the midline of the body.

Medial Longitudinal Fasciculus: Mixed spinal cord tract with both ascending and descending fibers. Responsible for the coordination of head, neck, and eyeball movements.

Medial Longitudinal Fissure: Runs along the midsagittal plane. Separates the right and left cerebral hemispheres.

Medulla: Carries descending motor messages from the cerebrum to the spinal cord, and ascending sensory messages from the spinal cord to the cerebrum. Located between the pons and the spinal cord.

Medullary Reticulospinal Tract: Descending extrapyramidal motor tract that inhibits antigravity muscles (inhibits extensor muscles).

Membrane Potential: The electrical charge that travels across the cell membrane. It is the difference between the chemical composition inside and outside the cell—in other words, the sodium potassium balance inside and outside the cell. If the membrane potential is strong enough, it causes an action potential.

Meninges: The meninges are located between the skull and brain and cover the spinal cord. They form a protective seal around the CNS. There are 3 layers of meninges: dura mater, arachnoid mater, and pia mater.

Mesolimbic System: The brain's reward system is called the *mesocorticolimbic*, or *mesolimbic*, *system*. This system consists of a complex circuit of neurons that evolved to encourage people to repeat pleasurable behavior that supports survival. The primary neural pathway of the mesolimbic system originates in the ventral tegmental area of the midbrain. This area sends projections to the nucleus accumbens, which is located deep beneath the frontal cortex. The primary neurotransmitter used by this system is DA. Almost all drugs of abuse have the potential to become addictive because of their ability to increase DA levels in the brain's reward system.

Metamorphopsia: Involves a visual-perceptual distortion of the physical properties of objects so that objects appear bigger, smaller, or heavier than they really are.

Micrographia: A sign of Parkinson disease in which handwriting becomes small and of poor quality due to movement decomposition.

Midbrain: The midbrain is the most rostral structure of the brainstem that sits atop the pons and is just inferior to the thalamus. Has a role in automatic reflexive behaviors dealing with vision and audition. Site of the reticular activating system; has roles in wakefulness and consciousness.

Midsagittal Plane: The midsagittal plane divides the left and right cerebral hemispheres. This plane divides the brain in half and runs along the medial longitudinal fissure.

Mononeuropathy: Involves damage to a single peripheral nerve; usually due to compression or entrapment.

Motor Association Area: (Also called the *prefrontal lobe*.) Has a role in the cognitive planning of movement.

Motor Homunculus: The cortical map that represents each body part's area for motor function. Location of M1—the precentral gyrus.

Movement Decomposition: Movement is performed in a sequence of isolated parts rather than as a smooth, singular motion. A sign of cerebellar damage. Also referred to as *dyssynergia*.

Multimodal Association Area: Cortical areas where sensory information merges for integration and interpretation. Two multimodal association areas: (1) anterior multimodal association area, located in prefrontal lobe; (2) posterior multimodal association area, located where the parietal, occipital, and temporal lobes converge.

Muscle Spindle: Proprioceptors that are located in the skeletal muscle. Provide a constant flow of information regarding length, tension, and load on the muscles.

Myelin: Axons are covered by a cellular sheath called *myelin*, an insulating substance composed of lipids and proteins. Myelin serves to conduct nerve signals. The more myelin the axon has, the faster its conduction rate.

Myotome: A group of muscles innervated by a specific single spinal nerve. The myotomes of the human body correspond closely to the dermatomes.

NE: See *Norepinephrine.*

Neostriatum: Collective name for the caudate and putamen (of the basal ganglia).

Neuron: The electrically excitable nerve cell and fiber of the nervous system. Composed of a cell body with a nucleus, dendrites, a main axon branch, and terminal boutons.

Neuropathy: A general term for pathology involving one or more peripheral nerves.

Neuroplasticity: Occurs when other areas of the brain assume the functions once mediated by regions that have been damaged. Human brains appear to possess a vast amount of brain matter that does not become active until damage occurs to other areas. At this time, those previously unused regions may become active and take over the function of damaged areas. It is possible that the same brain function may be shared by several, separate brain regions that lie dormant until injury/disease occurs. This may be the brain's evolutionary attempt at compensation. Neuroplasticity is most viable in children because the CNS is not fully mature, but rather is still developing.

Neurotransmitter: Chemical stored in the terminal boutons. Released into the synaptic cleft to transmit messages to another neuron.

Nociception: The detection and localization of pain.

Nodes of Ranvier: Spaces between the myelin—on an axon—where nerve signals jump from one node to the next in the process of conduction.

Norepinephrine (NE): A neurotransmitter essential in the production of the fight/flight response, fear, and panic.

Nystagmus: Involuntary back and forth movements of the eye in a quick, jerky, oscillating fashion when the eye moves laterally or medially to either the temporal or nasal extreme visual fields.

Occipital Lobe: Responsible for the detection and interpretation of visual stimuli.

Occipital Pole: Most posterior region of the occipital lobe. Site of V1, responsible for the detection of visual stimuli.

Oculomotor Nerve: CN 3. Responsible for extraocular eye movements. Lesion symptoms can include nystagmus and lateral strabismus.

Olfaction: Detection and perception of smell.

Olfactory Bulb and Tract: Also known as *CN 1*. The olfactory tract travels directly to the hippocampus, which accounts for the deep association between specific odors and long-term memories that have emotional significance.

Olfactory Nerve: CN 1. Responsible for smell.

Oligodendrocytes: Compose the myelin in the CNS. Because oligodendrocytes do not produce nerve growth factor, most nerve damage in the CNS cannot resolve.

Optic Chiasm: A cross-shaped connection between the optic nerves. Carries visual information from the optic nerves to the optic tracts.

Optic Nerve: CN 2. The optic nerves (one in each hemisphere) carry visual information from the retina, through the optic disk, to the optic chiasm. Visual information then travels from the optic chiasm to the optic tracts. Responsible for visual acuity.

Paleostriatum: Another name for the globus pallidus (of the basal ganglia) because of its striped appearance.

Parahippocampal Gyrus: Most medial and deepest gyrus in the temporal lobes. Folds back on itself at its anterior end to become the uncus. Relays information between the hippocampus and other cerebral areas, particularly the frontal lobes. The parahippocampal gyrus may function when humans compare a present event to an event stored in long-term memory to decide how to handle a present situation.

Parasympathetic Nervous System: A division of the autonomic nervous system. Responsible for peristalsis and the maintenance of homeostasis.

Paresis: Partial paralysis.

Paresthesia: The occurrence of unusual feelings, such as pins and needles.

Parietal Lobe: Responsible for sensory detection and interpretation.

Perception: The ability to interpret or attach meaning to sensory data from the external and internal environments. Perceptual impairment more often results from damage to the right hemisphere, which produces a distortion in the patient's perception of his or her physical body and environment.

Peripheral Nervous System (PNS): Composed of the CNs, autonomic nervous system, and SNS.

Phantom Limb Phenomenon: The sensation that an amputated body part still remains. If the sensation is painful, it is referred to as *phantom pain*. The cortical map of the body still retains the anatomical image of the amputated body part.

Photoreceptors: Sensory receptors that detect light on the retina of the eye.

Pia Mater: The deepest meningeal layer, located on the surface of the gyri and sulci of the brain and on the surface of the spinal cord. The pia mater of the spinal cord sends off 2 projections: the filum terminale and the dentate ligaments.

Pineal Gland: Innervated by the autonomic nervous system. Has a role in sexual hormonal functions and sleep-wake cycles.

Pituitary Gland: An endocrine gland that secretes hormones regulating growth, reproductive activities, and metabolic processes.

Plexopathy: A form of neuropathy involving damage to one of the plexus: brachial or lumbar. Involves multiple peripheral nerve damage.

PNS: See *Peripheral Nervous System*.

Polyneuropathy: A form of neuropathy involving bilateral damage to more than one peripheral nerve. An example is stocking and glove polyneuropathy. Usually caused by a disease process, such as diabetes.

Pons: Brainstem structure that acts as a relay system between the spinal cord, cerebellum, and cerebrum. It largely mediates sensorimotor information on an unconscious level, shifting weight to maintain balance and making fine motor adjustments in one's muscles to perform precise coordinated limb movement. Located between the midbrain and medulla. Site of the reticular inhibiting system; has roles in sleep states and unconsciousness.

Pontine Reticulospinal Tract: Descending extrapyramidal motor tract that facilitates antigravity muscles (ie, facilitates extensor muscles).

Position in Space Dysfunction: Involves difficulty with concepts relating to positions such as up/down, in/out, behind/in front of, and before/after.

Postcentral Gyrus: Located just posterior to the central sulcus; known as *SS1*, where sensory information from the contralateral side of the body is detected. Also referred to as the *sensory homunculus*, the cortical representation for each body part's sensory function.

Postcentral Sulcus: Sulcus located just posterior to the postcentral gyrus.

Posterior (or *dorsal*): Refers to the back of an organism.

Posterior Commissure: Located just superior to the superior colliculi. Allows information to travel between both diencephalic hemispheres.

Posterior Spinocerebellar Tract: Ascending sensory spinal cord tract. Carries unconscious information from the lower extremities to the cerebellum regarding proprioception.

Postpontine Fossa: Shallow depression located between the anterior aspects of the pons and medulla.

Postsynaptic Neuron: Second-order neuron. Receives the presynaptic neuron's neurotransmitter substance from the synaptic cleft.

Post-Tetanic Potentiation: Occurs in synapses that are frequently used. When the presynaptic bouton becomes excited, it releases greater amounts of neurotransmitter substance. The postsynaptic neuron then has prolonged and repetitive discharge after firing due to too much neurotransmitter release or too slow antitransmitter work.

Praxis: Motor planning. The ability to understand and implement the movements required for a specific activity.

Precentral Gyrus: Located just anterior to the central sulcus; considered to be M1, where voluntary movement (on the contralateral side of the body) is initiated. Also referred to as the *motor homunculus*, the cortical map that represents each body part's area for motor function.

Precentral Sulcus: Sulcus located just anterior to the precentral gyrus.

Premotor Area: Located just anterior to M1. Has a role in motor planning or praxis.

Prepontine Fossa: Shallow depression located between the anterior aspects of the midbrain and pons.

Presynaptic Neuron: First-order neuron. Releases its neurotransmitter into the synaptic cleft.

Primary Auditory Area (A1): Located within the insula in the temporal lobe. Responsible for detecting sounds from the environment.

Primary Motor Area (M1): Location of the precentral gyrus. Where voluntary movement (on the contralateral side of the body) is initiated. Also referred to as the *motor homunculus*, the cortical map that represents each body part's area for motor function.

Primary Somatosensory Area (SS1): Location of the postcentral gyrus. Where sensory information from the contralateral side of the body is detected. Also referred to as the *motor homunculus*, the cortical map that represents each body part's area for motor function.

Primary Visual Area (V1): Responsible for the detection of visual stimuli. Located at the most posterior region of the occipital lobe.

Primitive Reflexes: Reflexes that humans are born with or that develop and become integrated by the CNS in infancy and toddlerhood. These reactions facilitate gross motor patterns of flexion and extension. Primitive reflexes exhibited by an adult are signs of neurologic damage.

Procedural Memory: A type of memory involving the recall of steps involved in specific tasks. For example, knowing the steps involved in fabricating a wrist cock-up splint or knowing the steps involved in changing a flat tire.

Proprioception: The ability to sense one's body position in space. Proprioception occurs mostly on an unconscious level because it is primarily mediated by the cerebellum.

Proprioceptor: Sensory receptors located in the muscles, tendons, and joints of the body, and in the utricles, saccules, and semicircular canals of the inner ear.

Prosopagnosia: The inability to identify familiar faces because the individual cannot perceive the unique expressions of facial muscles that make each human face different from each other.

Protopathic Sensory Receptors: Adapted to identify gross bodily sensation rather than precise regions of sensation. Detect crude touch and dull pain rather than discriminative touch and sharp pain.

Putamen: A basal ganglial structure involved in stereotypic or automatic movement patterns. While the caudate nucleus works like a brake on motor activity, the putamen is an excitatory structure.

Pyramidal Decussation: The crossing-over point where motor fibers from the left cortex cross to the right side of the spinal cord. Motor fibers from the right side of the cortex cross to the left side of the spinal cord. This is why the right cerebral hemisphere controls the left side of the body and the left cerebral hemisphere controls the right side of the body.

Pyramids: Fiber bundles that carry descending motor information from the cortex to the spinal cord. The pyramids are 2 large structures on the anterior region of the medulla that are divided by the anterior median fissure.

Radiculopathy: Nerve root impingement that results from a lesion affecting the dorsal or ventral roots. Can result from herniated vertebral discs.

Rebound Phenomenon: The inability to regulate the action of opposing muscle groups. The patient is asked to resist the therapist's attempt to pull the patient's flexed elbow into extension. The therapist then releases the patient's forearm. Normally, the elbow would remain in approximately the same position due to the ability to regulate the speed of muscular contraction. Patients with cerebellar lesions are unable to regulate their opposing muscle groups, and their limb suddenly hits their torso. This occurs as a result of impaired proprioceptive feedback. The patient cannot regulate the speed and force of opposing muscle groups quickly enough to prevent the arm from hitting the torso.

Recent Memory: Considered to be a component of long-term memory. Recent memory refers to the ability to recall events/information that occurred hours to weeks ago.

Receptive Aphasia: A perceptual problem involving impairment in the comprehension of language.

Receptor Field: A body area that contains specific types of sensory receptor cells. Small receptor fields are located on body areas with the greatest sensitivity: lips, hands, face, soles of feet. Large receptor fields are located on body areas with less sensitivity: legs, abdomen, arms, back.

Referred Pain: Occurs when a specific body region shares its spinal nerve innervation with a separate dermatomal skin segment. The pain experienced by the body part is misinterpreted by the cortex as pain coming from a separate dermatomal skin segment.

Remote Memory: A component of long-term memory; refers to the ability to recall events/information that occurred in the distant past (eg, several years ago). Believed to be a function of the hippocampus and temporal lobe.

Resting Tremor: (Also called *nonintention tremors.*) Characteristic of Parkinson disease. Involuntary oscillating movements that occur in an extremity at rest. Resting tremors decrease with the intention of voluntary movement.

Reticular Formation: Two systems diffusely located in the brainstem: the reticular activating system and reticular inhibiting system. The activating system alerts the cortex to attend to important sensory stimuli and is involved in states of wakefulness. The inhibiting system is involved in states of unconsciousness such as sleep, stupor, or coma.

Retrograde Amnesia: A type of memory problem that involves the loss of one's entire personal past and occurs after injury or trauma. Memory of one's past is often recovered at some point after injury.

Reuptake Process: Process by which a neurotransmitter is reabsorbed into the presynaptic neuron's terminal boutons.

Right-Left Discrimination Dysfunction: Involves difficulty understanding and using the concepts of right and left.

Rigidity: Involves an inability to passively and/or actively move a joint on both sides of the joint. Example: cogwheel rigidity (commonly seen in Parkinson disease). Rigidity is velocity independent; that is, increased muscle tone exists whether an affected limb is passively moved slowly or quickly.

Rostral: Refers to the head of an organism. Also refers to structures that are above others.

Rostral Spinocerebellar Tract: Ascending sensory spinal cord tract. Carries unconscious information from the trunk and upper extremities to the cerebellum regarding proprioception.

Rubrospinal Tracts: Descending extrapyramidal motor tract. Facilitates antagonist of antigravity muscles (the flexors).

Saccule: One of the receptors of equilibrium in the inner ear. Responds to changes in head position. Part of the vestibular system.

Sagittal Plane: The sagittal planes run parallel to the midsagittal plane.

Sagittal Suture: The suture lines are areas where cranial bones have fused. The sagittal suture runs along the midsagittal plane and connects the 2 parietal bones.

Schwann Cell: The myelin in the PNS is composed of Schwann cells that produce nerve growth factor. This allows peripheral nerve damage to resolve (unlike damage in the CNS).

Secondary Somatosensory Area (SS2): Responsible for the interpretation of sensory stimuli from the contralateral side of the body.

Semantic Memory: A type of memory involving the recall of facts: dates of people's birthdays, state capitols, the names of presidents. Semantic memory includes the definitions of words and how to use the rules of grammar.

Semicircular Canals: Receptors of equilibrium that form a system of canals called the *bony labyrinth* in the inner ear. There are 3 semicircular canals; each responds to movement of the head. Part of the vestibular system.

Sensory Homunculus: The cortical representation for each body part's sensory function. Location of the postcentral gyrus, or SS1.

Sensory Receptor: A specialized nerve cell that is designed to respond to a specific sensory stimulus (eg, touch, pressure, pain, temperature, light, sound, position in space).

Septal Area: The region on either cerebral hemisphere that comprises the subcallosal area and the corresponding half of the septum pellucidum.

Septum Pellucidum: A sheath-like cover that extends over the medial wall of each lateral ventricle. May have a role in the processing of emotion.

Serotonin (5-HT): A neurotransmitter implicated in sleep, emotional control, pain regulation, and carbohydrate feeding behaviors (eating disorders). Low levels of serotonin are associated with depression and suicidal behavior.

Short-Term Memory: The ability to remember others and events encountered less than 1 hour ago.

Simultanagnosia: Involves difficulty interpreting a visual stimulus as a whole. Patients often confabulate to compensate for what they cannot interpret visually.

SNS: See *Somatic Nervous System.*

Somatic Nervous System (SNS): Part of the PNS. Responsible for the innervation of skeletal muscles.

Source Memory: A type of memory involving the recall of how information is learned. For example, an anatomist may recall that he or she learned specific information about the human shoulder joint from a specific dissection class. Often, people remember facts but cannot recall how they came to learn those facts.

Spasticity: Involves the inability to move a joint on one side of the joint. Usually, either the flexors or the extensors are spastic, but not both. Results from UMN lesions. Spasticity is velocity dependent; that is, spasticity can be elicited by passively moving an affected limb quickly. The same passive movement of the limb performed slowly may not elicit increased muscle tone.

Spinal Reflex Arc: A spinal reflex arc is mediated at the spinal cord level; there is no cortical involvement. A sensory receptor in the PNS sends a message along an ascending sensory spinal nerve that travels to the dorsal horn and synapses on an interneuron. The interneuron synapses with a motor cell body located in the ventral horn. The motor cell body in the ventral horn relays the message to a motor spinal nerve in the PNS, which sends the motor message to a skeletal muscle group for action in response to the initial sensory message.

SS1: See *Primary Somatosensory Area.*

SS2: See *Secondary Somatosensory Area.*

Staccato Voice: Broken speech; a sign of cerebellar damage. Because the modulation of speech is a proprioceptive function, patients with cerebellar damage may be unable to modulate the fluidity of speech.

Stereopsis: Depth vision.

Strabismus: Deviation of the eyeball laterally (lateral strabismus, also called *exotropia*) or medially (medial strabismus, also called *esotropia*).

Subarachnoid Space: Area beneath the arachnoid mater and above the pia mater. Contains CSF.

Substance P: Acts as a neurotransmitter in the nociceptive pathway, although it is classified as a peptide. The nociceptive pathway mediates the experience of pain.

Substantia Nigra: Located in the midbrain. The red nucleus and the substantia nigra of the midbrain form the inner coat of the cerebral peduncles. The substantia nigra produces DA, a neurotransmitter that functions in movement and mood regulation. The axons of the substantia nigra form the nigrostriatal pathway, which supplies DA to the striatum.

Subthalamus: A thalamic nuclei group located caudal to the thalamus. Contains cells that use DA. A key structure connecting feedback and feedforward circuits of the thalamus and basal ganglia.

Sulci (s., Sulcus): The valleys or crevices between the gyri.

Superior: Refers to the direction "above."

Superior Colliculi: A pair of relay centers for vision that communicate directly with the lateral geniculate nuclei of the thalamus. Located on the posterior region of the midbrain.

Supplemental Motor Area: Considered to be part of the premotor area. Located inside the medial longitudinal fissure. Has a role in the bilateral control of posture.

Sympathetic Nervous System: A division of the autonomic nervous system. Responsible for the fight/flight response and gearing the body up for action.

Synaptic Cleft: Space between a presynaptic neuron's terminal boutons and a postsynaptic neuron's dendrites. The terminal boutons release their neurotransmitter substances into the synaptic cleft.

Synaptic Delay: The time required for the neurotransmitter to diffuse across a postsynaptic neuron's membrane.

Synaptic Fatigue: Occurs as a result of a neurotransmitter depletion due to the repetitive simulation of a presynaptic neuron.

Synergy Pattern: A stereotyped set of movements that occur in response to a stimulus or voluntary movement. Involves pathology of muscle tone affecting joint position. Synergies are described as patterns because the involved joint positions occur consistently as a result of specific neurologic damage. Specific flexor and extensor synergies can be observed in the upper and lower extremities. Synergy patterns can change as the patient experiences stages of recovery, or they may continue if recovery of damaged brain structures cannot occur.

Synesthesia: A perceptual phenomenon involving the ability to combine senses in response to specific stimuli. For example, the ability to see colors when one hears music.

Tachykinesia: Speeded movement. Commonly seen in Tourette syndrome.

Tachyphrenia: Speeded thought. Commonly seen in mania.

Tactile Agnosia: The umbrella term for the inability to attach meaning to somatosensory data.

Tardive Dyskinesia: A movement disorder related to treatment with DA receptor antagonists (neuroleptics and antiemetics). The term *tardive* refers to the fact that this movement disorder occurs after chronic use of these drugs. Characterized by choreiform movements, dystonia, tics, and/or myoclonus. Example: tongue protrusions (orobuccolingual movements), chewing-type movements, facial grimacing, blepharospasm, lip smacking. Tardive dyskinesia is different from most disorders in that the discontinuation of the causative agent (the neuroleptic) does not result in the amelioration of the movement disorder.

Tectum: The tectum is the collective name for the superior and inferior colliculi (of the midbrain).

Tegmentum: The tegmentum is the inner coat of the cerebral peduncles (of the midbrain). The tegmentum is the collective name for the substantia nigra and the red nucleus.

Temporal Lobe: Responsible for the detection and interpretation of sounds and long-term memory.

Tentorium: The projection of dura mater that extends as a horizontal shelf between the occipital lobe and the cerebellum.

Terminal Boutons: Emerge from the end branches of the axon and contain the neurotransmitter substances.

Thalamus: An egg-shaped lobe (one in each hemisphere) that contains 26 pairs of nuclei that act as a relay system for sensory and motor information traveling to and from the cortex.

Thermal Receptors: Sensory receptors that detect changes in temperature.

Thermesthesia: The ability to perceive temperature (hot and cold).

Thermohyperesthesia: An increase in temperature perception (ie, hot and cold sensations become heightened).

Thermohypesthesia: A decrease in temperature perception.

Third Ventricle: Part of the ventricular system. The walls of the third ventricle are created by the thalamus and hypothalamus. The lateral ventricle connects to the third ventricle via the foramen of Monro. The third ventricle connects to the fourth ventricle via the cerebral aqueduct.

Tics: Repetitive, brief, rapid, involuntary movements involving single muscles or multiple muscle groups. Tics are caused by an increased sensitivity to DA in the basal ganglia. With increased sensitivity to DA, the caudate, which normally acts like a brake on extraneous movements, cannot suppress movements like tics.

Topographical Disorientation: Involves difficulty comprehending the relationship of one location to another.

Transverse Plane: (Also called *coronal* or *frontal plane*.) The transverse planes run perpendicular to the sagittal planes. Transverse planes divide the anterior aspect of the brain from the posterior aspect.

Tremor: Involuntary oscillating movement resulting from alternating or synchronistic contractions of opposing muscles. See also *Resting Tremor* and *Intention Tremor*.

Trigeminal Nerve: CN 5. Responsible for sensation of face, head, and inner oral cavity. Also innervates the muscles of the jaw for chewing.

Trochlear Nerve: CN 4. Responsible for extraocular eye movements. Lesion symptoms include nystagmus, diplopia, and vertical, medial strabismus.

Two- and Three-Dimensional Constructional Apraxia: A type of apraxia involving an inability to copy 2- and 3-dimensional designs or models.

Two-Point Discrimination: The loss of the ability to determine whether one has been touched by 1 or 2 points. An esthesiometer is the instrument used to assess 2-point discrimination.

UMN: See *Upper Motor Neuron.*

Uncus: The bulblike anterior end of the parahippocampal gyrus.

Unilateral Neglect: Involves the inability to integrate and use perceptions from one side (the affected side) of the body or environment.

Upper Motor Neuron (UMN): An UMN carries motor messages from the primary motor cortex to (a) the CN nuclei (in the brainstem), or (b) interneurons in the ventral horn. An UMN travels up to but does not actually enter the ventral horn. An UMN is considered to be part of the CNS.

Utricle: One of the receptors of equilibrium in the inner ear. Responds to changes in head position. Part of the vestibular system.

V1: See *Primary Visual Area.*

V2 and up: See *Visual Association Areas.*

Vagus Nerve: CN 10. Responsible for taste on the palate and epiglottis. Carries parasympathetic information to and from the heart, pulmonary system, esophagus, and gastrointestinal tract. Also responsible for innervating the muscles of the larynx, pharynx, and upper esophagus (the muscles of swallowing and speaking).

Ventral (or *anterior*): Refers to the front of an organism. Ventral means the belly of a 4-legged animal.

Ventral Horn, Root, and Rootlets: The ventral horn contains the cell bodies of the motor spinal nerves that innervate skeletal muscle. Descending motor spinal tracts travel from the cortex down to the spinal cord. In the ventral horn, the motor spinal cord tracts synapse on interneurons. These interneurons then synapse with motor spinal nerves that travel to skeletal muscles in the PNS. The motor spinal nerve exits the ventral horn through the ventral rootlets. The ventral rootlets then merge into the ventral root. The ventral horn, rootlets, and root are all considered to be within the PNS.

Ventricular System: Hollow spaces in the brain through which CSF flows. There are 4 ventricles: 2 lateral ventricles, 1 third ventricle, and 1 fourth ventricle.

Vermis: The midline structure of the cerebellum that may have a role in the integration of information used by the right and left cerebellar hemispheres. Some have also suggested that the vermis may have a role in emotion and the timing of appropriate affective responses.

Vestibular System: Functions to maintain equilibrium and balance, maintains the head in an upright vertical position, coordinates head and eye movements, and influences muscle tone through the alpha and gamma motor neurons and the vestibulospinal tracts.

Vestibulocochlear Nerve: CN 8. Responsible for hearing or audition, balance, and the position of the head in space.

Vestibulospinal Tract: An extrapyramidal tract (does not use the pyramids). Descending motor spinal cord tract. Facilitates antigravity muscles (extensors) that are responsible for posture and stance.

Visceral Sensory Receptors: Respond to pressure and pain from the internal organs.

Visual Acuity: The ability to see with accuracy.

Visual Agnosia: An umbrella term for the inability to identify and recognize familiar objects and people although the visual anatomy remains intact. Visual agnosia is a perceptual disorder involving the cortical visual association areas.

Visual Association Areas (V2 and up): Cortical areas in the occipital lobe that are responsible for the interpretation of visual stimuli.

Visual Perception: The ability to attach meaning to visual data.

Wernicke Aphasia: A language perceptual problem involving difficulty comprehending the literal interpretation of language.

Wernicke Area: Located only in the left hemisphere within the superior temporal gyrus. Responsible for the comprehension of the spoken word.

White Matter: Located beneath the gray matter in the internal regions of the cerebrum and cerebellum. Consists of myelinated fiber tracts or neuronal axons.

Withdrawal Reflex: A spinal reflex that works similarly to the spinal reflex arc. This reflex is a protective mechanism that allows reflexive withdrawal of a body part from physical danger, while simultaneously adjusting posture to avoid imbalance. The reflex works at the level of the spinal cord without cortical processing.

Working Memory: A subcomponent of short-term memory; involves moment-to-moment awareness. Also plays a role in the search and retrieval of archived information. Mediated by the frontal lobes.

Index

Printed in the United States
by Baker & Taylor Publisher Services